Everybody's Guide

to

Homeopathic

Medicines

Everybody's Guide

to

Homeopathic Medicines

THIRD REVISED EDITION

Safe and Effective Remedies
for You and Your Family

STEPHEN CUMMINGS, M.D.
DANA ULLMAN, M.P.H.

A Jeremy P. Tarcher/Putnam Book
PUBLISHED BY
G. P. Putnam's Sons
New York

Most Tarcher/Putnam books are available at special
quantity discounts for bulk purchases for sales promo-
tions, premiums, fund-raising, and educational needs.
Special books or book excerpts also can be created to fit
specific needs. For details, write or telephone Special
Markets, The Putnam Publishing Group, 200 Madison
Ave., New York, NY 10016; (212) 951-8891

A Jeremy P. Tarcher/Putnam Book
Published by G. P. Putnam's Sons
Publishers Since 1838
200 Madison Avenue
New York, NY 10016
http://www.putnam.com/putnam

Library of Congress Cataloging-in-Publication Data

Cummings, Stephen
Everybody's guide to homeopathic medicines : safe and
effective remedies for you and your family / Stephen
Cummings, Dana Ullman.—3rd rev. ed.
p. cm.
"Jeremy P. Tarcher/Putnam book."
Includes bibliographical references and index.
ISBN 0-87477-843-3 (alk. paper)
1. Homeopathy—Popular works. I. Ullman, Dana.
II. Title.
RX76.C94 1996
615.5'32—dc20 96-31021 CIP

Book design by Judith Stagnitto Abbate
Cover design by Susan Shankin
Front cover illustration © 1996 by Don Weller

Printed in the United States of America
1 3 5 7 9 10 8 6 4 2

This book is printed on acid-free paper. ∞

ACKNOWLEDGMENTS

WE WOULD LIKE to acknowledge the following people who reviewed all or part of this book: Maesimund Panos, M.D.; Edward C. Whitmont, M.D.; Randy Neustaedter; Jeff Gould, M.D.; Louis Klein; Jacquelyn Wilson, M.D.; Bob Stewart; Margaret Macasland; Fred Cagle; and Della Desrosiers. Janice Gallagher, the editor of the first edition of this book, did a phenomenal job bringing order to our initially massive manuscript and deserves special credit for making this book usable and understandable. Donna Zerner, the editor of this present edition, brought her considerable skills to further refine this book's value.

Heartfelt thanks also to our many friends and colleagues who helped us in one way or another: Liz Gregory; Greg Manteuffel, M.D.; Ina Gordon; Diana Jackson; Nancy Herrick; David Anderson, M.D.; Peggy Chipkin; Christine Ciavarella; Jack Guralnik, M.D.; Ray Rosenthal, M.D.; Kathleen Haley; Corey Weinstein, M.D.; Carole, Lisa, and Jason Morison; Marshall Cummings; Robert Bruce Moody; Sally and Sarah Aldinger; Alan Solares; Selden Cummings; Celia Cummings; Richard Grossinger; David Hoskinson; Marc Lappe; Harris Coulter; Burt Linnetz; Don Gerrard; Chris Mole; Jocelyn Stoller; Arnold Whitridge; and Dannon Lahey.

Dana Ullman: It is wonderful to have a father who is loving and supportive. It is a special privilege that he, as a physician and pediatrician, was also able to review our manuscript to assure that the book provided the most up-to-date medical information. My mother's continuous love and support also has been inspiring to me in my work and in helping me be the person that I am.

CONTENTS

FOREWORD

THE THEORY AND PRACTICE of homeopathy is strange to those of us who are accustomed to conventional Western medicine. Dr. Samuel Hahnemann, the nineteenth-century founder of homeopathy, believed that remedies which, in large doses, could create a particular set of symptoms, could, in minute doses—at times so small that no molecule of the original substance remains—relieve those same symptoms.

But if homeopathy is unfamiliar and at times seems incredible, it is not uncongenial. We look hopefully for medicines that offer answers to the chronic conditions afflicting so many of us and eluding the curative reach of conventional medicine. We want drugs that have fewer debilitating side effects. And we sense the rightness of a healing system that conceives of all symptoms as parts of a larger whole, that appears to stimulate the body's natural healing force, rather than attack its enemies. Homeopathy seems to work with us, not on us.

Everybody's Guide to Homeopathic Medicines is an enormously useful introduction to the theory and practice of homeopathy. It briefly traces the homeopathic movement from its heyday in mid-nineteenth-century America (when one in five American physicians in urban areas practiced homeopathy), through its eclipse by the American Medical Association, to its remarkable renaissance in the 1970s and '80s. It provides an introduction to the theory of homeopathic prescribing and casetaking. It offers a useful distillation of the extensive and usually overwhelming *materia medica* (the catalog of homeopathic medicines and their specific characteristics), a glossary of unfamiliar terms, and a list of references. The heart of the book is, however, a series of chapters on common ailments and their homeopathic treatments. This is appropriate; homeopathy always has been a practical and a participatory discipline. These chapters, with their descriptions of symptoms and their matching remedies, permit any careful reader to select the appropriate remedies—for fever, colds, skin problems, aches and pains, and other minor but distressing ailments. They invite us to participate in the evolution of the discipline, to see for ourselves if homeopathy works.

In presenting the material, the authors are careful to delineate the arena in which lay- or self-prescription is to be used. Each chapter makes clear those situations which are "Beyond Home Care" and which require consultation with a health-care professional. This is a valuable service— at once responsible and adventurous: responsible because it admonishes practitioners to appreciate the range of illness with which they can deal safely, and adventurous because it helps reconcile homeopathic and conventional health-care practice.

I believe the renaissance of homeopathy will continue. I know that many of those whom my homeopathic colleagues and I have treated have become enthusiastic advocates and students of homeopathy. At the same time, interest among young physicians and medical students is increasing. Cummings and Ullman's book will provide an entry point for those who would like to experience the challenge of homeopathic casetaking and treatment. It will whet the appetites of those who may eventually make the theoretical formulations and undertake the research that will help us come to terms with this little-understood but fascinating approach to health care.

JAMES S. GORDON, M.D.
Georgetown University School of Medicine

PREFACE

H OMEOPATHIC MEDICINE is becoming so popular throughout Europe that it is no longer considered an "alternative medicine." Homeopathy is instead becoming an integral part of mainstream medical care.

Currently, 32 percent of France's family physicians prescribe homeopathic medicines, and a similar percentage of the French population has used these natural medicines.[1] Homeopathy is gaining respect in England, as shown in a *British Medical Journal* survey, which indicates that 42 percent of British physicians refer patients to homeopathic physicians.[2]

The growth and increasing respectability of homeopathy has spread to the United States as well. Although the homeopathic movement is considerably smaller here than in Europe, more and more physicians are beginning to use homeopathic medicine, and more and more laypeople also are using homeopathy to treat themselves.

People have sought these natural remedies for their safety. But now AIDS and other immune-deficiency diseases have imprinted upon our minds the importance of having a strong and healthy immune system. A growing number of people seek homeopathy because it makes more

---

1. F. Bouchayer, "Alternative Medicines: A General Approach to the French Situation," *Complementary Medical Research* 4(2):4–8.
2. Richard Wharton and George Lewith, "Complementary Medicine and the General Practitioner," *British Medical Journal* 292 (7 June, 1986): 1498–1500.

sense to stimulate the body's own natural healing abilities, rather than use drugs that inhibit immune responses.

New research also has helped homeopathy gain greater credibility. Several dozen well-designed clinical and laboratory studies have been conducted and the results published in respected peer-review medical and scientific journals. For the most part, these studies have demonstrated the biological activity and therapeutic benefits of homeopathic medicines.[3]

Since the first edition of this book, research on homeopathic medicines has appeared in various prestigious medical journals, including *Lancet, British Medical Journal, British Journal of Clinical Pharmacology, Pediatrics, Human and Experimental Toxicology, The European Journal of Pharmacology, Phlebology,* and *The International Journal of Immunology.*

In 1991, three Dutch professors of medicine performed a review and analysis of clinical studies of homeopathy.[4] They uncovered 107 trials, 81 of which showed that homeopathic medicines were effective. Although many of these trials were flawed in various ways, the authors found 22 studies that met their criteria for scientific quality; of these, 15 showed that homeopathic medicines worked. In addition, homeopathic medicines were found to be effective in 11 of the best 14 studies. The authors of this review of research were not homeopaths, and noted, "The amount of positive evidence even among the best studies came as a surprise to us." They concluded, "The evidence presented in this review would probably be sufficient for establishing homeopathy as a regular treatment for certain indications."

In another, more recent analysis of clinical studies, which covered work published through 1995, a collaborative team of German and American physicians found more high-quality, controlled studies. An even higher percentage of these experiments showed homeopathy to be effective than did the earlier review.

In scientific studies, some of the conditions for which homeopathic medicines have been found to be effective treatment include allergic disorders, migraine headaches, rheumatoid arthritis, childhood diarrhea, influenza, respiratory tract infections, fibrositis, diabetic retinitis, labor and delivery, constipation after abdominal surgery, sprained ankles, and vari-

3. P. Bellavite and A. Signorini, *Homeopathy: A Frontier in Medical Science* (Berkeley: North Atlantic, 1995); K. Linde, W. B. Jonas, D. Melchart, et al., "Critical Review and Meta-Analysis of Serial Agitated Dilutions in Experimental Toxicology," *Human and Experimental Toxicology* 13 (1994) 481–92.
4. J. Kleijnen, P. Knipschild, and G. ter Riet, "Clinical Trials of Homeopathy," *British Medical Journal* 302 (1991): 316–23.

cose veins. In one example, a group of researchers at the University of Glasgow conducted three trials to test the efficacy of homeopathic medicines in allergic conditions. Two studies focused on treating hay fever, while the third examined allergic asthma. These trials showed such dramatic results from the homeopathic medicines that the researchers concluded that either homeopathic medicines work, or controlled clinical trials do not![5]

As research continues to verify the value of homeopathic medicines, more physicians are integrating them into their practices. And as increasing numbers of consumers are learning about homeopathy, they are using these medicines more frequently to treat common health problems.

We are pleased that sales for *Everybody's Guide to Homeopathic Medicines* have increased every year since its first publication in 1984, and we hope that this new edition continues to fill the need for practical and authoritative homeopathic and general medical information.

For this third edition, we have brought up to date again the medical information throughout the book. We also have updated all of the resources listed in part 4. In addition, we've added two new features to the heart of the book—the clinical chapters—designed to make it easier for the reader to choose the correct homeopathic medicine for a particular condition. These two new features, Casetaking Questions and Remedy Summaries, make the book even more user-friendly. By using the list of key questions to ask the sick person (or yourself) for each ailment, you will be able to collect enough information to find the correct remedy. Containing most of the same information as the narrative remedy descriptions, the Remedy Summaries will help you find the medicine more easily and rapidly. The Remedy Summaries also will help you commit to memory the key features of each homeopathic medicine, so that you can learn how to use these remedies without always having to look them up in the book.

As we begin to enter the twenty-first century, medical care will inevitably continue to develop its high-tech aspect. But alongside high-tech medicine will be "high-natural medicine"—the systematic and scientific use of natural medicines that can effectively help prevent and treat ailments. This integration of high-tech and high-natural medicine will be the next stage of medical care, and homeopathy will inevitably play an integral role in this medicine of the future. It is our hope that this book will help bring the health care of the future to you today.

5. D. Reilly, M. Taylor, N. Beattie, et al., "Is Evidence for Homeopathy Reproducible?" *Lancet* 344 (10 December, 1994): 1601–06.

WHY AND HOW TO USE THIS BOOK

Homeopathy is a two-hundred-year-old medical system you can use at home to help treat family members with a wide spectrum of acute health problems. It offers a way to gently stimulate your inner healing resources through recognizing and reinforcing the adaptive reactions of the body's natural defenses. By choosing the correct, individually suited homeopathic medicine from the plant, mineral, animal, or chemical kingdom, you can successfully stimulate the body's own defenses. Following our instructions, you can complement your family's efforts toward good health with these safe, natural medicines, which provide an effective, inexpensive alternative to conventional medicine.

The best reason to use homeopathic medicines in self-care is that they work. When the medicines are prescribed correctly, they act rapidly, deeply, and curatively, stimulating the body's defenses rather than simply suppressing symptoms.

Homeopathic medicines are exceptional, as they can greatly enhance deep healing without the harmful side effects so commonly caused by conventional medicines. What's more, the homeopathic medicines cost much less than conventional drugs. As violinist Yehudi Menuhin, president of the Homepathic Society in the United Kingdom—one of the largest homeopathic organizations in the U.K.—once said, "Homeopathy is one of the rare medical approaches which carries no penalties—only benefits."

Homeopathy works effectively in treating people with a wide variety of acute and chronic problems, including infectious disease, allergies, gynecological conditions, digestive problems, skin diseases, and even psychological and genetic disorders. The scope of effective homeopathic treatment is broad, but this book will not teach you to treat *all* health problems that you or your family can experience. The proper role of homeopathic medicine at home is in the treatment of people with mild-to-moderate acute conditions. Acute conditions for which homeopathic home care is appropriate are self-limiting accidents or illnesses that are short in duration, have a generally predictable course, and resolve without significant aftereffects. Using homeopathic treatment at home, you can speed healing of many such conditions. Of course, some acute conditions require medical supervision, and we alert you to potentially serious symptoms in the "Beyond Home Care" section of each chapter in part 2. Homeopathy may nevertheless lessen the severity of the problem and speed healing.

Chronic diseases, in contrast to acute ones, are long in duration, degenerative in nature, and do not tend to resolve spontaneously. Such illnesses are complex, and their care requires a great deal of knowledge of the medical sciences and of homeopathy. People with chronic disease need the care of an experienced homeopath, who can often help them feel stronger, experience less pain, and slow down the degenerative process.

Our book is divided into three main sections. Part 1 covers homeopathic history, principles, and practical methodology. We urge you to read this introductory material carefully before you undertake home treatment. To be consistently successful, you must understand the philosophies and principles that are the foundation of the homeopathic method.

In part 2 we cover a wide variety of acute conditions for which home care with homeopathic medicines is often appropriate. Our discussion of each condition in these "clinical" chapters is organized into several sections: a general description of the condition, advice on simple home-care measures, Casetaking Questions that are useful for individualizing the correct remedy, a Remedy Summary which highlights essential and confirmatory symptoms for each medicine, a description of possible homeopathic medicines and the symptoms each covers that are relevant to the condition, and "Beyond Home Care," a summary of warning signs that require professional care.

Part 3 consists of the *materia medica,* in which most of the medicines included in the clinical chapters are listed and their general characteristics described. Each medicine has a set of symptoms common to all conditions for which it may be properly used. The information in part 3 is complementary to the descriptions of the specific symptoms in part 2; part 3 gives you more information about the medicines you are considering and helps you choose among them.

It is our hope that this book will serve as the beginning of your involvement in homeopathy. Therefore, in part 4 we provide you with listings of homeopathic books, organizations, drug manufacturers, and Internet resources to help you obtain more information about homeopathic medicine.

The Chinese believe that the best doctors use no medicines and, instead, heal by giving guidance on healthful living. Strictly speaking, homeopathy is a system of giving medicines, and even natural medicines only temporarily can improve symptoms caused by continued exposure to personal or societal health stress (influences homeopaths call "obstacles to cure"). That said, if you are willing to put your powers of observation and judgment to use—and if you're treating others, your communications skills as well—you'll receive the most satisfying rewards by using homeopathic medicines at home; a greater understanding of your own and your family's health; and the knowledge that you're not only feeling better, but becoming truly healthier as well.

PART 1

UNDERSTANDING

HOMEOPATHIC

MEDICINE

CHAPTER 1

THE SCIENCE OF HOMEOPATHY

IN THE 1800s, homeopathy emerged as a highly systematic medical science through the efforts of German physician Samuel Hahnemann. Prior to developing homeopathic science, Hahnemann had been an esteemed physician and chemist. He was the personal physician to members of the German royalty, and the author of one of the most respected texts on chemistry in his day. Despite his successes, he left his own orthodox medical practice; he felt he was doing more harm than good with the routine use of bloodletting, poisonous doses of mercury and arsenic, and the other often harmful medical practices that were in vogue.

Hahnemann was a scholar of numerous languages, and because he had a family to support, he resorted to translating various medical and literary texts. While translating a work by William Cullen, a leading physiologist of the time, Hahnemann was startled by the author's claim that the bitter and astringent properties of Peruvian bark, which contains quinine, accounted for its effectiveness in treating malaria. Hahnemann proved Cullen wrong by preparing an even more bitter and astringent mixture which was useless against malaria.

Hahnemann decided to test the physiological effects of Peruvian bark by taking small doses himself. His body eventually reacted to the drug. To his surprise, he developed symptoms very similar to those of malaria. Hahnemann wondered whether the curative power of Peruvian bark resulted from its capacity to create symptoms similar to those of the disease.

By studying the records of accidental poisonings from other commonly used medicines of his time, such as mercury, arsenic, belladonna, and silver nitrate, and by testing these poisons on himself and others, he found that in overdose the "medicines" caused symptoms similar to those of the illnesses for which they were used. Mercury, used to treat syphilis, could cause syphilislike ulcers. Arsenic and belladonna were known to create certain types of fever and were given as medicines for fevers. Silver nitrate, applied for eye inflammation, caused severe irritation and discharge from the eyes.

THE LAW OF SIMILARS: THE BASIC PRINCIPLE OF HOMEOPATHY

To like things like, whatever one may ail; there is certain help.

—JOHANN WOLFGANG GOETHE, *FAUST*

Hahnemann coined the Latin phrase *similia similibus curentur* ("let likes be cured with likes") to describe his discovery that substances in small doses stimulate the organisms to heal that which they cause in overdose. He termed the medical system based on this principle *homeopathy,* from the Greek words *homoios,* for "similar," and *pathos,* for "suffering" or "disease." This principle, most commonly known as the "law of similars," states that any substance that can cause symptoms when given to healthy people can help to heal those who are experiencing similar symptoms.

The law of similars has been used throughout history and throughout the world, both in and out of health care.[1] In the fourth century B.C., Hippocrates wrote, "Through the like, disease is produced, and through the application of the like, it is cured." Paracelsus, a well-known fifteenth-century physician and alchemist, used the law of similars extensively in his practice and his writings. He affirmed, "You there bring together the same anatomy of the herbs and the same anatomy of the illness into one order. This simile gives you an understanding of the way in which you shall heal."[2]

---

1. Linn Boyd, *A Study of the Simile in Medicine* (Philadelphia: Boericke and Tafel, 1936); Harris L. Coulter, *Divided Legacy: A History of the Schism in Medical Thought* vols. 1–4 (Washington, DC: Wehawken, 1975–1994).
2. Harris L. Coulter, *Divided Legacy: A History of the Schism in Medical Thought.* vol. 1, *The Patterns Emerge: Hippocrates to Paracelsus (350 B.C.–1600 A.D.)* (Washington, DC: Wehawken, 1975) p. 432.

Part of the *similia* concept has echoes in conventional medicine as well. Since the time of Edward Jenner (1749–1823), small doses of agents that cause illness have been used to immunize patients against diseases. Radiation is a cancer treatment, though it can cause cancer. Ritalin, a stimulant, is often prescribed to hyperactive children. Gold is used to treat some types of arthritis despite the fact that it can cause joint pain. Although these and numerous other medical treatments are reminiscent of the fundamental principle of homeopathy, none of them obeys the other essential tenets of homeopathic practice: individualization of the drug to the person's total physical and psychological characteristics, the use of the single medicine at the minimum dose, and the unique homeopathic pharmaceutical process.

There has been some technical research in physics, biology, biochemistry, and other natural sciences to determine how the law of similars works.[3] Though important, a theoretical or technical explanation of this phenomenon is secondary to the success homeopathic medicines have brought to millions of patients and practitioners.

SYMPTOMS AS DEFENSES: APPRECIATING THE BODY'S HEALING PROCESS

Hahnemann's observation that a substance able to mimic a sick person's symptoms can help cure the patient prompted a revolutionary understanding of symptoms. Instead of assuming that symptoms represent illogical, improper, or unhealthy responses of the body and that they should be treated, controlled, and suppressed, Hahnemann learned that symptoms are positive, adaptive responses to the variety of stresses the body experiences. Symptoms represent the body's best effort to heal itself. Hence, instead of suppressing symptoms, therapies should stimulate the body's defenses to complete the curative process.

This understanding of illness was not without precedent in Western medical history. In Western culture, a long-held belief, dating from Hippocrates in 400 B.C., has been that symptoms benefit the organism

---

3. Paolo Bellavite and Andrea Signorini, *Homeopathy: A Frontier in Medical Science* (Berkeley: North Atlantic, 1995); P. C. Endler and J. Schulte (eds.), *Ultra High Dilution: Physiology and Physics* (Boston: Kluwer Academic, 1994); Dana Ullman, *The Consumer's Guide to Homeopathy* (New York: Jeremy P. Tarcher/Putnam, 1996); Roeland van Wijk and Fred A. C. Wiegant, *Cultured Mammalian Cells in Homeopathy Research: The Similia Principle in Self-Recovery* (Utrecht, The Netherlands: University of Utrecht, 1994).

by responding to the stresses impinging on it.[4] The Latin phrase *vis medicatrix naturae,* meaning "the healing power of nature," refers directly to the human organism's dynamic and powerful capacity to protect and heal itself.

Present-day physicians and scientists commonly acknowledge this "wisdom of the body." Hans Selye, internationally respected physician and scientist, noted, "Disease is not mere surrender to attack but also a fight for health; unless there is a fight, there is no disease. . . . Disease is not just suffering, but a fight to maintain the homeostatic balance of our tissues, despite damage."[5] (See also the important work of Williams and Nesse, 1994, who show how the symptoms of illness serve as sophisticated adaptations to stress or infection in human beings and other animals.)

In this context, symptoms are not the disease. Symptoms *accompany* disease. Symptoms are evidence of disease. But treating symptoms is like killing the messenger for bringing bad news. In fact, treating symptoms can suppress the body's natural responses and inhibit the healing process.

As a systematic observer of nature and healing, Hahnemann was savvy enough to recognize that the body makes amazing and impressive efforts to heal itself, but that it is not always strong enough to complete the healing process. Often it needs a catalyst to stimulate its defenses, particularly when battling serious acute infectious diseases, chronic illnesses, or genetic disorders. Using the law of similars, Hahnemann developed a highly systematic method to individualize the choice of the right catalyst by prescribing a substance that imitates the body's defenses.

Hahnemann strongly criticized conventional medical therapies of his day that simply suppressed symptoms. He frequently noted that the many "successes" of conventional medical treatments were only temporary and often harmful, since the symptoms often returned or more threatening symptoms manifested as the body sought to reestablish its internal harmony.

As Pulitzer Prize–winning scientist René Dubos said, "Western medicine will become scientific only when physicians and their patients have learned to manage the forces of the body and the mind that operate in *vis medicatrix naturae.*" Homeopathic medicine *is* this scientific method.

4. Harris L. Coulter, *Divided Legacy: A History of the Schism in Medical Thought* vols. 1–4 (Washington, DC: Wehawken, 1975–1994).
5. Hans Selye, *The Stress of Life* (New York: McGraw-Hill, 1978) pp. 12–13.

THE HOMEOPATHIC PROVINGS: ASSESSING TOXIC AND THERAPEUTIC PROPERTIES OF MEDICINES

Most drug experimentation conducted by orthodox medical researchers has been performed on sick people, on animals, or in laboratories. As an ever-innovative contributor to medical science, Hahnemann was the first to recommend giving medicinal drugs to healthy people to assess their physiological properties. These experiments, called "provings," involve giving the person small doses of the single substance on a daily basis until symptoms are elicited. The dose used is extremely small and is selected according to previous knowledge of the toxic properties of the potential medicine. Careful observations and records are made of the symptoms that occur. Each substance creates a variety of physical, emotional, and mental symptoms, unique to that substance.

Initially, Hahnemann used mostly herbs and heavy metals like mercury and arsenic for his provings, the drugs employed by orthodox practitioners of his day. Later he tested various herbs used in European folk medicine, and other homeopaths have since "proven" herbal medicines of many regions, and many other mineral- and animal-derived substances.

The homeopathic provings provide the experimental basis for learning what symptoms a substance causes and thus, according to the law of similars, what it cures. The provings allow the practitioner to individualize the choice of a medicine according to the totality of the patient's symptoms.

The detailed records of the symptoms produced during the provings are compiled in reference books known as *materia medica*. The *materia medica* (Latin for "materials of medicine") list the medicines used in homeopathy and describe in detail the specific psychological and physical symptoms of each medicine. *Repertories* catalog thousands of symptoms and are indexes to the information found in the *materia medica*. Under each symptom listed are all relevant homeopathic medicines, those medicines known to cause the symptom, and thus those that may be indicated in treating a person with that symptom.

Although most of the provings were done in the 1800s and early 1900s, the American Institute of Homeopathy started a program of re-proving the medicines in the 1940s. This effort ended when the institute discovered that the medicines caused the same symptoms previously listed. The homeopathic reference books are as valuable today as when they were first published. However, numerous investigators are conducting provings at present to discover the therapeutic applications of new medicines.

THE TOTALITY OF SYMPTOMS

As far back as 180 years ago, long before the terms "alternative medicine" and "holistic health" were coined, homeopaths recognized the inseparability of body and mind. Homeopaths always have stressed the importance of assessing the totality of the person.

Hahnemann found that many of the substances he tested in provings provoked common symptoms such as fever, diarrhea, cough, restlessness, irritability, and so on. Still, each created a unique overall pattern of physiological and psychological change. Hahnemann determined he needed to match the total pattern of a substance's toxic symptoms with all the sick person's own symptoms to effect a cure. These matchings had to be precise and individualized. Matching only a few common symptoms or prescribing medicines routinely—giving Peruvian bark to everyone with malaria, for instance—was not effective.

The homeopathic definition of the term "symptom" encompasses the physical and psychological, the obvious and subtle, the common and the unusual. Even if the person has a main symptom that is causing much discomfort, the homeopath also must assess all other physical and psychological symptoms. Characteristic emotional states, changes in the person's energy level, sensitivity to heat or cold, and numerous other factors all must be considered.

The assumption is that no matter what combination of conditions, complaints, and sufferings the patient experiences at any one time, all are manifestations of a single "disease," an internal physiological disorder that is unique to the individual. The homeopath believes that no one organ of the body can be sick without affecting the person as a whole. Therefore, all symptoms must be taken into account; all are part of the body's effort to heal. It is crucial to understand that, in spite of the homeopath's desire to know all the minute details of the patient's symptoms, he or she does not *treat* symptoms. Instead the symptoms guide the homeopath to the medicine that can best stimulate the person's defenses.

Just as no isolated part of the body can be sick alone, the various recurrent symptoms people experience throughout their lives evolve from one enduring "constitutional" weakness. Such an underlying constitutional weakness or susceptibility is best treated by an experienced homeopath, whether the prominent symptoms in evidence are chronic or acute flare-ups of a recurrent problem. This approach is called *constitutional homeopathy*. Often, however, the most pronounced symptoms of an acute illness are the body's response to a specific set of acute stresses—infection, psychological stress, exposure to extremes of weather or to toxic substances, lack of sleep, and such. During true acute illnesses, the body mounts a strong healing defense against these particular acute stresses and devotes most of its healing resources to the effort. These are the illnesses that can be treated at home by the lay homeopath, who can choose the medicines on the basis of the prominent acute symptoms alone.

THE SINGLE MEDICINE

A homeopath does not prescribe one medicine for a person's headache, another for her stomachache, and another for her depression. The use of a single medicine at a time is a basic principle of classical homeopathy. As we've said, the homeopath assumes that, although a person may have numerous physical and psychological symptoms, he or she has only one disease, an underlying susceptibility. Using the one medicine right for that time in the person's life, whether the condition is acute or chronic, effectively stimulates the person's natural defense system, helps heal the current illness, and raises the general level of health.

One value of the single medicine in healing is that the practitioner and patient know the effect of treatment. Research has shown that hospital patients receive an average of nine medicines. The side effects of individual drugs are often startling, but the unknown, synergistic effects of numerous medicines given together to an already disordered physiology may be frightening.

Mixtures of homeopathic medicines, also known as "combination remedies," often are sold for specific symptoms or conditions. We'll have more to say about their use later in this chapter under "Variations of Homeopathic Practice."

THE MINIMUM NUMBER OF DOSES

Another essential precept in homeopathy is the principle of the minimum number of doses. Hahnemann believed in the importance of this principle and felt that a person's inherent healing powers are so strong that only a small stimulus is needed to begin the healing process. In fact, Hahnemann and numerous other homeopaths have asserted that once the healing process begins, it is best to do nothing more but let the process continue in its own way. Another dose of medicine may be required at some future time, but classical homeopaths are adamant about prescribing no other medicine or dose until the first has completed its action. Since the medicines act as a catalyst to the body's own defenses, continual repetition is not needed. In the treatment of chronic illnesses, months or sometimes years may pass before reintroducing a medicine. A special benefit of the minimum-dose principle is its discouraging the obsession with treatment in the process of finding the best, most efficient, and deepest-acting medicine.

THE POTENTIZED DOSE:
HOMEOPATHY'S PHARMACEUTIČAL PROCESS

When Samuel Hahnemann first began applying the law of similars in his medical practice, he obtained impressive results. However, he noted that patients sometimes developed toxic symptoms as a result of an overdose of the medicine. Hahnemann began to experiment with the size of the dose to see how little medicine he could give that still would cause a sustained healing response. After years of rigorous study, he found a method of diluting substances that minimized the toxic properties and at the same time magnified the potential to cure. He called this pharmaceutical process "potentization."

Potentization consists of a process of successive dilution. If the medicine is soluble, 1 part is diluted in 99 parts water or alcohol, and the mixture is mixed vigorously by striking the bottle against a firm surface. If the medicine is insoluble, it is finely ground, or *triturated,* in the same proportions with powdered lactose (milk sugar). One part of the diluted medicine is then diluted again in the same manner, and the process is repeated as many times as necessary to achieve the desired final dilution strength. The most common strengths have been diluted as often as 3, 6, 30, 200, 1,000, 10,000, 50,000 or 100,000 times. The medicines that are diluted 1 part to 99 parts are called *centesimal* potencies and may be labeled 6c, 30c, and so on, though often the *c* is omitted. Sometimes the dilution factor is 1 part medicine to 9 parts diluent, and these *decimal* potencies are always labeled 6x, 30x, and so on. By convention, the more times a medicine has been diluted, the "higher" its potency. Most homeopaths refer to medicines diluted 15 or fewer times (pharmacies typically sell the 3x or 3c, 6x or 6c, and 12x or 12c dilutions) as "low potencies." Anything up to the thirtieth dilution (30x or 30c) is a medium potency, while dilutions greater than 30 are high potencies.

Potentization is different from simple dilution. Homeopaths have found that the medicines do not work if they are simply diluted repeatedly without vigorous shaking or if they are just diluted in vast amounts of liquid. Nor do the medicines work if they are only vigorously shaken. It is the combined process of dilution and vigorous shaking that makes the medicine effective, when the symptoms of the medicine are similar to those of the ill person.

That tiny amounts of various substances can cause significant physiological changes is not new to medical science. A milligram of acetylcholine dissolved in 500,000 gallons of blood has long been known to lower the blood pressure of a cat, and even smaller amounts affect the beat of a frog's heart.[6] Florey, the codiscoverer of penicillin, reported in 1943 that pure penicillin can inhibit the development of sensitive microorganisms in the laboratory at dilutions of 1:50,000,000 to 1:100,000,000. The human body manufactures only 50 to 100 millionths of a gram of thyroid hormone per day, and the concentration of free thyroid hormone in normal blood is just 1 part per 10,000 million parts of blood plasma.[7] Yet this hormone is a powerful regulator of metabolic rate.

There have been numerous other experiments in the fields of botany, zoology, bacteriology, and physics that attest to the power of microdoses, including homeopathic potencies more dilute than 12c.[8] Double-blind clinical and laboratory studies also have provided evidence that the medicines act even though the dose is infinitesimal. (See the Preface for a short summary of key scientific studies and a bibliography of the best scientific investigations of homeopathy, as well as their references.)

Homeopaths have found, in fact, that generally the more a substance is potentized, the deeper it acts, the longer it acts, and the fewer number of doses are required in treatment. Although the higher potencies—those that have been diluted and shaken more—are generally more powerful than the lower potencies, all have a place in clinical practice. Since the higher potencies are particularly powerful, they must be used very judiciously. Homeopaths recommend that laypeople and beginning students of homeopathy not use potencies higher than 30c.

Potentization is probably the most controversial part of the homeo-

6. J. McKean Cattell (ed.), *Science* 72 (1930): 256.

7. Ernest Starling and Sir Charles Lovatt Evans, *Principles of Human Physiology* 14th edition (London: J & A Churchill, 1968) pp. 1493–94.

8. Paolo Bellavite and Andrea Signorini, *Homeopathy: A Frontier in Medical Science* (Berkeley: North Atlantic, 1995); P. C. Endler and J. Schulte (eds.), *Ultra High Dilution: Physiology and Physics* (Boston: Kluwer Academic, 1994); Dana Ullman, *The Consumer's Guide to Homeopathy* (New York: Jeremy P. Tarcher/Putnam, 1996); Roeland van Wijk and Fred A. C. Wiegant, *Cultured Mammalian Cells in Homeopathy Research: The Similia Principle in Self-Recovery* (Utrecht, The Netherlands: University of Utrecht, 1994).

pathic method. Most scientists believe that no medicine diluted more than the 12c potency could have any biochemical effect, since it is improbable that any molecules of the original substance remain. Many observers suggest that, in fact, the benefits of homeopathic treatment are due to the placebo effect. Evidence to the contrary is the impressive clinical successes homeopaths have had treating serious infectious illnesses such as cholera, yellow fever, and whooping cough. Homeopathic literature also records many successes in the treatment of seriously ill infants and all kinds of animals, presumably not responsive to the placebo effect. In addition, carefully conducted provings using the high potencies have produced patterns of symptoms similar to provings done with the low potencies.

Homeopathic medicines thus have physiological activity, though we still do not understand how or why they act. Practicing homeopaths use the medicines because they work, and await further research for the explanation.

HERING'S LAWS OF CURE

Homeopaths define health as a state of freedom existing on three interrelated levels: the physical, the emotional, and the mental. A healthy person experiences physical vitality and freedom from physiological malfunction, emotional peace and freedom of expression, and mental clarity with creativity. The most serious symptoms affect the deeper, more vital parts of the person. When evaluating a patient's overall state of health, the homeopath views the mental state as most important, followed by the emotional state, and then the physical state.

A homeopath is not content to hear that the symptom for which the patient originally came to be treated has improved. The practitioner needs to know what else has changed, for better or worse, and whether the person's overall vitality has increased or decreased. If, for instance, a skin problem has improved but a chest infection has developed, the homeopath may conclude that the therapy has actually made the person worse.

Experience with homeopathic treatment has shown that, following the administration of the correct medicine in the treatment of chronic disease, symptoms on the deeper levels improve while those on more external levels often temporarily worsen. It has come to be expected that the cure will progress from inside out, and this progress can be used to validate the success of treatment. Details of the important changes in posttreatment symptoms were codified by Constantine Hering, a German homeopath who emigrated to the United States in the 1830s and who is considered the father of American homeopathy. The three general principles of the homeopathic healing process are known as Hering's laws of cure or Hering's guides to cure.

According to the first of Hering's laws, healing progresses from the deepest part of the organism—the mental and emotional levels and the vital organs—to the external parts, such as the skin and extremities. A cure is in progress when a person's psychological symptoms lessen and the physical symptoms increase (so long as the physical symptoms are not severely pathological). Eventually, as this healing moves outward, even the superficial symptoms are alleviated. On the other hand, if physical symptoms improve but the psychological state worsens, the person's state of health is thought to be deteriorating.

Within each of the three broad levels of the defense system, symptoms that affect more vital functions are the deepest and most threatening to health. George Vithoulkas, a respected contemporary homeopath, has outlined the varying depths of symptoms from each level in descending order of depth, symptoms, and their impact on one's state of health.[9]

PHYSICAL	EMOTIONAL	MENTAL
Brain ailments	*Suicidal depression*	*Complete confusion*
Heart ailments	*Apathy*	*Destructive delirium*
Endocrine ailments	*Sadness*	*Paranoid ideas*
Liver ailments	*Anguish*	*Delusions*
Lung ailments	*Phobias*	*Lethargy*
Kidney ailments	*Anxiety*	*Dullness*
Bone ailments	*Irritability*	*Lack of concentration*
Muscle ailments	*Dissatisfaction*	*Forgetfulness*
Skin ailments		*Absentmindedness*

The exact location of these symptoms in the table is not critical, but the outline serves as a guide for evaluating the patient's progress according to Hering's first law.

Hering's second law states that as healing progresses, symptoms appear and disappear in the reverse of their original chronological order of appearance. Homeopaths have consistently observed that their patients briefly reexperience symptoms from past conditions, even those

9. George Vithoulkas, *The Science of Homeopathy* (New York: Grove, 1980) p. 24.

conditions that occurred many years before the present treatment. These observations, of course, pertain more to patients being treated for chronic conditions, but even during an acute illness, a retracing of the development of the symptoms may be noticeable after the medicine is given.

According to Hering's third law, healing progresses from the upper to the lower parts of the body. For instance, a person is considered to be on the mend if the arthritic pain in his neck has decreased although he now has pain in the finger joints.

As the symptoms change in accordance with Hering's laws, it is common for individual symptoms to become worse than they had been before treatment. These aggravations are welcomed by the knowledgeable homeopath, provided there is corresponding improvement in the symptoms on deeper levels, of more recent onset, and higher on the body. If healing is truly in progress, the patient feels stronger and generally better in spite of the aggravation. Before long, the symptoms of the aggravation pass and leave the person healthier on all levels.

Hering's laws are extremely valuable tools in the holistic assessment of health, for they provide a way to evaluate the person's total state of health, not only the person's main complaint. Sometimes, however, the three guidelines of Hering's laws as observed in a patient may not conform to the classic pattern. For instance, the symptoms may move from within outward, in accordance with the first law, but also travel upward, violating the third law. Whenever the progress of healing is difficult to interpret, the final judgment depends on whether the person experiences an overall increase in health and freedom. Violating one law may be insignificant if the symptoms that arise are minor. It is most important that the other laws are observed and the person's general state improves.

Homeopaths are not the only practitioners who have observed the existence of Hering's laws. Acupuncturists have witnessed aspects of these laws for thousands of years. Psychotherapists and healers utilizing various natural therapies also have noticed this phenomenon.

The main use of Hering's laws for you will be in home-treatment situations. You'll want to know whether the medicine you have given is helping. That the medicine is working is usually obvious. In acute situations, the homeopathic healing response is usually rapid and complete, and the progress of symptoms as it follows the laws often will be too rapid to notice. Whenever you are in doubt about a person's response, however, consider the changes in symptoms in light of Hering's laws.

THE HOMEOPATHIC VIEW OF INFECTIOUS DISEASE

Most commonly, the illnesses you will treat at home with homeopathy are the acute infectious diseases. An infectious disease is the disruption of normal body function that occurs when a microorganism enters the body, multiplies, and thrives where it is not normally present.* The signs and symptoms of the illness result from the interaction between the germ, which injures or poisons the tissue, and the person's inherent physiological defenses, which respond to the infection.

Although many today think of homeopathy as useful mostly for psychosomatic conditions or other chronic problems, the rapid spread of the treatment in the early 1800s resulted from its superior record in fighting deadly epidemics of cholera, typhoid, scarlet fever, yellow fever, and other infectious diseases. You won't be treating such serious illnesses at home, but homeopathy remains an effective therapy for people with all types of infections.

Homeopaths do not assume that germs are the primary cause of infections. In order to determine the "cause" of an infectious disease, it is necessary to take into account both the virulence of the infecting agent *and* the resistance of the person's defense system. This broader view of infectious disease explains how, in the same environment and exposed to the same germs, some people get sick and others do not. Biologists and homeopaths refer to these phenomena as "states of susceptibility" and "host resistance."

Indeed, homeopaths see the presence of microbes as the *result* of disease, and they understand the "disease" to be the preexisting susceptibility of the person to infection—the constitutional weakness previously discussed. For instance, that a throat culture shows *Streptococcus* bacteria growing in a child's throat does not necessarily mean the germ *caused* the illness. The problem is that the child's defense system is not as strong as it could be, and this weakness created an environment conducive to the growth of bacteria.

In fact, strep bacteria often live harmlessly in the throats of people who have no symptoms and who are resistant to the infection. Medical tests frequently show that individuals have various bacteria, viruses, and

*In 1832, at least thirty years before scientists recognized the existence of germs, Hahnemann noted that the cholera epidemic was caused by a "brood of . . . excessively minute, invisible, living creatures," further evidence that Hahnemann was ahead of his time.

other pathological agents in their bodies yet are not ill. Usually it is only when the person's defenses are significantly weakened by some type of stress, whether it be malnutrition, lack of exercise, mental or emotional stress, or exposure to chemical or environmental dangers, that the pathological agents are able to multiply easily enough to make the body vulnerable to disease.

Certainly some microbes are so virulent that few individuals can build resistance to them. Widespread epidemics have often been related to social upheavals, malnutrition, poor hygiene, and the like, but in some cases they have decimated apparently healthy populations. Epidemics and virulent infections aside, the overall resistance of the person and his or her exposure to stress are of primary importance in dealing with ordinary illnesses.

The homeopathic approach to infectious disease assumes that most people have sufficiently strong physiological resources to overcome infecting organisms and restore good health. Homeopathic medicines strengthen and rally these inherent resources, and those treated homeopathically not only recover faster, but become more resistant to other infections as well.

Since homeopathic medicines do not kill germs directly, it makes little difference which agent is associated with the illness, be it bacteria, virus, fungus, or other microbe. The sometimes difficult process of diagnosis and the inability of conventional therapies to treat viral conditions are not impediments to homeopathic treatment. No germ will remain a major problem for the person whose defenses are sufficiently strong.

Most medical research concerning infectious disease has focused on how to kill germs or inhibit their growth rather than how to stimulate the body's own defenses. Antibiotics, the main group of drugs used to combat bacterial infection, may help rid the body of certain bacteria, but they don't change the various factors that led to the infection. As Dr. Marc Lappé, pathologist and associate professor at the University of Illinois, wrote in his powerful book *When Antibiotics Fail,* "A basic truism of antibiotic treatment is that it will not work under most circumstances unless the body can mount its own attack against invading bacteria."[10] In fact, the person for whom antibiotics are prescribed may become more susceptible to further infections if the antibiotic inhibits the growth of beneficial bacteria, those that aid digestion and protect the skin and mucous membranes. Resistance to infection may even be lowered when cer-

---

10. Marc Lappé, *When Antibiotics Fail* (Berkeley: North Atlantic, 1986) p. 173.

tain patients experience side effects caused by antibiotics. Dr. Lappé cites a study that showed that certain antibiotics can actually depress the body's immune responses.[11]

There is no question that there is growing resistance to antibiotics and that antibiotics attack and destroy beneficial bacteria. Something must be done to curb the overdose of these drugs, and it seems clear that infectious diseases should, when possible, be treated with less ecologically disturbing treatments.

Despite such drawbacks, antibiotics can literally be lifesaving when serious infections of vital organs occur. Most infections, however, are not life-or-death situations, so when you or your child has an illness that might respond to antibiotic treatment, deciding whether or not to use antibiotics may be difficult. You should consult your health practitioner to discuss such factors as the severity of the illness, the person's vitality, and the possible alternatives, including homeopathy.

If you or your child receives antibiotic treatment for an infectious illness, we strongly recommend you follow the prescription's instructions carefully. Take the drug for the entire time prescribed, even if symptoms diminish rapidly. Even if you are receiving antibiotic treatment, we recommend you take an appropriate homeopathic medicine concurrently. While antibiotics may interfere with the action of the homeopathic medicine to some degree, we have often observed that people being treated with antibiotics tend to improve more rapidly after administration of the homeopathic remedy. People often continue to have symptoms of their illness even after the antibiotic treatment is complete, and when this occurs, homeopathic treatment is again appropriate.

VARIATIONS OF HOMEOPATHIC PRACTICE

A number of variations on classical homeopathy are popular. The practice of using multiple homeopathic medicines simultaneously is especially widespread. This style of practice is common in Europe and Latin America, and also has been adopted by some homeopaths in the United States.

Similarly, many pharmacies and health-food stores sell over-the-counter "combination" medicines labeled for specific conditions, such as colds, insomnia, or headaches. Intended primarily for home use by non-professionals, each of the combination medicines consists of a mixture of

11. Ibid., p. 178.

several homeopathic medicines commonly used in a given condition. Some people find that using combination medicines is easier than carefully selecting each remedy, a process required in classical homeopathy. Using combination medicines may make sense when choosing the single correct remedy is difficult, or when the indicated single remedy isn't immediately available. At any rate, many people report good results with them when treating common, minor ailments, accidents, and injuries, and several scientific studies have shown their value for such conditions.[12]

However, classical homeopaths generally are critical of giving more than one medicine at a time. They point out that the effects of a mixture of medicines are likely to be different than the additive effects of the individual medicines, which may interact unpredictably in the body. Another concern is that the indiscriminate use of many medicines might change a person's symptoms and make the selection later on of the single correct remedy more difficult. In the case of the combination medicines, they are not chosen on the basis of the sick person's unique pattern of symptoms, and therefore aren't as likely to be deeply curative.

"Cell salts," also called the "twelve tissue salts," are commonly used medicines often thought of as being similar to homeopathy. They were developed in the 1870s by a German physician, Dr. W. H. Schussler, who found these simple mineral substances to be the most abundant constituents of cremated human remains. Schussler's theory is that these simple minerals are largely responsible for harmonious function of physiological processes, and that disease results when the body is deficient in these minerals or when their metabolism is disordered. He thought that such problems could be corrected by supplying the appropriate mineral, homeopathically prepared.

These theories of disease appear antiquated and simplistic in light of modern understanding of physiology. While minerals and their proper balance are vitally important to homeostatic processes, there are many complex physiological systems that depend as well on thousands of biochemicals, not simply twelve inorganic minerals.

Although the cell salt theory may not be accurate, potentized cell salts certainly have effects on organisms. All cell salts are used by classical homeopaths for the specific physical and psychological symptoms that they create in provings. Most users of cell salts, however, prescribe them on very limited physical symptoms. Also, since many cell salt users take

---

12. Dana Ullman, *The Consumer's Guide to Homeopathy* (New York: Jeremy P. Tarcher/Putnam, 1996).

more than one medicine at a time, the criticisms previously stated of such practice are applicable here too.

Some practitioners use electronic devices that measure skin resistance at specific acupuncture points to determine which homeopathic medicines the patient needs. These practitioners claim good results in a wide variety of acute and chronic ailments. However, the technique is not compatible with the principles of classical homeopathy, because the selection of the remedy isn't based on symptom analysis, and multiple medicines are typically prescribed at the same time.

The Bach Flower remedies were developed by Edward Bach, a British bacteriologist and homeopath. Based on his observance of ailing animals licking the dew from various flowers, Bach intuited the healing properties of thirty-eight flowers. He believed that each flower suited a specific emotional state. Accordingly, the Bach Flower remedies are given solely on the basis of emotional and psychological symptoms—the person's physical symptoms aren't considered in the choice of the remedy. Since Bach, practitioners have extended his system, adding new remedies from flowers native to other parts of the world.

Although Bach was for some time a homeopath, his system of flower remedies is clearly not in accord with classical homeopathy. For one thing, the indications for the remedies came primarily from Bach's tests on himself and his intuition, not provings on multiple individuals. For another, in Bach's process, multiple remedies are usually given at the same time, and frequent repetition is the rule.

HISTORICAL NOTES, AND THE STATUS OF HOMEOPATHY TODAY

Although rejected by the medical establishment of the nineteenth century, homeopathy spread rapidly throughout Europe and then to the United States in the years following Hahnemann's announcement of his discoveries, largely because of its medical successes with dread epidemic illnesses. In 1900 a comparison of mortality rates among homeopathic and conventional medical patients throughout the United States and Europe showed that two to eight times as many homeopathic patients with life-threatening infectious diseases survived, as compared with those receiving conventional medical care of the day.[13]

---

13. Thomas Lindsay Bradford, *The Logic of Figures or Comparative Results of Homeopathic and Other Treatments* (Philadelphia: Boericke and Tafel, 1900).

The history of homeopathic medicine in America is fascinating. Few people, including doctors, are aware that the first national medical association in the United States was the American Institute of Homeopathy, founded in 1844. By the turn of the century, fully 20 to 25 percent of all physicians in urban areas identified themselves as homeopaths. There were twenty-two homeopathic medical schools, and more than a hundred homeopathic hospitals. Many well-known people were patrons of homeopathy, including William James, Harriet Beecher Stowe, Henry Wadsworth Longfellow, John D. Rockefeller, Louisa May Alcott, and Daniel Webster. William Cullen Bryant, noted journalist and poet, was the president of the Homeopathic Medical Society of New York City and County.

Since the turn of the century, however, homeopathy declined to the point that few people outside the health professions had even heard the word. Some of the reasons for this decline included: (1) Strong opposition from the AMA. The AMA Code of Ethics prohibited members from consulting with homeopathic physicians, even if conventional medical treatments were failing. Orthodox physicians influenced legislation that limited homeopathic training and practice; (2) the advances of modern medicine. Although the orthodox treatments of Hahnemann's day were largely ineffective and often caused immediate suffering or even death, the twentieth century saw a rapid growth in treatments that were at least superficially successful. Powerful painkilling drugs and other suppressive medicines seemed to work magically, though they merely checked symptoms and often created new problems in time. Potent antimicrobial drugs further enhanced the reputation of conventional medicine; (3) the cultural effects of the Industrial Revolution. Homeopathic medicine is impossible to practice successfully in the medical "assembly line" so common in the doctors' offices of this century; and (4) infighting among homeopaths. Several severe doctrinal and political splits impaired the homeopathic community's ability to respond to the challenges of conventional medicine and cultural transitions.

In the United States, the long period of declining interest in homeopathy and of attrition in the ranks of practitioners ended in the early 1970s. A sharp resurgence of homeopathic activity began then, and homeopathy has continued to grow since.

As of 1996, there are several thousand practitioners in the United States who specialize in the practice of homeopathy. This total includes 1,000 to 2,000 medical doctors and osteopathic physicians, 750 to 1,000 naturopathic doctors, 500 veterinarians, 300 to 500 dentists, 200 to 400 chiropractic physicians, and 300 to 500 acupuncturists. In addition, several thousand conventional physicians prescribe homeopathic medicines occasionally. There are also hundreds of physicians' assistants, nurse practitioners, nurses, and midwives who practice homeopathy and regularly prescribe these natural medicines.

While homeopathy continues to grow in the United States, it is much more popular in other parts of the world, particularly in Europe and parts of Asia and Latin America. In France, approximately 36 percent of the public and 32 percent of the physicians use homeopathic medicines. In Germany, 10 percent of the physicians specialize in homeopathy, and another 10 percent occasionally prescribe homeopathic remedies. In the United Kingdom, 42 percent of physicians refer patients to homeopathic doctors, and homeopathic training is the most popular postgraduate training program.

Although illegal in much of Eastern Europe during the Communist period, homeopathy has become increasingly popular since the Iron Curtain fell. The Hungarian Homeopathic Medical Association had only 11 members in 1990, but membership had grown to 302 by 1994. In Slovakia, where the last homeopathic physician died in 1967, the homeopathic medical organization formed in 1990 grew to 800 members by 1993.

Homeopathy is practiced even more widely in India, where there are 125 four- and five-year homeopathic medical colleges, and more than 100,000 homeopathic physicians.

Understanding the basic principles of homeopathy we've presented in this chapter prepares you for "taking a case," that is, observing and recording information to help you prescribe the appropriate remedy.

CHAPTER 2

HOMEOPATHY IN PRACTICE

THERE ARE FIVE BASIC STEPS you'll follow when putting homeopathy into practice at home.

1. Casetaking: collecting complete and accurate information about the illness
2. Case analysis: evaluating the information you've gathered
3. Selecting the homeopathic medicine that best suits the person and his or her illness
4. Administering the remedy
5. Observing the reaction to the treatment and deciding whether to repeat or change the medicine

Before you even begin this process, you must be able to recognize situations that are beyond your level of skill. More and more people are becoming well educated about medicine and health, and certainly you can learn to decide whether an illness can be treated at home or consultation with your health professional is necessary. The "Beyond Home Care" section included with each of the various illnesses and conditions in part 2 describes symptoms that require immediate or timely consultation with your practitioner. There are also many books covering conventional home medical care. Perhaps the most helpful are *Take Care of*

Yourself, by James Fries and Donald Vickery, and *Taking Care of Your Child,* by Robert Pantell, James Fries, and Donald Vickery. These books contain concise descriptions of all the common injuries and illnesses people encounter, along with clear instructions for determining whether home treatment is safe and how soon to see a professional.

If you do require a visit to your health-care provider, he or she may still decide that the illness is not serious enough to require conventional therapies. You can then go ahead and use homeopathic treatment.

CASETAKING

In preparation for casetaking, it is a good idea to keep a home medical record for each member of the family. This could include pregnancy and birth history, a record of immunizations and serious illnesses or injuries, and a description of any allergies or other reactions to foods, medications, or environmental factors. You might want to jot down what you consider possible reasons for the illnesses' onsets as well as comments about their severities, durations, and so on.

Should you choose homeopathy to treat a particular illness, we strongly recommend you *write down* your findings as you assemble the homeopathic case. The record will ensure completeness and accuracy, and you'll have the whole case available to study at a glance. Keeping this record may also prove helpful if a similar illness occurs later, for you'll want to know how effective your earlier prescriptions were. An example of such a case record is given in the section "A Sample Casetaking" later in this chapter.

Since homeopathic medicines are chosen to match the symptoms the sick person experiences, successful homeopathic prescription requires an accurate description of the symptoms. The homeopathic definition of a "symptom" is broader than the strict medical use of this term. For our purposes it means any change that is experienced or observed during the course of an illness. Symptoms of pain (sore throat, headache, or stomachache), physical changes (fever, flushed skin, runny nose, or skin eruptions), unusual reactions to environmental conditions or food, and the predominant emotional and mental state during the illness all are important homeopathic symptoms. Each symptom must be described in as much detail as possible for the prescriber to better understand that individual's unique state of psychophysiological balance.

In order to recognize the important symptoms for your casetaking, you should be aware of homeopathy's distinctions among symptoms. For instance, "particular symptoms" are distinguished from "general symptoms." Particular symptoms refer to local symptoms associated with a specific part of the body (for example, burning pain in the throat, cold feet, throbbing pain in the back of the head). General symptoms are those felt by the entire body (exhaustion, coldness of the whole body, restlessness). Emotional and mental characteristics are considered general symptoms, too, since they are felt and experienced by one's entire being. General symptoms are usually more valuable in choosing the correct medicine, since these symptoms represent the reaction of the whole body to some type of stress and, as such, represent a deeper response of the organism in its effort to reestablish health.

Homeopaths also make note of "peculiar symptoms"—that is, symptoms that do not occur in most people with a similar illness or that are simply unusual. Such idiosyncrasies sometimes are even more valuable in individualizing the choice of medicine.

The method you ultimately use for taking the case will vary, depending on whether you treat yourself, another adult, or a child. If you are treating yourself, you need only run through the steps of the casetaking process outlined in this chapter. Treating others requires careful observation in addition to thoughtful questions.

Casetaking begins with a general exploration of the illness and its most obvious symptoms. Next, find out if there are symptoms affecting any other parts of the body and solicit details about how the person as a whole is reacting to the condition. As much as possible, use *the patient's own words* to record the symptoms in the outline format we show in "A Sample Casetaking" later in the chapter. Assemble a complete description of the overall illness and its separate symptoms as follows.

CONTRIBUTING CAUSES: First, decide whether there is any apparent cause for the illness or the particular symptom. Possible stresses that made the individual susceptible to illness (other than exposure to someone who was sick) include loss of sleep, dietary indiscretions, exposure to adverse weather, or emotional stress. You may discover that a particular symptom has resulted from a different cause than the illness as a whole. For instance, after staying up late one too many nights, a person might come down with a cold and then develop a cough only because she went out in the rain a few days later.

ONSET: Describe the onset of the illness and the individual symptoms. How rapidly did the symptoms develop, and how quickly do they come and go? In what order did the symptoms appear?

CHARACTER OF SYMPTOMS: Try to describe the sensations that are felt in as much detail as possible. You want to know whether the pain feels sharp, dull, bruising, cutting, burning, or is of some other type. Sensations like tingling, numbness, and so forth also should be noted.

LOCATION OF PARTICULAR SYMPTOMS: Write down the location of the pain, discomfort, or physical symptom. Be precise. Often, for example, an inflamed throat is sore on only one side, and many ear infections involve only one ear.

MODALITIES OF SYMPTOMS: Describe any factors that aggravate or improve each symptom. These descriptions are essential to an adequate homeopathic casetaking. You must find out what makes each symptom better or worse. These factors are called the "modalities" of the symptom in homeopathic terminology. The more definite the positive or negative effect on the symptom, the more valuable the modality is in the choice of the remedy. It is not unusual to find that the modalities of a symptom are the opposite of what you expected. For instance, a sore throat may be improved by swallowing, and a person with a fever may feel better in a warm room. Also, the factors that aggravate one symptom may improve another, so be sure you get the specific details right. We have found from experience that almost anything may turn out to make a symptom better or worse in a particular case. See the accompanying "Outline for Casetaking in Acute Care" for a list of possible modalities to look for while casetaking.

GENERAL SYMPTOMS: Once you've gathered information about each individual symptom, find out how the person has been affected generally by the illness. In many cases the initial investigation of the most prominent symptoms already touched upon general symptoms such as fever, energy level, and so on. General symptoms you'll want to know about include overall energy, general response to temperature, change in thirst or appetite (unusual craving or distaste for particular foods or drinks), perspiration level, change in sleep pattern, and change in emotional and mental state during the illness. The distinct modalities of each general symptom should be noted. Again, for an exhaustive list of possible general symptoms, see "Outline for Casetaking in Acute Care."

For most of the illnesses and other conditions covered in part 2, we provide Casetaking Questions, a list of the most important questions to answer regarding the specific symptoms of that condition. To avoid repetition, the Casetaking Questions don't address all the general information you should gather in every illness. Use them in conjunction with the material in this section to be sure you've covered all the bases.

CASETAKING HINTS

You may be your most difficult patient. Acute illness can make concentration hard, and it is hard to be objective about oneself even when well. If there is no one else in the family able to treat you, though, go ahead with the treatment process on your own.

When you take another person's case, let the patient describe his symptoms in his own way. Limit most of your questions to the likes of "What else?" or "Tell me more about that." It is best to keep him talking without putting words in his mouth. Should he run out of things to say on his own, begin asking more specific questions about each of the symptoms, as outlined above. Make your questions as open-ended as possible, and try especially to phrase them well, to avoid yes or no answers. For instance, asking "How does your throat feel?" or "What makes it worse?" is preferable to saying "Does it hurt when you swallow?" or "Is it worse in the morning?" If the patient can't think of what makes a symptom better or worse, try offering a group of alternatives ("Is your cough affected by exertion, by time of day, by warm or cold air, or by position?"); or ask about a specific modality in an open-ended way ("How is your headache affected by moving around?"). If he's having trouble describing a particular sensation, give examples ("Does it feel like a pounding hammer, like an electric shock, or like a vise?").

Try to get a sense of how reliable and definite the ailing person's statements really are. You'll want to be sure of his symptoms before you use them to choose the correct medicine.

Sick people, and particularly children, may not be able to give you exact descriptions of their symptoms. Your own careful observations are meant to supplement the verbal information you collect, but sometimes they are your only source. You should note the person's *appearance*. Does she look pale or flushed; are her pupils dilated or constricted; do her eyes look puffy or heavy? Her actions should give you clues about the nature of her discomfort. She may be protecting one part of her body by covering it or by adopting a particular position. She may cry when she swallows or urinates, or she may rub or tug at her ears. Watch closely to determine the modalities of the symptoms. Observe whether factors such as time of day, temperature or weather, food or drink, or motion make the symptoms better or worse. How has the sick person's *behavior* changed? Is she more irritable, restless, sleepy, or weepy than usual? Your familiarity with her normal personality should make it easy to discern the emotional changes that accompany the illness.

OUTLINE FOR CASETAKING IN ACUTE CARE*

The following information should be obtained in acute care:

Description of the Onset of the Symptoms
Possible factors that may have led to the illness (for example, exposure to heat or cold or wet weather, stress or a specific emotion, overindulgence, loss of sleep)

Description of the onset of illness—how quickly the symptoms developed, and in what order

Particular Symptoms
Character of pain or any sensation (dull, aching, pulsating, pressing, shooting, numb, tingling, etc.); location, extension, and radiation of the pain or sensation

Patterns of symptoms that occur at regular intervals or that alternate with one another

Description (color, thickness, odor) of any discharge from the body; changes in urine or stool

Factors that make each symptom better or worse (modalities):

Time: hour; day or night; morning, afternoon, or evening; before or after midnight
Temperature and weather: wet, dry, cold, or hot weather; weather changes; storms or thunderstorms (before, during, or after); sun, wind, fog, or snow; open air, warm rooms, changes from one room to another, or stuffy or crowded places; drafts; warmth of bed; heat of stove; uncovering
Bathing: hot, cold, or sea bathing
Rest or motion: slow or rapid; ascending or descending; while turning in bed, exerting oneself, or walking; upon first motion, after moving awhile, while moving, after moving, during passive motion in a car or boat
Position: standing; sitting with knees crossed, rising from sitting, stooping; lying on painful side, back, right or left side, abdomen, ly-

*Adapted from *A Brief Study Course in Homeopathy,* by Elizabeth Wright Hubbard (St. Louis: Formur, 1977).

ing with head high or low, rising from lying; leaning head backward, forward, sideways; closing or opening eyes; any unusual position such as knees against chest
External stimuli: touch (hard or light), pressure, rubbing, constriction (clothing, etc.), jarring, riding, light, noise, conversation, odors
Eating or drinking: during or after eating something hot or cold; swallowing solids or liquids, empty swallowing after eating any particular food; eating in general
Sleep: before or during sleep, during first part of sleep, on waking
Urination or defecation: before, during, or after
Sweat or other discharges: during or after
Coition, continence, masturbation
Emotions: anger, grief, mortification, fear, shock, consolation, apprehension of crowds, anticipation, or suppression of these emotions

General Physical Symptoms
Strength and energy level: exhaustion, sleepiness, muscular weakness, disinclination to move; increased energy, restlessness

Temperature reactions: effects of exposure to heat or cold, hot or cold air, other warm or cold environments, damp or dry air, or changes of temperature

Sleep: ability to fall asleep and stay asleep, degree to which sleep is refreshing, feelings upon waking, sleeping position

Thirst and appetite: intensity of thirst and strong preferences for hot, cold, or iced liquids; food cravings and aversions (not just likes or dislikes but actually what the person craves or hates); appetite; food aggravations—any foods that cause general symptoms (Note: a craving for sweets in children is not considered a symptom unless it is unusually strong.)

Sweat: its odor; when it occurs; where it occurs—on covered or uncovered parts of the body, etc.

How do the modalities listed under particular symptoms affect each of these general symptoms?

General Psychological Symptoms
Describe all marked mental and emotional states just prior to and during the illness: fearful, anxious, sad, weepy, timid, hurried, irritable, jealous, moody, impatient, quarrelsome, obstinant, restless, obsessive, absentminded, confused, dull, anguished, lacking confidence or exhibiting

bravado, impulsive, indecisive, easily offended, easily startled, excitable, highly critical, lazy, malicious.
It is also important to know:

- Does the person want to be alone, or in the company of others?
- Does the person like or dislike sympathy?
- How is the person affected by noise, music, or being touched?
- Is the person unusually messy or tidy?

Be sure to get as specific information as possible. For example, if the person has fears, what is he or she fearful of: being alone, being in crowds, darkness, night, animals, illness, robbers, heights, the future, death?

CASE ANALYSIS AND REMEDY CHOICE

Complete and accurate casetaking is crucial to successful homeopathy, but evaluation and interpretation of the symptoms you collect is probably the most challenging part of homeopathic practice. Once you've completed an accurate analysis, choosing the correct medicine is fairly simple, for you'll have a clear and reliable picture of the person's overall physical, emotional, and mental symptoms.

Finding one medicine that fits each and every symptom is usually impossible. Fortunately, this is not necessary for the successful use of homeopathy. In essence, you attempt to match the symptoms to the medicine rather than the medicine to the person. In this process you first evaluate the key symptoms of the person and then assess the total symptom picture.

Case analysis consists of understanding the illness by determining which symptoms are more serious from a homeopathic perspective. Rather than focusing all your attention on a runny nose, a bad cough, or even a high fever, the important question to ask is: Which symptoms are most limiting to the person's optimal physical and psychological functioning? Sometimes a sick person feels fine generally, and only an irritated, congested nose causes him distress. But other times that runny nose is just the most obvious symptom, not the most important one—exhaustion or irritability may be causing much more misery than the sniffles.

A more analytical and mechanical step-by-step method will help you make sense of the formidable amount of information you've probably collected during casetaking. Also it will help you avoid the mistake of trying to find medicines for individual symptoms or of simply picking the medicine that matches the most symptoms. As your familiarity with homeopathy grows, you'll be able to dispense with the formal analysis, as long as you remember the guidelines for symptom evaluation and case analysis. Use the following steps for case analysis.

1. *Evaluate intensity of symptoms.* The simplest test to use when evaluating the symptoms is to rank their intensity or strength. What is the most definite change the person is experiencing with this illness? How strongly does each symptom affect the patient?

One way to gauge intensity is to consider how easy it was for you to recognize each symptom. If you're treating a family member, did the person complain to you about the problem (verbally or nonverbally), or did you have to ask what was wrong and observe him or her closely? Of course, these judgments depend on how expressive the sick person is and whether the illness has weakened him enough to limit clear communication.

Another way to evaluate symptom intensity is to ask yourself how much each symptom limits normal function. If the function of the affected body system seems all right, the symptom cannot be very intense. Of course, direct statements from the individual, or your own observations, greatly help determine which symptoms are stronger, more definite, or simply worse.

We suggest you rank the intensity of each symptom on a scale of 1 to 3, using 1 to describe apparently genuine symptoms about which you're not certain or that don't seem to bother the person much, and 3 to describe intense or glaringly obvious symptoms. A commonly used method for indicating ranks is underlining the recorded symptoms one to three times, but feel free to use any method you prefer.

2. *Evaluate depth of symptoms.* Once you have evaluated the intensity of each symptom, you must next determine its "depth," or "level." As we pointed out earlier, the homeopathic understanding is that general symptoms of the body or symptoms that affect the organs crucial to survival are more significant manifestations of the disease imbalance. *Assuming equal intensity,* symptoms are ranked by depth from deepest to most superficial.

- Mental and emotional symptoms of deviations from the norm rank as 3.
- Physical general symptoms, including the person's energy level, sleep, fever, perspiration, thirst, and appetite, along with the effects

of time, temperature, and other factors in general well-being, rank as 2. Factors associated with the onset of an illness, if definite, should be considered important general symptoms. The pace of the illness is also included in this category. Symptoms that are similar in character and that occur in different localized parts of the body may be grouped together and considered a general symptom. For example, burning pains occurring in the throat, stomach, and rectum during a digestive illness are considered one general symptom, "burning pain." The widespread muscle aches that accompany fever or the flu also can be considered a general symptom, since the aches affect the whole person (refer to the preceding "Outline for Casetaking in Acute Care" for a more detailed listing of general physical symptoms).

- Particular symptoms, such as runny nose, nausea, diarrhea, throat pain, or other localized discomforts, should be given a 1.

Within each category, rank the symptoms according to level. These judgments don't have to be exact, but use the chart of symptom levels presented in the section "Hering's Laws of Cure" in chapter 1 to help you decide where each symptom fits. Among the particular symptoms, those involving the lungs, kidney, and liver are of greater importance than those of other less vital internal organs, which, in turn, are more important than those of the muscles, joints, nose, and throat. Particular skin symptoms are of the least importance.

3. *Total points given each symptom for both intensity and depth categories.* List them in order of decreasing point totals for both rankings.

4. *Note idiosyncratic symptoms.* Mark symptoms on the list that you consider peculiar or unexpected. Unusual symptoms might include contradictory states, such as lack of thirst in spite of a high fever, vomiting that seems improved by eating, or a sensation of burning that is relieved by application of heat. Symptoms that aren't normally a part of a common illness pattern are included, too. Of course, you may not have enough medical background to know with certainty when a symptom is atypical of the illness, but anything that seems to fit this description should be noted.

5. *Evaluate modalities.* Once your symptom list is complete, add the modalities beside each symptom. Again, rate each modality according to how strongly it affects the symptom for better or worse on a scale of 1 to 3. Modalities do not require a ranking for level, since they are evaluated only in relation to symptoms of known level. By convention, homeo-

paths use the symbols ">" to indicate "made better by" and "<" to indicate "made worse by" in a summary list of symptoms.

6. *List "key symptoms" of the case.* From the list you've made, select four or five symptoms of higher rank and any pronounced, unusual symptoms. Note the one or two more definite modalities of each of these symptoms. This list of key symptoms will be used to begin the process of medicine selection.

Case analysis is now complete. Collect your original casetaking notes and the list of key symptoms, and you're ready to choose the medicine.

SELECTING THE RIGHT MEDICINE

Choosing the right medicine is essentially a matching process; you match the symptoms the sick person has with those that the medicine is known to cause in healthy people. The information we provide in this book is not as detailed as that in the reference *materia medica*s for professionals, but the main symptoms of the more commonly used medicines are listed. Each clinical chapter contains the pertinent symptoms of the homeopathic medicines more commonly used for people with that condition. The general symptoms of each medicine, along with other symptoms, are described in the *materia medica* in part 3.

The process of choosing a medicine also can be broken down into a number of steps.

1. *Read the appropriate clinical chapter(s).* If there are several symptoms (a cough and a sore throat, for example), read all pertinent chapters. Try first to match the key symptoms you listed during case analysis. Find all the medicines that fit at least one or two of these symptoms. For most conditions, we provide a Remedy Summary, which highlights the key symptoms of each medicine and helps you narrow down the list of possible medicines. In the Remedy Summary, symptoms listed under each remedy as "Essentials" are the more characteristic of that medicine and *must* be present for you to select it. The presence of any "Confirmatory symptoms" makes the choice of that medicine more certain, but these symptoms aren't critical. Then read the *materia medica* descriptions of any medicine that matches the key symptoms for more details on the medicine.

2. *Make a table.* Keep track of your progress by listing key symptoms and possible remedies in a table. Check off the appropriate column for every symptom matched by the medicine being considered (see the example, in the section "A Sample Case"). When you've finished the table, it will be easy to find the two or three medicines that cover the greatest number of key symptoms.

3. *Study the totality of symptoms.* At this point you should go back to the original complete case and compare *all* the symptoms with those of the medicines still under consideration. The process of selecting the right medicine requires more than mechanical matching. Subjective and even intuitive judgments can be decisive, especially as your experience grows. The key symptoms of the case are still more important, but you may now find that some aspect of one of the medicines just doesn't describe the remaining symptoms particularly well. Note these impressions in the table you made earlier.

4. *Choose the medicine.* Be flexible in making your final choice. Try to find a medicine that stands out as a nearly perfect match, or at least one that fits most of the key symptoms and seems to cover the overall picture. At this point, you'll have to dispense with numerical rankings and rely on reading the descriptions carefully.

As we have said, the medicine you choose does not have to cover every symptom. If, however, it has symptoms that are contradictory to key symptoms, you should consider other choices. For example, people who need *Pulsatilla* are usually gentle, mild, and yielding individuals. A child who is willful and stubborn and who throws angry temper tantrums would almost never be given *Pulsatilla,* even if she had other typical symptoms that medicine covers.

Finally, if you feel that two or more medicines fit the key symptoms equally well, or that none fits them particularly well, you may have to rely less on the key symptoms and more on matching the greatest number of symptoms from the complete case. Use this method only after you've tried the other approaches.

Important note: Even after careful study, sometimes you still can't find a medicine that clearly matches the sick person's symptoms. In the Remedy Summary for each condition, we have put a star next to the medicine that you should give under these conditions. The starred medicine is a "fall-back" choice, *not* the one you should always give first. In some cases, two or three medicines are starred when each is best given at a different stage of the illness.

ADMINISTERING THE MEDICINE

For the home prescriber, we recommend the use of the lower potencies: 6x, 6c, 12x, 12c, 30x, or 30c. When used according to the principles we've outlined, these potencies work well in stimulating the healing process. The 30x or 30c strengths generally act more deeply and quickly than the lower potencies, but they require more precise prescriptions than the lower potencies. If you feel uncertain about your prescription, we encourage you to use the 6x, 6c, 12x, or 12c.

In the clinical chapters of this book, we will occasionally recommend the use of specific potencies. If you have the medicine but not the potency recommended, do not delay giving the medicine to the ill person. Homeopaths have found that choosing the correct medicine is more critical than finding the best potency.

Homeopathic medicines are manufactured in several forms, which generally are available in all potencies. Sometimes you can obtain the liquid dilution of the medicinal substance. More often this liquid has been poured over sucrose pills of various sizes, from tiny "cake sprinkle" granules (#10 pellets) to larger spherical pills the size of buckshot or small peas (#35 pellets). Lactose is used to prepare cylindrical tablets when the medicine has been made by the trituration process described in chapter 1.

Depending on the form in which you have your homeopathic medicines, a dose consists of one drop of liquid, ten to twenty of the tiny #10 pellets, or one to three of the larger #35 pills or tablets. Medicine bottle labels often recommend somewhat larger doses, but they are not necessary. Since the medicines are already in such dilute form, their action does not depend on a large quantity of the substance being present, and the exact amount of the dose is not critical. Giving more in no way increases the strength of the body's response. The frequency of the dose's repetition is important, however, so follow the general rules below as well as the instructions in the chapter on the specific illness.

Before opening the medicine bottle, be sure there are no strong odors in the room; recap the vial as soon as you've poured out the dose. To avoid contaminating the medicine and to prevent receiving an accidental dose, you should not touch it. Pour it from the bottle onto a clear piece of white paper or into the bottle's cap, then tip the dose directly onto or under the tongue and allow it to dissolve in the mouth. Don't give the medicine with water. The best results occur when no taste of food, drink, or other flavors, such as toothpaste, is in the mouth. As a rule of thumb, avoid eating or drinking for fifteen to twenty minutes before and after administration of the dose.

Since the beginnings of homeopathic practice, certain substances and treatments have been found to reverse, or "antidote," the action of homeopathic medicines, and this causes the person's symptoms to return. Even relatively small amounts of substances such as camphor or coffee sometimes cause this antidoting effect. We recommend that you avoid coffee and products containing camphor or related substances during the period of homeopathic treatment and for forty-eight hours after the last dose.

Camphor is found in aromatic balms and cosmetics, including lip balms, Ben-Gay, Vick's, Heet, Campho-Phenique, Tiger Balm, Noxema, Caladryl, and some lipsticks, nail polishes, and other cosmetics. Substances containing mint or menthol, or the oils of eucalyptus, rosemary, pennyroyal, or other strong-smelling herbs also are best avoided, as are mouthwashes, cough drops, and the like.

If, for some reason, you do drink coffee or have contact with camphor or the like, you should continue treatment according to the guidelines in the following section, if no obvious changes in the symptoms occur. Since these substances do not always antidote homeopathic medicines, do not assume that they have created any problems unless you personally experience them. If the symptoms improved but suddenly return after the antidoting, the original medicine should be repeated. If the symptoms have changed significantly, a new medicine may be necessary, so study the case carefully.

Homeopathic medicines maintain their strength indefinitely when they are handled and stored properly, but their potency may be lost if they are treated incorrectly. The following guidelines for proper care, handling, and storage of the medicines should be observed.

- Prevent medicines from exposure to sunlight or other intense light, temperatures higher than 100°F, or odors of camphor, mothballs, perfumes, or other strong-smelling substances. Avoid storing them where such substances are kept, even when the medicines are tightly capped.
- Keep the medicines in their original container. They certainly should not be transferred to any other bottle that has previously contained other substances.
- Be careful not to contaminate the bottle cap, and try to replace it in the shortest time possible.
- Never open more than one bottle at a time in the same room. Cross-potentization may result if this precaution is not observed.

- If more than the desired number of pills are shaken out of the bottle, throw the excess away.
- If a medicine does become accidentally contaminated, simply replace it.

REPEATING AND CHANGING THE MEDICINE

How often you repeat the dose is crucial to effective homeopathic home care. The fundamental rule in classical homeopathy is: *Give no more medicine until the previous dose has ceased to act, no matter how long or short a time that may take.* Therefore no hard-and-fast schedule exists for dose repetition (ignore the recommendations printed on bottle labels); close observation of the response to treatment is the best way to tell when to repeat the medicine.

Often the person treated begins to improve markedly right after the first dose of the medicine or within an hour or two, and from there he continues to get better. Further treatment is unnecessary in these cases. Other times, however, the patient seems to pick up after the remedy is given, or a key symptom becomes less intense, and then no further improvement can be observed, and the condition gets worse again. This is an indication that repetition of the medicine is needed. You certainly should not wait until the symptoms are as bad as they were before the treatment to begin repetition.

Such close observation can be difficult. Moreover, the symptoms of acute illnesses tend to vary in the course of a few hours even without treatment. It therefore may be hard to decide exactly when to repeat the medicine. If improvement is dramatic, you should stop giving the medicine. If it's not dramatic, you may give it on a flexible schedule. Each chapter on individual ailments contains our recommended schedule of dose repetition for people with that condition (these recommendations are usually located in the Remedy Summary box). In general, follow these guidelines.

1. *The more severe the person's acute symptoms, the more often the medicine should be repeated.* If the person suffers from very high fever, extremely intense pain, or other significant symptoms, or if the person is severely ill and life is threatened, medicines can be given as often as every ten to fifteen minutes (of course, in these situations, obtaining medical care should be your first priority and you should use homeopathic medicines only while en route to emergency care or with the permission of your

health practitioner). As the person's symptoms diminish in intensity, reduce the frequency of dosage to every one to four hours.

For illnesses that are less extreme but still have intense symptoms—high fever, bad cough, severely painful throat—you can give the medicine every three to six hours. For even less severe illnesses, such as skin problems and run-of-the-mill colds or flus, two or three doses a day are all that's usually necessary.

2. *Continue the medicine for no more than two or three days.* This should suffice if the correct medicine has been chosen. If the medicine helped at first but the symptoms returned after the first two days, you'll probably need to find another medicine.

3. *Allow enough time for the medicine to act before changing to a new remedy.* There is sometimes a delayed response, so you should give the medicine according to the schedule recommended in the relevant clinical chapter for at least twelve to twenty-four hours.

4. *Don't try too many medicines for any one illness.* Do your best to find the right medicine, but stop after you've tried two or three different remedies without success.

A SAMPLE CASE

Now we can apply the steps of the homeopathic method to a hypothetical case. The case will be presented first as one person would tell it to another, and then in the outline form you would actually use while taking the case.

Our patient is eighteen-year-old Craig. Yesterday he came down with a sore throat that developed gradually. When he first woke up, he noticed his throat was scratchy. None of his friends or family members had been ill, and he hadn't been out in the cold. By yesterday evening he was beginning to feel quite sick, with a fever higher than 102°F. Now he describes the sore throat as a raw, burning pain. It became much worse as the fever increased. The pain had grown somewhat worse during the night, especially on the right side. Swallowing and talking aggravate it the most, although his throat feels better for a short time when he swallows warm liquids.

Craig is also having some trouble with diarrhea. He has had two or three very liquid stools over the past twenty-four hours and has felt weaker each time, but he doesn't feel any extreme urge to move his bowels, and there is no pain.

In general, our patient's fever makes him chilly. In spite of his high temperature, he needs to bundle up with lots of blankets and can't stand a draft or cold air. He feels agitated, internally restless, and notices that his left foot is constantly tapping and wiggling. Despite the restlessness, he is so weary he can't get out of bed. He experiences some body aches, but mainly he's just very tired and sick. All these general symptoms were worse during the night, and he perspired heavily sometime after midnight, after he was fully awake this morning, and he's still sweating lightly. He is about as thirsty as he normally is.

Craig feels unusually anxious, though he doesn't want to show it. He is worried that his illness might get worse, and when he woke up during the night, he couldn't help thinking that he might have a deadly disease. The anxiety and restlessness he experiences make it difficult for him to concentrate while reading his favorite magazine. He doesn't really care whether anyone else is around today, but during the night he got up and looked in on his parents to make sure they would be there if he suddenly got worse. He doesn't particularly seek sympathy, but when his mother comes in to see how he's doing, he doesn't mind her attention. Ordinarily, he leaves his records in a jumbled pile by the stereo. But earlier today when he felt a little better, he just had to get up and put them away in alphabetical order.

When he looks in the mirror he sees a pale, tired face. His throat is bright red, and there are a few tiny white spots on the right tonsil. He notices that some of the lymph nodes in his neck are a bit swollen.

That completes our description of Craig's case. The outline format you'll actually use when writing down the symptoms as you take the case will be organized in sections divided into parts of the body and the general and mental symptoms. Though you will want to be brief as you make note of the symptoms, you should write down the symptoms in the patient's own words. The case outline allows you to see all the symptoms at a glance. It's much easier to indicate the intensity of a symptom or modality by underlining and to make further notes if necessary. Here's how the case outline might look.

Main Concern: sore throat and fever since yesterday morning

Throat: had scratchy feeling in throat on waking yesterday, got worse in the evening when his fever went up, now intense <u>burning</u> raw pain—

worse on <u>right side</u>, at night, <u>swallowing, speaking</u>

better from <u>warm drinks</u> (a little while)

Digestion: diarrhea—liquid stools 2 to 3 times only since yesterday

no pain, no urging between movements

General: <u>chilly, worse drafts of air, cold air</u>—wants to bundle up
<u>felt sicker during the night</u>

<u>restless</u>, left foot keeps tapping and wiggling; person has difficulty read-
ing—with the restlessness he is very tired and has to lie still in bed

no apparent reason for onset—no exposure to cold, has been sleeping and
eating well

Mind: <u>anxious, worried that the disease will get worse</u>—during the
<u>night was scared of having a deadly disease</u>

doesn't especially want company now, but during the night had to make
sure that parents were there "in case"

put away records that are usually lying around in piles

indifferent to company and sympathy today

Examination: temperature is 102.5°, face pale
throat red and swollen with white spots on right tonsil

Let's try to make sense of all this information from the homeopathic
perspective. Much of the work has been done already by this point if
you've followed the pattern of the sample chart.

Now, with the help of the underlining you did while taking the
case, use the method we described in the section on case analysis: rate the
symptoms of the mind, the general symptoms, and the individual physical symptoms by intensity and depth. A reminder: each symptom is rated
1 to 3 on the basis of intensity; for ranking the depth, symptoms of the
mind earn 3 points, general symptoms 2, and particular physical symptoms 1 point. Add these two evaluations together to determine the overall rank of each symptom. Modalities are rated only according to how
definite or intense they are and are grouped with the symptom they pertain to. Going back over the sample chart, we can add the ratings of each
symptom to the outline (Figure 2-1).

		RATING (INTENSITY/DEPTH = TOTAL)
Throat:	*burning sore throat*	*3/1 = 4*
	worse on right side	*2*
	worse swallowing	*3*
	worse talking	*3*
	better warm drinks	*2*
	worse at night	*1*
Digestion:	*diarrhea*	*1/1 = 2*
General:	*chilly*	*3/2 = 5*
	worse at night	*2/2 = 4*
	restless	*3/2 = 5*
Mind:	*anxious, worried about the illness*	*3/3 = 6*
	more tidy than usual	*1/3 = 4*
Examination:	*red tonsils with small white dots*	*1/1 = 2*

Figure 2-1

Now we reorganize the symptoms, listing them in order of their ratings (Figure 2-2). Note that symptoms of equal total rating are placed in order of their level, "deeper" symptoms appearing higher on the list (we may want to alter this order later).

Remember, these numerical listings are not iron-clad, and the overall case should be referred to whenever there is doubt. Still, we are ready to choose the key symptoms that we'll use for remedy selection. In this example, the first five or six symptoms qualify for key-symptom status. All have overall ratings of 4 or more, and all except the unusual tidiness are fairly well marked.

We first compare the key symptoms to those of the remedies in chapter 8 on sore throats, also consulting the *materia medica* entries in part 3. We then make a table of the medicines and the symptoms they cover as we go.

SYMPTOM	RATING
Anxious, fearful	6
Chilly	5
Restless	5
Tidier than usual	4
Generally worse at night	4

Burning sore throat	4	
worse speaking	3	
worse swallowing	3	modalities
worse on right side	2	
better warm drinks	2	
Spots on tonsils	2	
Diarrhea	2	

Figure 2-2

The highest-ranking symptom is anxiety and fear, and this symptom is a notable feature of four medicines: *Aconite, Arsenicum, Lycopodium,* and *Rhus tox.* General chilliness is found in symptoms of *Hepar sulph.* and three of the four medicines, but not *Lycopodium.* Marked restlessness is also characteristic of *Arsenicum, Aconite,* and *Rhus tox.* Only *Arsenicum* covers the patient's unusual tidiness. All three of these medicines cover the nighttime aggravation, but only *Arsenicum* is noted for the particular after-midnight increase of symptoms. All also apply to sore throats, but burning sore-throat pain is a pronounced characteristic of *Arsenicum* only. Our new table of key symptoms now looks like this (Figure 2-3).

So far *Arsenicum* is clearly the leading candidate, but *Aconite, Rhus tox.,* and *Lycopodium* all cover at least three of the key symptoms. It's time to look for confirmatory symptoms. The modalities of the throat pain should help. However, all the sore-throat medicines covered here worsen during swallowing, and none is listed for aggravation from talking. Sore throat on the right side is covered by *Lycopodium* and *Belladonna.* Relief brought by warm drinks is a symptom of *Arsenicum, Rhus tox., Hepar sulph.,* and *Lycopodium.*

	ANXIOUS	CHILLY	RESTLESS	TIDY	WORSE AT NIGHT	BURNING THROAT PAIN
Aconite	x	x	x		x	
Arsenicum	x	x	x	x	x	x
Hepar sulph.		x				
Lycopodium	x	x	x		x	
Rhus tox.	x	x	x		x	

Figure 2-3

Diarrhea is a minor symptom in this case, but referring to the section on diarrhea shows that, of the medicines that look more promising, only *Arsenicum* is listed as appropriate.

Now compare the overall case to the pictures of each of the possible remedies. This is usually when the choice of the correct medicine becomes more clear. *Aconite* is best given in the earliest stages of acute illnesses that suddenly bring intense anguish and fearful restlessness. *Arsenicum* covers conditions that have progressed a little further and that are characterized by anxiety and restlessness accompanied by a greatly weakened state. These conditions also include a desire for reassuring company and a special tendency to be concerned about tidiness. The associated pains are more often burning in character, and are relieved by warmth. Digestive symptoms, especially vomiting and diarrhea, are common. *Rhus tox.* is also suited to anxiety and restlessness, but pass when the person is moving about, a characteristic that is not listed for the other medicines. *Rhus tox.* conditions typically arise after exposure to cold and damp weather, and the symptoms improve with warmth.

Based on these comparisons, we can eliminate *Aconite.* Our patient's illness did not begin suddenly, and the inflammatory symptoms did not come on with great force. *Hepar sulph.* is for someone more irritable, and *Lycopodium* is for those less chilly and thirsty. Only *Arsenicum* and *Rhus tox.* are really in the running. While almost all the symptoms of the case are covered by both medicines, *Arsenicum* fits most of the details of the case better, and some of its characteristic symptoms—restlessness with weakness, burning pains, tidiness—are present. Important characteristic symptoms of *Rhus tox.* that might confirm its choice are missing.

Now we must review the original case to see if we have left anything out. One detail is interesting: the patient says he doesn't care whether he has company, but when he felt afraid during the night, he had to get up to see if his parents were there. This may in fact be evidence of the *Arsenicum* tendency to seek company for reassurance.

Based on the results of this analysis, we choose *Arsenicum* as the medicine and administer it according to the guidelines in "Administering the Medicine" and the specific instructions in chapter 8. After several hours we evaluate the case again and decide whether the medicine is helping. Our next action regarding whether or not to repeat or change the medicine will be based on the guidelines in "Repeating and Changing the Medicine." If the symptoms are essentially unchanged after giving *Arsenicum* a fair try, *Rhus tox.* will be a good medicine to try next.

Well done. The clinical chapters in the following part will mean more to you now that you've experienced your first homeopathic case.

PART II

HOME CARE WITH HOMEOPATHIC MEDICINE

Before you begin to use the specific chapters, please glance through the following listing of homeopathic remedies to be found in this book, and familiarize yourself with their names and abbreviations.

TABLE OF MEDICINES

An asterisk (*) signifies those medicines we recommend be included in your home medicine kit. The dagger (†) signifies second-choice medicines for your home medicine kit; depending on the health problems you and your family experience, other medicines also may be included.

Aconite (Acon.)—monkshood*
Allium cepa (Allium cepa)—onion*
Anacardium (Anac.)—marking nut
Antimonium crudum (Anti. c.)—black sulphide of antimony
Antimonium tartaricum (Anti. t.)—tartrate of antimony and potassium
Apis mellifica (Apis)—bee venom or the honey bee*
Arnica montana (Arnica)—mountain daisy (internal and external preparations)*
Arsenicum album (Arsenicum/Ars.)—white arsenic; arsenious acid*
Belladonna (Belladonna/Bell.)—deadly nightshade*
Bellis perennis (Bellis)—English daisy
Berberis vulgaris (Berberis)—barberry
Borax (Borax)—borate of sodium
Bryonia alba (Bryonia/Bry.)—wild hops*
Calcarea carbonica (Calc. carb.)—calcium carbonate or carbonate of lime†
Calendula (Calendula)—marigold (an external preparation)*
Cantharis (Cantharis)—spanish fly*
Carbo vegetabilis (Carbo veg.)—vegetable charcoal†
Caulophyllum (Caulo.)—blue cohosh
Causticum (Caust.)—potassium hydrate
Chamomilla (Cham.)—chamomile*
Cheladonium majus (Chel.)—celandine
Chimaphilla umbellata (Chim.)—pipsissewa
China officinalis (China)—peruvian bark or cinchona
Cimicufuga racemosa (Cimic.)—black snakeroot
Colocynthis (Coloc.)—bitter cucumber†
Croton tiglium (Croton)—croton oil seed
Cuprum metallicum (Cuprum)—copper
Drosera (Drosera)—sundew

Dulcamara (Dulc.)—bittersweet or woody nightshade
Equisetum (Equisetum)—scouring rush
Eupatorium perfoliatum (Eup. perf.)—boneset or thoroughwort†
Euphrasia (Euphrasia)—eyebright†
Ferrum phosphoricum (Ferrum phos.)—phosphate of iron*
Gelsemium (Gels.)—yellow jessamine*
Glonoine (Glon.)—Nitroglycerine
Graphites (Graph.)—graphite†
Hepar sulphuricum (Hepar sulph.)—Hahnemann's calcium suphide*
Hydrastis (Hydrastis)—goldenseal
Hypericum perforatum (Hypericum or Hyper.)—St. John's wort (internal and
    external preparations)*
Ignatia imara (Ign.)—St. Ignatius bean*
Ipecacuanha (Ipec.)—ipecac root*
Iris versicolor (Iris.)—blue flag
Kali bichromium (Kali bi.)—bichromate of potash*
Kreosotum (Kreos.)—beechwood kreosote
Lachesis (Lach.)—venom from the bushmaster or surucucu snake*
Ledum palustre (Ledum.)—marsh tea*
Lycopodium (Lyc.)—club moss*
Magnesium phosphorica (Mag. phos.)—phosphate of magnesia*
Mercurius (Merc.)—quicksilver or mercury*
Mezereum (Mez.)—spurge olive
Natrum muriaticum (Nat. mur.)—sodium chloride or table salt†
Natrum sulphicum (Nat. sulph.)—salicylate of sodium
Nitric acid (Nitric acid)—nitric acid
Nux vomica (Nux)—poison nut*
Petroleum (Pet.)—crude oil
Phosphorus (Phos.)—phosphorus*
Phytolacca (Phyto.)—pokeroot
Pilocarpinum (Pilo.)—pilocarpine
Podophyllum (Podo.)—mayapple†
Pulsatilla (Puls.)—windflower*
Ranunculus bulbosus (Ran. bulb.)—buttercup
Rhus diversiloba (Rhus div.)—poison oak†
Rhus toxicodendron (Rhus tox.)—poison ivy*
Ruta graveolens (Ruta)—rue bitterwort†
Sabadilla (Sabadilla)—cevadilla seed
Sanguinaira (Sang.)—bloodroot
Sarsaparilla (Sars.)—smilax
Sepia (Sepia)—inky juice of the cuttlefish*

Silica (Silica)—silica or flint*
Spongia tosta (Spongia)—roasted sponge†
Staphysagria (Staph.)—stavesacre†
Sulphur (Sulphur)—sulfur*
Symphytum (Symph.)—comfrey*
Tabacum (Tabacum)—tobacco
Tellurium (Tell.)—tellurium
Thuja occidentalis (Thuja)—arbor vitae or the tree of life†
Urtica urens (Urtica)—stinging nettle†
Veratrum album (Veratrum alb.)—white hellebore
Wyethia (Wyethia)—poison weed

CHAPTER 3

FEVER AND INFLUENZA

F EVER IS NOT A DISEASE, but it so commonly accompanies many kinds of illnesses that we have covered it separately here. Influenza, on the other hand, is a specific type of viral infection. We include it in this chapter because fever often is one of the only symptoms of the flu. We also include a brief description of Reye's syndrome, a rare but very dangerous condition associated with viral illnesses including influenza.

FEVER

Fever can accompany almost every type of infection and occurs in other illnesses as well. Fever may be the only apparent symptom of an illness, especially in the early stages. But if symptoms other than fever also are present, consult the chapter that covers those symptoms as well.

Don't be frightened by the fever itself—fever is usually a beneficial phenomenon. Not only is it a valuable warning that an infection is taking place, but the fever is itself part of the body's defense against the infection. Ancient physicians, such as Hippocrates and Celsus, considered fever a means by which the body "cooks," separates, and eventually eliminates the disease. In more scientific terms, the ability to increase body temperature has come to be understood as a basic defense shared by all organisms that can regulate their own internal temperature.[1]

Fever may help fight infection in various ways. Simple elevation of temperature reduces the growth of or even kills some disease-causing organisms. More indirect effects of fever include enhancement of such innate immune defenses as increasing the production of interferon (a substance made by the body that inhibits viral reproduction) and increasing white blood cell mobility and activity. Fever, indeed, is an important positive response of the body.

WHAT YOU SHOULD KNOW ABOUT FEVER

Fever is defined somewhat arbitrarily as a rise in body temperature to above 99.5°F (measured orally). Actually, normal body temperature varies from person to person and, for each person, with time of day, activity level, and other factors. The traditionally normal reading of 98.6°F (37°C) is only an approximate average; your own temperature may range from a little higher than 96°F to about 99°F when you're perfectly healthy. Also, temperature elevations (as high as 103°F in children) can occur after exercise or from being overdressed.

The body's regulatory mechanisms limit fevers to a maximum of 105°F to 106°F during simple acute illnesses in normal individuals. Higher temperatures can be harmful, but unless there is something else complicating the acute illness, a fever rarely gets so high that it threatens health. Dehydration that results from fever can be dangerous, especially in children and the elderly, but it can be prevented by making certain that extra liquids are consumed (see chapter 9).

High fevers also sometimes cause seizures in children. Such "febrile seizures" usually occur while the temperature is rising rapidly, and end once it has reached its peak. They are most likely to occur in boys between six and twenty-four months old. In children who are otherwise healthy, the seizure tends to affect the whole body, not just one part or one side, and to last no more than twenty minutes, usually much less. Any deviation from this pattern may indicate an underlying neurologic disor-

---

1. Matthew J. Kluger, "Fever," *Pediatrics* 66 (November 1980): 720–24; Matthew J. Kluger and Barbara A. Rothenburg, "Fever and Reduced Iron: Their Interaction As a Host Defense Response to Bacterial Infection," *Science* 203 (26 January, 1979): 374–76; Matthew J. Kluger and Barbara A. Rothenburg, "Fever, Trace Metals, and Disease," in *Fever*, edited by J. M. Lipton (New York: Raven, 1980).

der. Although all children who have seizures during a fever need to be medically evaluated, simple febrile seizures tend to happen only once or twice and cause no lasting ill effects. They are not uncommon and generally do not represent a serious health problem.

What all this means is that the fever accompanying an acute illness is not ordinarily a cause for concern. Instead of worrying about the fever, you should pay attention to the illness responsible and try to aid the healing efforts of the body. So long as it is not too high, the fever is best left to continue its work as part of the body's effort to heal.

GENERAL HOME CARE

Rest and plenty of liquids (to replace the body fluid lost due to sweating) are still important in the care of a person with a fever. It is normal for fever to be accompanied by a diminished appetite, so don't force-feed the patient. Since heat is dissipated through the skin, allow for good air circulation in the room and make certain the patient isn't heavily covered or dressed—clothing should be the minimum necessary to prevent chilliness. Often these steps are all that's necessary to relieve a mild fever. We don't recommend treatment with either conventional or homeopathic medicines for minor fevers.

Sometimes bringing the fever down is a worthwhile goal in itself—if the temperature is 103.5°F or higher for more than an hour, if at any time it climbs above 105°F, if the patient is a child who has had febrile seizures, or if the fever simply has lasted long enough to be exhausting or really uncomfortable. But remember, fever is a protective response, and you should consider suppressing a fever only for the reasons just mentioned.

Although there is some controversy about its efficacy, sponge bathing is recommended by many clinicians as an effective, drug-free way to bring down fevers of mild or moderate illnesses. If the patient can put up with some discomfort, sponge bathing works more quickly than and for just as long as conventional medicines. Actually, research shows that sponge bathing works best in combination with acetaminophen given to reset the body's "thermostat" about a half-hour before—but if you've decided to use conventional medicine, you probably won't need to bother with a sponge bath.

In any case, here's the technique: Just have the person sit in a basin or tub in waist-deep, lukewarm water (don't use alcohol). Gradually lower the water temperature by letting a little cold water run into the tub. Use a wet sponge or washcloth to bathe all exposed skin, including the face, and get the hair wet as well. Continue for ten or fifteen minutes. Then pat-dry the largest drops of water and allow the skin to air-dry in a cool room, protecting the person from drafts.

When fever is too high, too uncomfortable, or has lasted too long, and if the homeopathic medicines are not working rapidly enough, you may want to use medication such as acetaminophen, aspirin, ibuprofen (Motrin, Advil), or naproxen (Aleve, Naprosyn). All of these drugs work, but each has its pros and cons and should not be used with any other. In general, we prefer acetaminophen if one of these drugs must be used. In any case, you must be absolutely certain they are stored in a safe place so accidental poisoning cannot occur. Seek medical advice before giving any of these medicines to a baby younger than two.

When used correctly, acetaminophen is safe and rarely causes side effects, and it is easier to give to children because it is available as a liquid and as suppositories. However, overdoses can cause serious poisoning with potentially irreversible liver damage. *Be especially careful to follow package directions when using the liquid forms of acetaminophen.* The drops meant for babies are much more concentrated than the liquid intended for older children, which has led to poisonings when parents confused the two forms.

Aspirin should not be given to children or teenagers because it has been implicated in Reye's syndrome, a rare but often fatal disease. Aspirin also can produce side effects and allergic reactions in relatively low doses. Still, it's inexpensive and time-tested, and a good choice for adults who are not allergic to it.

The newer over-the-counter drugs ibuprofen and naproxen work much like aspirin and share its most serious side effects, although they are less likely to cause ringing in the ears. Their effects last longer than acetaminophen's, so you can take them less often—but this is a disadvantage when you're trying to minimize your interference with the body's natural healing process.

CASETAKING QUESTIONS FOR FEVER

Character of the symptoms:
- Did the symptoms seem to begin after a particular stress? For example, from exposure to cold air or wind, loss of sleep, or overindulgence in food or drugs?
- How recently did the fever start? Within the last 12 hours, or earlier than that?
- How quickly did the symptoms begin?
- Is the face flushed?
- What is the person's mental condition—is he dull or confused, delirious, restless and anxious, irritable, or clingy and tearful?

Modalities:
- Does the person feel warm or chilly? How do external heat and cold make him feel?

HOMEOPATHIC MEDICINES

If you decide that the illness should be treated and fever is the only obvious symptom, consult the homeopathic information in this chapter for help with choosing the right medicine. If there are other symptoms as well (sore throat, earache, and so on), consult the appropriate chapter for relevant homeopathic medicines.

A homeopathic medicine should be given every two to six hours depending on the severity of the symptoms. Generally, the ill person will recover quickly or at least after one night's rest. If the fever isn't gone or much lower by the next morning, you'll probably want to try another medicine.

Belladonna and *Aconite* are the best medicines to try during the first stages of a sudden fever. *Belladonna* is by far the most commonly given medicine for people with simple fever. It's the medicine to give first unless another is clearly indicated.

The classic picture of the *Belladonna* fever includes a red flushed face, intensely hot skin, reddened mucous membranes, and glassy eyes with dilated pupils. The skin can be so hot that you notice the heat lingering on your hands after you touch it. Although *Belladonna* patients are mentally dull and may not fully comprehend what's going on around them, they may well be restless and agitated. Children may even hit, bite, tear at things, or exhibit strange behaviors such as speaking incoherently about scary or violent hallucinations. Of course, most people who need *Belladonna* don't have these extreme symptoms. Still, they often do show some nervous excitability and their senses often are more acute. As the illness progresses, they may develop muscle twitching, which, like many of the *Belladonna* symptoms, comes and goes suddenly.

Choose *Aconite* when fever comes on suddenly and the patient is anxious, restless, and fearful, especially if the illness begins after exposure to dry and cold air or wind. The *Aconite* patient is mentally alert—unlike *Belladonna*—but frightened, and he may toss in his sleep or throw off his covers or clothes. In the classic case, he has dry skin, dry mouth (perhaps with unquenchable thirst for cold drinks), and a dry cough. The pupils may be constricted.

Ferrum phos. is another medicine to consider early in the course of a fever. Choose this remedy when symptoms develop gradually, rather than all of a sudden as in *Belladonna* and *Aconite.* You can give *Ferrum phos.* also when *Belladonna* seems indicated but doesn't work after two or three doses.

The chief indication for *Nux vomica* during a fever is that the patient feels extremely chilly. The chills are worsened by uncovering or even slightly moving the blankets—she can't move under the covers without setting off a wave of chilliness. The symptoms of *Nux* patients often begin after overeating, going without sleep, or using too much alcohol or drugs of any type. The person also may have various digestive symptoms, such as constipation or nausea, and may have a sensation of heaviness of the head. The symptoms are worse in the morning and in the open air. Irritability is typical.

Although *Pulsatilla* is more often used when there are clear symptoms of a cold or ear infection, you can give it when fever is the only symptom. Choose *Pulsatilla* when the characteristic mental and general symptoms of this medicine are evident (see the *materia medica* section). Individuals who need *Pulsatilla* are weepy and clingy, craving affection. Their moods are changeable. They may be irritable, but the irritability is more whiny than angry or strong. They are intolerant of external heat, and they feel much worse when warmly covered or in warm rooms. The symptoms often begin after the patient has eaten too much rich or fatty food, and tend to get worse at night. Classically, the *Pulsatilla* patient isn't thirsty, even with a fever.

REMEDY SUMMARY FOR FEVER

Give the medicine: Every 2 to 4 hours at first, gradually less frequently as the patient improves, for up to 3 days.

When to try another medicine: If there is no significant improvement within 2 hours (if the fever is high and the person is quite ill) to 24 hours (in mild illnesses).

BELLADONNA★

Essentials
- The most common medicine for the early stage of fever (first 12 to 24 hours), especially with sudden onset
- Red flushed face, reddened mucous membranes, glassy eyes

Confirmatory symptoms
- Skin very hot, heat lingers when you touch the skin
- Mental dullness, confusion, agitation

ACONITE

Essentials
- Also indicated during the early stages of a sudden fever
- Acute fever accompanied by anxiety, fear, restlessness

Confirmatory symptoms
- Symptoms come on after exposure to cold air or wind

FERRUM PHOS.

Essentials
- Early in fevers when the symptoms develop gradually
- Patient is more alert, less restless or anxious than with *Belladonna* or *Aconite*
- If no remedy seems clearly indicated, try this if *Belladonna* hasn't helped (see p. 53 for instructions on how long to wait before switching remedies)

Confirmatory symptoms
- Flushing of the face may be confined to circular patches

NUX VOMICA

Essentials
- Great chilliness, worse from uncovering or from moving the blankets

Confirmatory symptoms
- Symptoms beginning after overindulgence, overwork, loss of sleep
- May be accompanied by queasy stomach
- Irritability

PULSATILLA

Essentials
- Weepy, clingy mood, craving affection; changeable moods *and/or*
- Worse in warm rooms or when warmly covered; unusually little thirst

Confirmatory symptoms
- Symptoms may have started after eating rich food

BEYOND HOME CARE

See "Beyond Home Care" following the section on influenza below.

INFLUENZA

Though illnesses such as colds, digestive upsets, and other maladies are often called "the flu," technically influenza is an acute infection of the respiratory tract associated with a particular group of viruses. Practically speaking, the diagnosis is influenza if acute respiratory symptoms like runny nose or cough are accompanied by marked fever, general weakness, and muscular aching. The person with the flu looks and feels more ill than he would with just a common cold.

Though uncomfortable, influenza ordinarily lasts only three to five days in most healthy people. However, the severity of the illness varies from person to person and from year to year. Influenza can be a life-threatening disease among young children, the elderly, and those debilitated by chronic illnesses—especially because severe bacterial infections such as pneumonia can develop when the system is weakened by the flu virus (ear and sinus infections also may occur). Also, the flu viruses mutate rapidly, and some strains have been much more virulent than others.

GENERAL HOME CARE

Home treatment for people with influenza is the same as for those with fevers and colds (see chapter 4). Avoid aspirin, especially when treating children, since its use for influenza is associated with Reye's syndrome. Antibiotics are unnecessary and actually can be harmful; they should be avoided unless a secondary bacterial infection has developed.

CASETAKING QUESTIONS FOR INFLUENZA

Character of the symptoms:
- Which are the more bothersome symptoms—tiredness, a heavy feeling, or aches and pains? (If fever is a predominant symptom, see the previous section; if there is significant runny nose or cough, see chapter 4.)
- Is there a headache, and if so, where is it located and what sort of pain does it cause? (If headache is severe, see chapter 11.)
- Does the person have chills?
- Is the person restless, or does she prefer to lie still?

Modalities:
- How does moving about affect the pains?
- How do heat and cold affect the body aches, and do they make the person feel better or worse in general?

HOMEOPATHIC MEDICINES

One of the great success stories of homeopathic medicine concerns its superb treatment of epidemic influenza during the 1917–18 flu season. Records maintained by government medical officers at the time show that proportionally, far fewer patients treated homeopathically died from the flu or its complications than those who received conventional medical treatment.

To decide on a homeopathic medicine when flu symptoms strike, review the remedies described in this chapter as well as those discussed in chapter 4 on colds and coughs. Among appropriate flu medicines covered in other chapters are *Aconite, Belladonna, Arsenicum, Pulsatilla,* and *Nux vomica.*

In many ways, the symptoms of *Gelsemium* represent the classic picture of flu—this is the medicine to give if you can't find a better fit. The person mainly feels tired, weak, heavy, and sick. Generally, *Gelsemium* patients want to be left alone, not because they're especially irritable, but simply because it's too much work to interact with people. They don't feel restless, and although motion isn't painful, the patient just lies still because she's so weak. The eyelids look heavy and droopy, and the face may appear dull and lacking in expression. A *Gelsemium* flu is characterized by chills, which often run up and down the back. Typically, there is little thirst in spite of the fever. The nose may be runny and the throat may burn. Headaches are common, usually in the back of the head and extending to the top or forehead. More striking symptoms, however, are general weakness and tiredness.

There are two main symptoms that should lead you to choose *Bryonia* instead of *Gelsemium:* irritability with aversion to company, and physical aggravation from motion. If either or both of these are present, give *Bryonia.* Like the *Gelsemium* patient, someone who needs *Bryonia* doesn't want to be disturbed, but the *Bryonia* patient is truly irritable. He may snap when asked questions or refuse to answer them altogether. He may be preoccupied with worries about his business or other ordinary affairs. Motion makes *Bryonia* patients worse, and they feel better when lying still. They are likely to have generalized muscle and joint aches that are definitely more painful from motion. The patient lies still because it hurts to move, not just because he's too tired. A common *Bryonia* symptom is a headache that grows worse with motion, from walking, or even from moving the eyes. Light touch, eating, stooping, and talking also may make headaches worse, while applying firm pressure and lying still may relieve them. *Bryonia* patients generally feel worse in warm rooms and better in the cool air. They may have an intense thirst for cold drinks. A dry, hacking, often painful cough may accompany the flu symptoms. Constipation is also typical of *Bryonia.*

In contrast with *Bryonia* patients, people with a *Rhus tox.* influenza are restless. The muscles become stiff and achy if the patient lies still for any length of time. Paradoxically, her pain feels most severe when trying to move after a period of rest, but it improves as soon as she moves about and limbers up. She may be unable to sleep, because it's so uncomfortable keeping still. The *Rhus tox.* patient is likely to be chilly and feel worse in cold, wet weather, improving in warmth and with applied heat. Exposure to damp weather or overexertion may have brought on the illness. The patient is thirsty, sometimes only for sips of water at a time, and may sweat profusely. Mentally, she may be anxious, apprehensive, irritable, or depressed. Dry mouth and lips, dry sore throat, and hoarseness often accompany the general symptoms.

Severe aching and pain that feels as though it comes from deep inside the bones is the most distinctive symptom of *Eupatorium perfoliatum.* There is a bruised soreness all over the body, and the bones, especially in the back, feel as though they would break. Symptoms that confirm the choice of this medicine—but that aren't necessarily present—include a sudden nasal discharge with sneezing and redness in the eyes preceding the onset of the body aches. *Eupatorium* patients are subject to chills, especially in the morning between 7 and 9 A.M. Typically they have great thirst for ice-cold drinks, but liquids may cause digestive disorders. A dry, hacking cough that shakes the body also is characteristic.

One medicine to try early in the illness when there are few distinguishing symptoms is *Oscillococcinum.* Research published in the *British Journal of Clinical Pharmacology* shows that *Oscillococcinum* is considerably more effective in treating influenza than a placebo.[2] *Oscillococcinum* has become the most popular flu medicine in France and is quickly gaining popularity in the U.S. It is most effective when given within forty-eight hours of onset of flu symptoms.

REMEDY SUMMARY FOR INFLUENZA

In addition to the medicines listed here, consider those covered in the sections on fever (if fever is the primary symptom) or colds (if a runny or stuffy nose is prominent).

Give the medicine: Every 6 to 8 hours for 2 to 3 days, stopping when there is definite improvement.

When to try another medicine: If there is no significant improvement after 24 hours.

2. J. P. Ferley, D. Zmirou, D. D'Admehar, et al., "A Controlled Evaluation of a Homeopathic Preparation in the Treatment of Influenza-like Syndrome," *British Journal of Clinical Pharmacology* 27 (March 1989): 329–35.

GELSEMIUM ★

Essentials
- Tired, weak, heavy sensation of the body
- Lies still and wants to be left alone because of tiredness

Confirmatory symptoms
- Chills running up and down the spine
- Little thirst
- Headache beginning in the back of the head or neck and extending upward

BRYONIA

Essentials
- Motion aggravates the pain and other symptoms
- Irritable and doesn't want people around

Confirmatory symptoms
- Thirsty for cold drinks
- Feels worse in warm rooms, better in cool air
- Headaches worse from motion, walking, or moving the eyes

RHUS TOX.

Essentials
- Restlessness
- Aches and pains while lying still; worse when first starting to move but get better with continued motion

Confirmatory symptoms
- Chilly, feels worse in cold and damp air
- Thirsty for sips of water
- Dry mouth, dry sore throat

EUPATORIUM PERFOLIATUM

Essentials
- Severe aching pain, feels like the bones are breaking

Confirmatory symptoms
- Runny nose, sneezing, and red eyes prior to the body aches
- Chills, especially in the morning
- Thirsty for ice cold drinks

OSCILLOCOCCINUM

Essentials
- Can be given during the first 48 hours of a flulike illness when few distinguishing symptoms are present

BEYOND HOME CARE

See also the section on dehydration in chapter 8. If other symptoms (earache, sore throat, cough, etc.) accompany the fever, be sure to consult "Beyond Home Care" in the chapters that cover those symptoms.

GET MEDICAL CARE IMMEDIATELY:

- for *any* fever in a child less than 4 months of age;
- for fever of 106°F or higher (orally or rectally) in any age group;
- if, with any illness whether or not there is fever, there is extreme irritability, lethargy, or mental confusion; stiffness of the neck; seizures; rapid, shallow, or labored breathing; recurrent, prolonged vomiting; or simply if the person looks terribly sick;
- for fever accompanied by a rash that is purple, looks like blood or a burn, or does not blanch when pressed.

GET MEDICAL CARE TODAY:

- for any fever in a child 4 to 6 months old;
- for fever of 103.5°F or higher (orally) that does not respond within 6 hours to home care measures, including sponge bathing, homeopathic medicine, or conventional medicine. Adults and older children who feel all right in general may wait longer;
- if fever below 103.5°F has lasted longer than 24 hours in children 6 to 24 months, or longer than 72 hours in older individuals.

SEE YOUR PRACTITIONER SOON:

• if you have any doubts about the severity of the illness.

Note: The exact temperatures we refer to are somewhat arbitrary, and when deciding to seek medical advice, you must always consider the severity of the person's general illness, your experience in caring for sick people, and the patient's previous history with similar illnesses.

REYE'S SYNDROME

Reye's syndrome is a rare but potentially deadly disease that usually follows a viral respiratory illness, especially influenza or chicken pox. Children younger than eighteen are most often affected, but anyone can get it. Reye's syndrome affects the liver and brain, along with other vital organs. Symptoms include vomiting that occurs after the onset of a viral illness, irritability, and sleepiness or disorientation progressing to coma. Diarrhea or rapid, shallow breathing may occur. Fever may or may not be present. Unlike gastrointestinal infections, Reye's syndrome causes unexpected vomiting that is remarkable because it begins some time after the initial symptoms of the viral illness. Vomiting is usually recurrent and prolonged, though this is not always the case, and it may be entirely absent in young children. Reye's syndrome is an immediate, life-or-death medical emergency.

CHAPTER 4

COLDS, COUGHS,
AND RELATED CONDITIONS

THE SYMPTOMS of the common cold are the body's way of responding to a viral infection of the upper respiratory tract. Through nasal discharge, sneezing, coughing, and fever, the body expels and "burns out" the infecting viruses. Thus, these symptoms reveal the body's efforts to reestablish health, and they should not be suppressed unless truly necessary. Don't cure a cold—let a cold cure you.

Medicines such as nasal sprays, cough suppressants, and fever reducers may offer temporary relief from the symptoms of a cold, but they do so by hindering the body's own defenses. Nasal sprays and cold capsules slow down mucus production and therefore inhibit healing, since mucus serves to cleanse the tissues of the virus and to protect them from further infection. Cough medicines block the body's cough reflex, which can be problematic, since coughing helps clear breathing passages. Fever also is an important defense the body has against infection, and aspirin or acetaminophen interferes with this protective response (see chapter 3 on fever). Instead of relying on these suppressive medications, support the body's efforts by taking homeopathic medicines.

In this chapter we review the many symptoms associated with colds and coughs, and describe home-care measures that support the body's own efforts to return to health rapidly. The list of homeopathic medicines useful for cold symptoms is quite long, so we provide an index of symptoms to help you find possible medicines more quickly. (Each symptom is followed by a list of the medicines which fit that symptom.) This chapter also includes separate, brief sections on sinus congestion and conjunctivitis, or "pinkeye." These conditions are closely related to colds, but we cover them individually because they may require specific home-care and homeopathic treatment measures.

COLDS AND COUGHS

The symptoms of a cold—runny or stuffy nose, sneezing, and watery eyes, sometimes accompanied by mild sore throat or earache—are familiar to everyone. Some swelling of and tenderness in the lymph nodes is common during a cold. Most people feel tired or just plain bad, and moderate fever is fairly common. Some loss of appetite often occurs; bowel movements may be affected, becoming either less frequent or loose.

If earache or sore throat is at all marked, you should consult chapters 6 and 7. When weakness, fever, or swollen glands is the predominant symptom, the illness may be influenza, mononucleosis, or something else other than a cold. See chapter 3 on influenza, and the section on mononucleosis in chapter 7 for advice.

COUGHS

During a cold, cough occurs when the body reacts to viruses infecting the lower airways, including the throat, trachea, or bronchi. Whether the cough is shallow or deep, dry or loose, depends on the location and severity of the infection and in turn on the strength of the person's healing defenses. A cold virus rarely invades the lungs themselves, and although coughs tend to drag on longer than head colds, the person almost always gets well on his own with time. On the other hand, a cough is sometimes evidence of a more serious condition such as bacterial infection, allergy, or a foreign body in the air passages.

A variety of conditions and symptoms may affect the lower respiratory passages. The most common include the following.

CROUP: Caused by viral infection of the larynx (voice box) and the breathing passages of the upper chest. Croup occurs most commonly in children three months to three years old and is characterized by a cough that sounds harsh, loud, barking, and ringing. The child is often hoarse.

Because of the swelling caused by the infection, the breathing passages become more narrow and the child breathes rapidly, forcefully, and noisily as air moves through the constriction.

Croup must be differentiated from epiglottitis, which can cause sudden, complete obstruction of breathing and is a medical emergency. See chapter 7 on sore throats for details. Epiglottitis is rarely accompanied by a cough, but the other symptoms can be similar to those of croup.

LARYNGITIS: Inflammation of the larynx and upper-chest airways that accompanies viral infection. Symptoms include a harsh, dry, barking cough low in the throat, and hoarseness. The breathing difficulty characteristic of croup is absent; otherwise this is a similar illness.

BRONCHITIS: Technically, bronchitis is the term for inflammation of the bronchi, the larger breathing tubes that lead from the trachea to the lungs. Therefore, any deep, chesty cough that is not pneumonia can be considered bronchitis. The term is used loosely but usually applies to deep, lingering coughs or to those fairly severe ones accompanied by fever but not diagnosed as pneumonia.

BRONCHIOLITIS: Infection of the bronchioles, the smaller breathing tubes that fan out from the bronchi throughout the lungs. It occurs mostly in infants no older than six months, though children as old as two years may be affected. Swelling and constriction of the bronchioles make it hard for the infant to *exhale*. These babies breathe quite rapidly and with much more effort. They look sick and anxious. Though somewhat alarming, bronchiolitis is usually self-limited and can be treated at home under medical supervision.

PNEUMONIA: Any inflammation of the lung tissues themselves that causes fluid to form in the tiny air sacs at the ends of the breathing tubes. The fluid interferes with oxygen's entering the lungs and, in turn, the bloodstream. Symptoms include a bad cough, fever, and marked lethargy, and they vary with the cause and the person's health.

Pneumonia is only a descriptive term for fluid in the lungs. It may be caused by many different microorganism infections, inhalation of foreign substances, or other diseases. It is a serious illness and must be diagnosed and cared for by your health practitioner.

WHEEZING: High-pitched squeaking or whistling sounds heard during breathing. It is caused by air flowing through constricted breathing tubes in the chest. Narrowing of the airways may be caused by swelling of the tubes' linings during infection, accumulation of secretions in the tubes, or spasms in the muscular walls of the passages. The person who wheezes feels short of breath and usually has particular trouble exhaling. Marked wheezing most often accompanies asthma, which we cover in chapter 12 on allergies, but wheezing also may occur during any type of chest infection or when a foreign body has been inhaled.

Sometimes a cold will set off an allergic reaction in the susceptible individual, so the situation can get complicated. If a cold or cough develops after exposure to pollen, dust, animal fur, or certain foods, if colds are recurrent, or if the cough is associated with wheezing or shortness of breath, allergy is a likely cause.

GENERAL HOME CARE

For ordinary head colds and coughs, our recommendations are simple and old-fashioned.

• Get plenty of rest. Enforced bed rest is not necessary, and children can be allowed to go outdoors, but the more energy used up, the less available for healing. Psychological stress often delays healing longer than physical activity, so try to take a break from deadlines and responsibilities.

• Drink plenty of fluids. Liquids are the best expectorant for loosening mucus and helping the body to discharge it. Illness also causes increased loss of body fluids, which must be replaced. Over the short term, there is no need to eat if you are not hungry.

• Blow your nose and cough phlegm out of the chest regularly. Teach children to do this at an early age.

• Use a cool-mist humidifier or vaporizer if available, and if not, try a closed bathroom with a steamy shower running. Water vapor may also help liquefy sticky mucus, making it easier to expel.

• A rubber-bulb syringe may help babies too young to blow their own noses. Use the syringe to gently suck mucus from the nose and throat. Two or three drops of salt solution (one level teaspoon in a quart of water) put into the nose will loosen thick, sticky mucus for easier removal.

• Avoid overexposure to extreme cold or heat. The energy expended in adapting to temperature stress is better used for healing.

• Although vitamin C has not been clearly proven to be effective in treating the common cold, many people who have tried it say it seems to make colds less lasting and severe. The recommended dose during a cold is one to five grams a day. You can also try zinc: Dissolve a 25 mg zinc gluconate tablet in the mouth every two hours for up to a week.

Again, see chapters 3 on fevers and influenza, 6 on earaches, 7 on sore throats, and 8 on digestive problems for further home-care information if the cold is accompanied by any of these symptoms.

FOR CROUP: Croup sounds frightening, but it can usually be treated at home. Using a humidifier or taking the child into the bathroom and turning on the hot shower is especially important. If the steam doesn't begin to relieve the symptoms within twenty minutes, or whenever the child has severe breathing difficulty, emergency care is needed.

FOR BRONCHIOLITIS: Infants should be kept as calm as possible, for they need to conserve their energy. Cuddle them gently. A humidifier may help.

FOR INHALATION OF A FOREIGN BODY: Inhalation of a foreign body or substance is a relatively common cause of coughing in children, especially in toddlers who are always putting things into their mouths. For children under six years of age, inhaling a foreign body is one of the most common causes of accidental death in the home. Parents should take special care to prevent this. Young children must not be given small objects to play with, and older children should be taught not to hold things in their mouths. Peanuts and other hard, smooth foods should not be given to children under four. Hot dogs also are notorious for causing choking. All children should be kept from walking, running, or playing while eating.

Inhalation of a foreign body can cause obvious symptoms like choking, difficult breathing, and panic. However, if the object is small enough to become lodged more deeply in the chest, or if the substance inhaled is liquid or powdery, there may be no immediate sign of a problem. Unexplained coughing or wheezing that develops suddenly or without fever (fever may occur later) should alert you to the possibility that your child has inhaled a foreign object. X rays or bronchoscopy (a direct examination of the airways through a tube) may be necessary to make the diagnosis.

CASETAKING QUESTIONS FOR COLDS

Character of the symptoms:
- At what stage is the illness: early (within the first 24 hours), late (after a week or so), or in between?
- Which are the more bothersome symptoms: runny or stuffy nose, watery eyes, laryngitis, or cough?
- Do the symptoms alternate?

- Describe the color and consistency of the nasal discharge. Do the tears or discharge irritate the skin?
- Is the patient hoarse? Does he have a constant need to clear the throat?
- Is the cough dry, or wet and rattling? Where is the "tickle"? What is the color and consistency of any coughed-up mucus, and is there any blood in it? How hard is it to raise the mucus?
- Describe any pain or other sensations (such as tightness or pressure) in the chest.

Modalities:
- At which time of day is each symptom more or less bothersome?
- How is each symptom affected by external warm or cold, warm or cold drinks, motion, swallowing, or touch?
- Is the cough related to sleep? Does it come on just before or during sleep, or when first awakening? Does it wake the patient from sleep?

Other symptoms:
- Is there a nosebleed? Any skin eruptions? A headache?
- Has the patient lost the sense of smell or taste?

HOMEOPATHIC MEDICINES

Colds are usually mild illnesses and don't require treatment with medicines of any kind. We suggest you treat yourself or family members with homeopathic medicines only if the cold or cough is particularly severe or lingers more than a few days. A homeopathic medicine should be given between three to four times a day, depending on the intensity of the person's symptoms. Generally, its effects will be noticed after one or two nights' rest, although sometimes it takes longer. If no changes are observed after forty-eight hours, you can consider taking another homeopathic medicine if it adequately fits your symptoms.

Aconite is indicated when the cold symptoms come on suddenly, often after exposure to cold weather or cold, dry wind. *Aconite* is indicated only in the first twenty-four hours or so of the illness. *Aconite* patients become violently ill within a few hours, experiencing high fever, anxiety and restlessness, sensitivity to light, and thirst. Though feverish and fearful, they are not delirious. A watery runny nose may be accompanied by violent headache or bright-red nosebleed. *Aconite* also is indicated during the early stages of suddenly appearing coughs, especially croup. The child may wake early in the night with a dry, choking, croupy cough and sit up in bed and grasp his throat, feeling that he is choking. He may look frightened or even panicked, and may toss about with anxiety. The cough may be dry, or there may be expectoration of a little watery mucus.

The colds of *Belladonna,* like those of *Aconite,* come on suddenly, and this medicine also is indicated early in the course of the illness. Symptoms include high fever, leaping pulse, and flushed but dry face. While many medicines cover flushed skin, *Belladonna* is particularly suitable when fever produces bright redness (especially of the face) and intensely hot skin. The person may experience pounding or throbbing in the head, and you may be able to see pulsations of the arteries in the head and neck. As the fever first comes on, the *Belladonna* patient is likely to be agitated, excited, or even destructive, and her senses may be hyperacute, causing irritatability and sensitivity to light, noise, odors, and so on. She is mentally dull, however, and as the illness progresses she pays little conscious attention to the environment. *Belladonna* patients may be anxious but also delirious, and have fears of imaginary things. In contrast, *Aconite* patients are alert and fear death or the dark. The pupils usually are dilated and the skin is dry during a *Belladonna* fever. The nasal discharge is thin and watery. The nose feels dry and hot, and there may be much sneezing. Sometimes the discharge dries up suddenly, bringing on severe throbbing pain in the head or face. The throat often feels raw and sore and is very red, and there may be a bad earache. There may be a dry, clutching sensation in the throat or larynx that leads to painful, scraping, spasmodic coughing from the upper chest or throat. Sometimes the cough hurts so much that a child may start to cry as soon as the urge to cough is felt. The cough sounds croupy, barking, and short. It is worse at night and may wake the individual from sleep. Only a little thin mucus is coughed up.

Like *Aconite* and *Belladonna, Ferrum phos.* is useful during the early stages of respiratory illnesses. Those who need *Ferrum phos.* are less restless than *Aconite* patients and more alert than *Belladonna* patients. The skin may be flushed with fever but not so intensely hot as it is with *Belladonna* patients. They are not delirious, and do take notice of everything going on around them. *Ferrum phos.* is indicated particularly when flushing of the face is confined to well-demarcated, circular patches, where the *Belladonna* face typically is more uniformly red. During the early part of an acute respiratory infection that has few unique symptoms accompanying high fever, we recommend you give *Belladonna* first and then try *Ferrum phos.* if the former has failed.

Allium cepa (raw onion) is an easy medicine to remember since we all have had experience with the symptoms it creates. With the *Allium cepa* cold, there is a clear, *burning* nasal discharge that irritates the nostrils and upper lip. There is also a profuse tearing of the eyes that does not cause irritation of the skin, though the eyes themselves may be red and burning. Both of these symptoms grow worse in warm rooms, indoors, and in the evening, and both are better in open air. Those suffering from frequent sneezing also feel better in the open air. There is often a tickling in the larynx that may lead to a dry cough so painful it makes the person grasp the throat while coughing. Though there is not much fever, the patient may be quite thirsty. Mood changes are not pronounced.

Euphrasia colds include a nonirritating, watery nasal discharge and copious, burning tears—the opposite of *Allium cepa*'s symptoms. The nasal discharge is worse in open air, in the morning, and while the patient is lying down. There may be a loose cough, but it is usually not too deep or severe. Large amounts of mucus formed in the upper airways may be coughed up. The cough is worse during the day and may occur only during the daytime. It is relieved at night by eating and by lying down, though lying down makes the nasal symptoms worse.

Natrum mur. can be a good medicine for those with colds, but it has few distinguishing symptoms. You should consider this medicine when the most striking symptom is simply a copious nasal flow of clear to slightly whitish mucus. The discharge is thicker and stickier than water, and it may look like raw egg whites or boiled starch. The mucus may run down behind the nose and collect in the throat. There may be sneezing spells, and smell and taste may be lost. A symptom that can help confirm your choice of this medicine is tiny blistery eruptions around the mouth and nose that break open to form thin crusts, such as cold sores. The lips may be dry and cracked. *Natrum mur.* patients tend to be depressed and weepy, but they don't want attention and may be made worse if you try to comfort them or offer sympathy.

Nux vomica is a valuable remedy for some people with colds, particularly with illnesses brought on by exposure to cold or to cold, dry weather. The onset of the cold is not especially sudden, and typically it does not have the violent symptoms or early high fever of the *Aconite* cold. *Nux* corresponds well to the dry, tickling, and scraping sensations in the nose. Initially the nose is stuffy and dry, but as the cold develops, a watery, often irritating discharge begins, accompanied by frequent sneezing. Often the nose is alternately stuffed up and runny. Stuffiness predominates at night and outdoors, runniness in warm rooms and during the day. The cold symptoms in general are made worse by eating. The throat feels raw and rough, and there may be a tickling in the larynx with a teasing, dry cough that causes soreness in the chest. The cough is worse in the morning (especially upon waking), between midnight and daybreak, in cold air, after eating, or after mental work. It gets better after warm drinks. *Nux* patients tend to be chilly and can't get warm even when they pile on the covers and turn up the heat. Every little motion of the covers causes new chills. *Nux* is appropriate for those who are irritable, oversensitive, and easily offended.

Gelsemium colds tend to come on gradually. The person may feel less energetic for two to three days while a tickling in the nose or the back of the mouth gradually increases. When the runny nose finally starts, the discharge is watery and irritating. Particularly characteristic of a *Gelsemium* illness is the great tiredness and the sensation of heaviness felt throughout the body. The illness is often accompanied by chills running up and down the back, or by a headache above the nape of the neck.

Arsenicum is useful for both head colds and coughs. There is a profuse, watery nasal discharge that burns the skin. Even though the nose runs freely, it feels stopped up. There is irritation and tickling in the nose and frequent, violent sneezing that doesn't relieve the irritation. In time the nasal discharge may become thick and yellow. A dull, throbbing headache in the forehead may accompany the nasal symptoms. *Arsenicum* is suited for various types of coughs. The cough may come from tickling in the larynx or from deep in the chest, and it may be loose or dry. It tends to be worse during the night (especially between midnight and 3 A.M.), in cold air, or when the person becomes cold, is lying down, is moving, or is drinking cold liquids. The person may cough at the sight of strangers. The cough is better after something warm to drink. Often the air passages are constricted, and the patient may wheeze, especially at night. There may be chest pain, often of a burning character, especially during deep breathing. *Arsenicum* patients are very chilly, but unlike *Nux* patients, they eventually feel better if the room is made warm enough. The classic mental symptoms include restlessness, anxiety, and fear. Despite being weak from the illness, they may be preoccupied with tidiness.

Kali bichromium should be considered during the later stages of a cold. This medicine suits a thick yellow or greenish discharge that is often distinctively ropy or stringy. It may be so thick that it can barely be blown from the nose and comes out in long strings. Crusts and mucus plugs form in the nose, and the discharges may smell offensive. A thick postnasal drip is characteristic. Sinus headaches frequently accompany the cold symptoms, often with a pressing pain at the root of the nose.

Bryonia is one of the more common medicines for people with coughs. This medicine is indicated during a cold only after it has moved down into the chest. The *Bryonia* patient's cough is usually dry and spas-modic, and it is worse when he moves or breathes deeply as well as dur-ing the day, after eating or drinking, and in warm rooms. Open air or a swallow of warm water relieves the cough temporarily. The cough is of-ten quite painful and may cause soreness in the larynx, chest, abdomen, or back. The person may need to press his hands against his head or chest to limit painful motion while coughing. Since deep breathing and mov-ing around also may cause chest pain, the person wants to lie perfectly still on the painful part—pressure on the sore area feels good. He wants to sigh and breathe deeply, but it hurts to do so, and respirations are shal-low and panting. There is usually little expectoration; what comes up may be mucous, yellow, or streaked with a little blood. The *Bryonia* pa-tient is thirsty and may feel too warm or too cold. He is likely to look sick, tired, and heavy, and to have a dusky, dark complexion. He is irrita-ble and wants to be left alone.

Phosphorus is another common medicine for treating people with various types of coughs. Like *Bryonia,* generally it is not used for simple head colds. The *Phosphorus* cough may be dry or loose, croupy or deep. If the person brings up phlegm, it may be of any color or consistency, from watery mucus to thick yellow or green pus, and may be streaked with blood. Chest pain may occur, and as with *Bryonia,* the pains worsen with motion and get better with pressure (*Bryonia* is a better choice if these are the only symptoms you have to work with). The chest pain is worse when the patient lies on the left side. There may be a sense of tightness, constriction, or weight in the chest. Characteristically, cold or cold air, laughing, talking, and eating worsen the cough, as does lying down, es-pecially on the left side. The cough also may be provoked by strong odors. It may occur at any time of the day or night, less frequently from after midnight until morning. It often comes on as the person goes to sleep, or it may wake her from sleep. Liquids in general and cold drinks in particular aggravate the cough. The cough may be accompanied by any type of nasal discharge.

Phosphorus is an important remedy for those with laryngitis and hoarseness, especially when the symptoms are worse in the morning or evening. *Phosphorus* patients are chilly and crave ice-cold drinks. They are more alert than *Bryonia* patients and get nervous when they're alone or in the dark. They enjoy company and reassurance.

Causticum is another first-line medicine for people with laryngitis, especially if there is a constant desire to clear the throat. During coughs, choose *Causticum* when the person must keep trying to cough more deeply in an effort to dislodge the mucus deep in the chest. The cough may be better from cold drinks but worse from cold air or when bending forward. In some cases it is much less severe during the day than at night; in others, it is especially bad on first waking. The patient is chilly in general but may feel much better in cloudy or rainy weather.

Pulsatilla is indicated when the mucus has become thick and yellow-green. It is bland and does not burn the skin. A fluent discharge may alternate with nasal congestion. The nose tends to run in the open air and in the evening, and to become stuffed up in a warm room. *Pulsatilla* matches both dry and loose coughs. Lying down, exertion, and warm rooms worsen the cough, while it is better in open air. Deep breathing may aggravate or relieve the cough. Sometimes the cough is dry at night and loose by day. It often wakes the person from sleep. Spasms of coughing may end in gagging or vomiting (*Bryonia, Arsenicum, Drosera, Kali carb., Hepar sulph., Ipecac.,* and *Lachesis* all have this symptom). The mental and general symptoms may be critical in the choice of this medicine (see the *materia medica* section for details).

Spongia is probably the most important medicine for a croupy or harsh cough (*Aconite* and *Hepar sulph.* are other strong possibilities for croup). A loud, dry cough and hoarse rasping are typical of croup. Some homeopaths have compared the sound of the *Spongia* cough to that of a saw being driven through a dry pine log. The cough may wake the *Spongia* patient from sleep, often before midnight, with suffocative constriction of the throat. Excitement, talking, lying down, alcoholic beverages, and ice-cold drinks worsen the cough, but drinking fluids that aren't so cold, as well as eating, may bring relief. The nose may be dry and obstructed or runny, but these symptoms are less important than those of the cough.

Drosera is another medicine for people with dry, spasmodic, croupy coughs. Probably the most distinguishing feature of the cough is a barking or ringing sound. The larynx is inflamed and irritated, there are clutching or constricting sensations (which sometimes get better when the patient is walking), and a tickling or roughness excites the cough. Or the cough may be in the chest, sometimes even feeling as though it is coming from the abdomen. Spasms of coughing, especially after midnight, may follow one another quickly and may end in retching or vomiting. The person may have to support the chest or abdomen while coughing to reduce pain. The *Drosera* cough is worse also while the patient is lying down, and may come on even as soon as his head touches the pillow. It is made worse also by eating and particularly by drinking. Though for the most part the cough is dry, there may be some mucus or yellowish sputum.

The cough of *Rumex*, or yellow dock, is dry (like those of *Drosera* and *Spongia*), but the *Rumex* cough is not so croupy or barking. It is shallow and is set off by tickling in the airways, particularly in the "throat pit" just above the breastbone. Inhaling cold air especially aggravates the cough, so the person may keep the covers pulled up over his head to keep the air he is breathing warm. Even the minute temperature differences from one room to the next may cause renewed coughing. Any little irregularity in air flow also may incite the cough, so he tries to keep his breathing as shallow as possible. In fact, the *Rumex* patient may not want to talk or even listen to conversation, for he fears it might break his concentration on regulating his breathing. The cough is worse also in the evening before midnight (often around 11 P.M.) or on first waking, and when the patient is lying down. Touching the throat also may bring on the cough (as with *Lachesis*). A fluent, watery nasal discharge with much sneezing may accompany the cough.

Lachesis is characteristically indicated by short, dry, choking coughs and violent tickling in the larynx. What little phlegm there is in the chest is brought up only with great effort. Whatever the type of cough, it is likely to be made worse after falling asleep, during sleep, or right after waking up. Exposure to cold or open air, rising from a lying position, and the slightest pressure on the throat (even from clothing) may aggravate the cough. A *Lachesis* patient experiences suffocative constriction of the larynx just on entering a deep sleep, or later during sleep, and he wakes with a choking and coughing spell. He may have trouble swallowing even liquids. (Anyone who has genuine difficulty with swallowing during an acute illness may have epiglottitis, and emergency care may be necessary; see the section on epiglottitis in chapter 7.) A bad sore throat may accompany the cough. The *Lachesis* patient may be unusually excitable, impulsive, talkative, and sometimes inappropriately jealous or suspicious.

Hepar sulph. is more often indicated during the later stages of a cold. The symptoms may have begun several days earlier with a watery runny nose, but by now a thick, yellow, and sometimes offensive-smelling discharge is present. These patients may sneeze at the slightest exposure to cold. After exposure to cold dry air, a croupy throat cough may be present, but the cough is less dry and more rattling than that of *Aconite* or *Spongia*. Also there may be much deep, wet coughing of thick yellow phlegm. Cold air, eating cold foods, and exposure to the wind worsen the *Hepar* cough. Uncovering brings on the cough to such an extent that the *Hepar* patient may cough if she puts a hand or foot out from the covers. The cough is aggravated also in the evening before midnight and by deep breathing. *Hepar* patients are irritable, sensitive to touch and cold, and they feel better in warm, moist weather.

Ipecac. is especially valuable in treating infants' bronchitis or bronchiolitis, although older individuals often need this medicine, too. These illnesses come on fairly rapidly, spreading from a simple head cold down into the chest within a day or two. By the time the person needs *Ipecac.*, the cough is deep and wet, marked by coarse, loud rattling and accumulation of much mucus in the chest. The phlegm and the spasmodic cough cause choking and suffocation, and the patient may have trouble getting her breath. Phlegm comes up with difficulty. As is typical during bronchiolitis, breathing out may be harder than breathing in. Spasms of nearly incessant coughing may occur, ending in retching, gagging, or vomiting. *Ipecac.* should be considered even for dry coughs if gagging or vomiting is severe, whether or not the patient is nauseated. Usually the cough is worse in a warm room. There may be a stuffy nose and sneezing, and sometimes bright-red nosebleeds. Mentally, the *Ipecac.* patient may be full of desires but doesn't really know what she wants, and she may reject things she has asked for when she gets them. *Ipecac.* children often are quite irritable.

Like *Ipecac.*, *Antimonium tartaricum* is indicated when the person has a rattling cough and a chest full of mucus. The symptoms of this medicine come on more slowly than those of *Ipecac.*, however, and *Antimonium tart.* usually is given during the later stages of a progressively worsening cough. In these cases the sputum is not difficult to raise, but the person is just too weak to cough effectively and can't clear his chest. Breathing sounds rattling, and as the mucus builds up, the patient becomes short of breath. He is quite ill and exhausted and may look drowsy and pale, sometimes with sunken features and slightly bluish skin (these symptoms require medical evaluation).

The *Rhus tox.* cold or cough symptoms usually include a congested nose with a thick yellow or green discharge, a red and scratchy throat, and a dry cough with tickling behind the upper part of the breastbone. Hoarseness is common. The cough worsens in cold rooms or in cold, wet weather, with the slightest uncovering, during deep breathing, when lying down, after bathing, and in the evening or during the night. The cough may prevent sleep or come on during sleep, sometimes waking the person. Motion may make the cough better. In general, the person is restless and feels better when moving about.

A patient can develop the symptoms of *Dulcamara* during or after exposure to cold and wet weather, when wet or chilled, or when experiencing a sudden temperature change from hot to cold. If the onset of the illness is related to this kind of exposure, and if there aren't enough symptoms to indicate another medicine, you should try this one. All kinds of nose and cough symptoms are covered by this medicine. Sometimes the cold symptoms are accompanied by neck pain and stiffness from the cold damp weather.

The *Kali carbonicum* cough, whether dry or wet, is violent, spasmodic, and particularly severe in the early morning hours, between 2 and 5 A.M. Needlelike pains in the side commonly accompany the cough. The pains are worse during breathing and coughing, but are not particularly aggravated by motion. They tend to be worse on the right side of the chest. The cough itself is made worse by the patient's breathing cold air, becoming cold, moving or exerting energy, and lying down, especially in the evening or at night. There may be choking, retching, or vomiting along with the cough. The sputum may be difficult to bring up even though at times there is a lot of it. It may look thick and yellow. The throat may feel as though a splinter or fish bone is caught in it (also a symptom of *Hepar sulph.* and *Lachesis*). The person is usually thirsty and chilly and is often sweaty. He may be irritable and yet want company, and often he is full of fears.

REMEDY SUMMARY FOR COLDS

See the text for descriptions of other medicines not listed here that may be helpful during a cold.

See also the descriptions of *Belladonna, Aconite,* and *Ferrum phos.* in chapter 3; these medicines often are indicated in the earliest stages of a cold.

Give the medicine: Three to 4 times a day, less frequently as symptoms improve.

When to try another medicine: If no changes are observed after 48 hours.

ALLIUM CEPA ★

Essentials
- Clear, burning nasal discharge irritating the nostrils and upper lip
- Profuse tearing of the eyes that does not cause irritation of the skin, though the eyes themselves are red and burning

Confirmatory symptoms
- Symptoms worse in warm rooms, indoors, and in the evening; better in open air
- Frequent sneezing better in the open air
- Tickling in larynx causing dry, painful cough; person grasps the throat while coughing
- Thirst

EUPHRASIA

Essentials
- Nonirritating, watery nasal discharge
- Copious burning tears

Confirmatory symptoms
- Nasal discharge worse in open air, in the morning, and when lying down
- Loose cough, worse during the day, better at night, from eating and by lying down; patient coughs up mucus from the upper airways

NATRUM MURIATICUM

Essentials
- Nasal flow of clear to slightly whitish mucus, thicker than water (may look like raw egg whites or boiled starch)

Confirmatory symptoms
- Mucus runs down behind the nose and collects in the throat
- Sneezing spells
- Loss of smell and taste
- Cold sores or other small blisters around mouth and nose
- Lips may be dry and cracked
- Patient depressed, weepy, but doesn't want attention; feels worse when comforted

NUX VOMICA

Essentials
- Dry, tickling, and scraping sensations in the nose
- Nose alternately stuffed up and runny; stuffy at night, runny in warm rooms and during the day
- Frequent sneezing

Confirmatory symptoms
- Colds developing after exposure to cold or to cold, dry weather
- Symptoms worse from eating
- Throat raw and rough
- Tickling in the larynx; teasing, dry cough causing soreness in the chest
- Cough worse in the morning (especially upon waking), between midnight and daybreak, in cold air, after eating, or after mental work; better after warm drinks
- Chilly patient; motion of the covers causes chills
- Irritable, easily offended

ARSENICUM (see also "Remedy Summary for Cough")

Essentials
- Profuse, watery nasal discharge that burns the skin (discharge may become yellow in time)
- Nose runs freely but feels stuffed
- Irritation and tickling in the nose and frequent, violent sneezing

Confirmatory symptoms
- Chilly patient, better from heat
- Patient anxious, restless, and fearful
- Dull, throbbing frontal headache
- Preoccupation with tidiness

GELSEMIUM

Essentials
- Symptoms develop gradually
- Nasal discharge watery
- Tiredness; body feels heavy

Confirmatory symptoms
- Chills running up and down the back
- Headache above the nape of the neck

KALI BICHROMIUM

Essentials
- Later stages of a cold with thick, yellow or greenish discharge

Confirmatory symptoms
- Nasal discharge ropy or stringy; crusts and mucus plugs form in the nose; offensive-smelling discharge
- Thick postnasal drip
- Sinus headaches; pressing pain at the root of the nose

PULSATILLA (see also "Remedy Summary for Cough")

Essentials
- Mental or general symptoms of *Pulsatilla* are pronounced (see *materia medica* section)
  and/or
- Nasal discharge thick, yellow-green, nonirritating

Confirmatory symptoms
- Nose alternately stuffed up and runny; runs more in open air and in the evening, becomes stuffed up in a warm room

---

REMEDY SUMMARY FOR COUGH

See the text for descriptions of other medicines not listed here that may be helpful during a cough.

Give the medicine: Three to 4 times a day, less frequently as symptoms improve.

When to try another medicine: If no changes are observed after 48 hours.

BRYONIA ★

Essentials
- Dry, spasmodic cough, worse from motion, deep breathing
- Cough painful; person may press hands against chest while coughing to limit painful motion

Confirmatory symptoms
- Cough worse during the day, after eating or drinking, and in warm rooms; better from open air or warm drinks
- Chest pain better from pressure
- Breathing shallow, panting
- Thirst
- Irritable, wants to lie still and be left alone

RUMEX

Essentials

- Dry, shallow cough set off by tickling in the airways, especially in the "throat pit" just above the breastbone
- Cough worse from inhaling cold air or from any irregularity in air flow; patient breathes shallowly to prevent cough

Confirmatory symptoms

- Cough worse lying down; in the evening, before midnight, or on first waking; from touching
- Fluent, watery nasal discharge; sneezing

ARSENICUM

Essentials

- Restless, anxious patient
- Weakness
- Chilly, improved in warmth

Confirmatory symptoms

- Cough from tickling in the larynx or from deep in the chest
- Cough worse during the night (especially between midnight and 3 A.M.); worse from cold air, drinking cold liquids, lying down, motion
- Cough better from warm drinks
- Wheezing at night
- Chest pain, often of a burning character, worse from deep breathing

PHOSPHORUS

Essentials

- Any type of cough, especially with:
  —chills
  —mental alertness; nervousness when alone or in the dark; patient enjoys company and reassurance
  or
- Laryngitis and hoarseness, especially when the symptoms are worse in the morning or evening

Confirmatory symptoms

- Blood-streaked phlegm
- Craving for ice-cold drinks, which may worsen the cough
- Chest pain worse with motion and better with pressure; worse lying on the left side
- Tightness, constriction, or weight in the chest
- Cough worse from cold or cold air, laughing, talking, eating, drinking, lying down, or strong odors
- Cough begins on going to sleep or wakes the patient from sleep

PULSATILLA

Essentials

- Mental or general symptoms of *Pulsatilla* are pronounced (see *materia medica* section)
  and/or
- Cough with thick, yellow-green phlegm

Confirmatory symptoms

- Cough worse from lying down, exertion, and warm rooms; better in open air
- Cough dry at night, loose by day

LACHESIS

Essentials

- Short, dry, choking cough with violent tickling in the larynx
- Cough worse after falling asleep, during sleep, or just after waking up; and/or worse from slightest touch or pressure on the throat (even from clothing)

Confirmatory symptoms

- Cough worse from cold or open air, rising from a lying position
- Difficulty swallowing, even liquids (see section on epiglottitis if this symptom is present)
- Excitable, impulsive, talkative; sometimes inappropriately jealous or suspicious

IPECAC.

Essentials

- Deep, wet cough with coarse, loud rattling sound and much mucus in the chest
- Sensation of choking and suffocation, with trouble catching the breath

Confirmatory symptoms

- Illness began rapidly (over 1 to 2 days)
- Spasms of nearly incessant coughing ending in severe retching, gagging, or vomiting (other medicines also have this symptom but it is very marked in *Ipecac.*)
- Phlegm coughed up with difficulty
- Bronchitis or bronchiolitis in infants; expiration most difficult
- Cough worse in a warm room
- Person feels as though she wants something but doesn't really know what it is; rejecting things she has asked for
- Stuffy nose and sneezing; nosebleeds with bright-red blood

ANTIMONIUM TART.

Essentials

- Rattling cough and a chest full of mucus
- Patient quite ill, exhausted; too weak to raise the phlegm

Confirmatory symptoms

- Symptoms developed gradually

CAUSTICUM

Essentials

- Cough with sensation that patient can't cough deeply enough to reach the mucus
  or
- Laryngitis, especially if there is a constant desire to clear the throat

Confirmatory symptoms

- Continuous cough
- Cough worse from cold air; when first waking up
- Cough better during the day; from cold drinks
- Patient chilly; may feel better in cloudy or rainy weather

RHUS TOX.

Essentials
- Dry cough with tickling behind the upper part of the breastbone

Confirmatory symptoms
- Cough worse in cold rooms or in cold, wet weather, or with the slightest uncovering; worse from deep breathing, while lying down, after bathing, in the evening, or at night
- Cough prevents sleep or comes on during sleep; may wake the patient
- Cough better from motion
- Hoarseness
- Congested nose with thick yellow or green discharge; red and scratchy throat
- Patient restless, feels better when moving about

KALI CARBONICUM

Essentials
- Cough in spasms most severe between 2 and 5 A.M.

Confirmatory symptoms
- Cough worse from cold air, becoming cold, moving or exerting energy, and lying down
- Needlelike pains in the side with the cough, worse on the right and during breathing and coughing
- Sputum difficult to bring up
- Throat feels as though a splinter or fish bone is caught in it
- Patient thirsty, chilly, sweaty

REMEDY SUMMARY FOR CROUP

See the text for descriptions of other medicines not listed here that may be helpful during croup.

Give the medicine: In early croup, give *Aconite* every 1 to 2 hours at least twice. If it hasn't helped, or if you begin treatment more than 12 hours after the onset of symptoms, select another medicine and repeat it 3 to 4 times per day.

When to try another medicine: In early croup, if there is no improvement after 2 doses of *Aconite*. Later, with other medicines, switch to a new medicine after 12 to 24 hours if symptoms are stable; if symptoms are getting worse, switch after 6 hours.

ACONITE ★

Essentials
- Very first stages of croup, with dry, raspy cough just developing

Confirmatory symptoms
- Fear, anxiety, restlessness
- Symptoms appear suddenly
- Sitting up in bed, grasping the throat

SPONGIA ★

Essentials
- Give if *Aconite* fails, or if symptoms have been present for more than about 12 hours
- Loud, dry cough with hoarse, raspy sound

Confirmatory symptoms
- Cough sounds like sawing of a log
- Cough wakes the patient from sleep with constriction of throat
- Cough worse from talking, cold drinks, excitement

HEPAR SULPH.

Essentials
- For later stages of croup when cough is more rattling

Confirmatory symptoms
- Irritable mood
- Symptoms worse from cold or cold air; uncovering brings on the cough
- Cough worse from deep breathing and before midnight

DROSERA

Essentials
- Dry cough with a barking or ringing sound

REPERTORY FOR COLD AND COUGH SYMPTOMS

Since there are so many medicines to consider when treating a person with a cold or cough, the following index of symptoms, or repertory, will help you find the medicines most likely to cover the case. After taking the case, compare the patient's main cold and cough symptoms to those listed in the repertory, writing down the medicines listed under each symptom. Then, to make your final choice, read the remedy summaries (or the text descriptions) of the medicines that match most of the symptoms. You may want to consult the *materia medica* section as well. Medicines printed in all capital letters in the repertory are those most strongly indicated for that particular symptom.

I. Head Colds
Early stages of a cold: ACON., BELL., FERR. P.
More common medicines for head colds: ALLIUM, ARS., BELL., EUPHR., GELS., KALI BI., NAT. M., NUX, PULS.

Nasal Discharge
Green: Bry., KALI BI., Kali C., Phos., PULS., Rhus
Offensive: HEP., KALI BI., Kali C., Lach., Phos., PULS.
Ropy or Stringy: KALI BI., Phos., Spong.
Thick: ARS., Hep., KALI BI., Kali C., Nat. M., Phos., PULS., Rhus, Spong.
Watery: Acon., ALLIUM, ARS., Bry., EUPH., Kali Bi., Nat. M., NUX
White mucus: Ars., NAT. M., Nux, Phos., Puls.
Yellow: Ars., HEP., KALI BI., Kali C., Lach., Nat. M., Phos., PULS.

Nasal Discharge Modalities
Worse in the morning: Acon., Euph., NUX
Worse at night: Kali Bi., Rumex
Congested at night: Nux
Worse in open air: Dulc., Kali Bi., Phos., PULS.
Better in open air: Allium, NUX, Puls.
Nasal discharge with chilliness: Acon., Ars., Bry., NUX, Puls., Spong.
Fluent discharge with cough: Allium, Ars., BELL., EUPH., Ferr. P., Gels., IPEC., Kali Bi., Nat. M., Phos., Rhus, Spong.
Fluent discharge with fever: Acon., Ars., Bell., BRY., Hep.
Fluent discharge with croup: Acon., Ars., Hep., Spong.

II. LARYNGITIS OR HOARSENESS: CAUST., PHOS., Rhus

III. COUGHS

More common medicines for coughs: ACON., ANTI. T., ARS., BELL., BRY., DROS., FERR. P., HEP., IPEC., KALI C., LACH., PHOS., PULS., RHUS, RUMEX, SPONG.
Dry cough: ACON., ARS., BELL., BRY., Dros., Dulc., Ferr. P., Hep., Kali Bi., KALI C., LACH., NAT. M., NUX, PHOS., PULS., Rhus, RUMEX, SPONG.
Loose cough: ANTI. T., ARS., Euph., Hep., Lach., Phos., PULS.
Croupy cough: ACON., Ars., Bell., DROS., Hep., Kali Bi., Lach., Rumex, SPONG.

Cough Modalities:
Worse after bathing: RHUS
Worse from cold: ARS., Bry., Dulc., HEP., Kali Bi., Kali C., Lach., NUX, PHOS., RHUS, RUMEX
Worse from bending forward: CAUST.
Worse from cold air: ARS., CAUST., HEP., Kali C., Lach., PHOS., RUMEX
Worse from cold drinks: ARS., Phos., Spong.
Better from cold drinks: CAUST.
Worse from cold foods: Hep.
Worse from cold wet weather: Dulc.
Worse in the day: Bell., Bry., EUPH., Ferr. P., Kali C., LACH., PHOS.
Better during the day: Caust.
Worse from deep breathing: ARS., Bry., DROS., Hep., Lach., Phos.
Worse from drinking: Ars., Bry., DROS., Hep., Lach., Phos.
Better from drinking: Bry., SPONG.
Better from warm drinks: ARS., BRY., NUX, RHUS, Spong.
Worse after eating: Ant., Ars., Bry., Ferr. P., Hep. Ipec., KALI BI., Kali C., NUX, RUMEX
Worse after exertion: Kali C., Nat. M., Nux, PULS.
Worse from laughing: Phos.
Worse from lying on the left side: Phos., Rumex
Worse from lying down: Ars., Bry., Dros., Dulc., Kali C., Lach., Phos., PULS., Rhus, RUMEX, Spong.

Worse in the morning: ARS., EUPH., KALI BI., KALI C., Nat. M., NUX, PHOS., PULS., RUMEX

Worse from motion: Ars., Bry., Kali C., Nux, Phos.

Worse at night: ACON., ARS., Bell., Dros., HEP., IPEC., KALI C., LACH., Nat. M., Phos., PULS., Rhus, Rumex, Spong.

Worse in the open air: Acon., ARS., Hep., Lach., PHOS., Rhus, RUMEX

Better in the open air: Allium, BRY., PULS.

Worse from talking: Bell., DROS., Euph., Hep., Lach., Phos., RUMEX, Spong.

Worse on first waking in the morning: Caust., KALI BI., NUX, RUMEX

Chest pains during cough: Acon., BELL., BRY., DROS., PHOS., PULS., RHUS, SPONG.

Throat pain during cough: Acon., ALLIUM, BELL., Bry., Hep., Kali Bi., Kali C., Lach., Phos., Puls., Spong.

BEYOND HOME CARE

Please also refer to "Beyond Home Care" in chapter 3 on fever and influenza. People with a common cold may be more susceptible to secondary bacterial infections like ear infections, sinusitis, strep throat, lymph node infections, and pneumonia. Check chapters 6 and 7 and the section on sinus conditions in this chapter for more information on how to treat such conditions and when medical care should be sought.

GET MEDICAL CARE IMMEDIATELY:

- if something is inhaled that can't be coughed out completely, even if there isn't any obvious breathing difficulty at first. This includes inhaling powders and liquids, though small amounts of water generally won't be a problem;
- if there is severe headache, extreme weakness, convulsions, or stiffness of the neck;
- if there is marked irritability or confusion;
- if there is severe breathing difficulty or chest pain.

CALL YOUR PRACTITIONER IMMEDIATELY:

• if vomiting begins unexpectedly during the course of the illness.

SEE YOUR PRACTITIONER TODAY:

• if fever has persisted. See chapter 3 for specific advice for each age group;
• if the symptoms have been accompanied by marked weakness and have lasted longer than a week or so;
• if there is breathing difficulty, shortness of breath, or much more rapid breathing than normal. Babies with any breathing difficulty must be examined. A respiratory rate of greater than 50 breaths per minute *at rest* in young children, above 40 in children older than 2, or more than 20 in individuals older than 10 should prompt at least a phone call to your practitioner;
• if any wheezing occurs for the first time or if there is moderate or severe wheezing at any time;
• if there is significant chest pain;
• if stools are very light in color, if urine is very dark, or if there is yellowing of skin or eyes.

SEE YOUR PRACTITIONER SOON:

• if mild cold symptoms have been persistent for more than 3 weeks.

SEE YOUR HOMEOPATH:

• if you get recurrent colds. Everyone gets an occasional cold, and children between 3 and 6 years of age get an *average* of 8 colds per year. As long as the illnesses clear up fairly quickly and aren't severe, you should not be concerned. Susceptibility to frequent or severe colds does indicate a weakness of the healing defenses, and constitutional homeopathic treatment can build strength and resistance.

SINUS PROBLEMS

The sinuses are cavities in the bones above the eyes and around the nose. Normally, they are filled only with air. During a cold or allergic reaction, the membranes that line the sinus cavities may swell and produce excessive mucus. If the openings from the sinuses into the nose are blocked by swelling, the pressure of the air trapped inside and the buildup of mucus cause sensations of stuffiness and fullness in the face. The nose is stuffed up. When the sinuses are involved during a simple cold but there is no bacterial infection, the condition is sometimes referred to as sinus congestion.

A true sinus infection results when bacteria enters a blocked sinus cavity, thrives and multiplies in the trapped mucous fluid. Inflammation increases and pus is produced, and throbbing and pressure in the sinuses increase. If the lower sinuses are involved, the teeth hurt or feel too long. Because of pressure and inflammation in the infected sinuses, the overlying parts of the face are tender to touch. A thick yellow-green nasal discharge is produced, but it may not be that profuse because of the blockage. Fever and tiredness usually accompany the illness, and the person can become very sick.

GENERAL HOME CARE

Sinus congestion and mild infections can be cared for at home. Home care is simple. Rest is essential. Drink plenty of liquids and use a humidifier to help thin and loosen the secretions.

HOMEOPATHIC MEDICINES

Consider first the medicines listed here when treating someone with a sinus infection. All of these remedies cover thick yellow to green drainage from the nose. You can consult also chapter 11 on headaches, and the medicines covered earlier in this chapter for colds and coughs in general. Give a dose of the medicine every eight hours or so, stopping if there is improvement. Switch to another remedy if the symptoms aren't getting better after a day.

Kali bi. is one of the most helpful medicines for people with sinus pain and congestion. It's especially indicated when pain or pressure is worse above the root of the nose and when the discharge is particularly thick, stringy, or tough. Pain may occur also in the forehead, often over one eye or shooting to the outer angle of an eye. The pain may be confined to small, particularly localized spots. The symptoms generally begin in the morning, get worse by noon, and go away in the late afternoon. Cold weather, stooping, motion, and walking make them worse. Pressure, warmth, and warm drinks help relieve the pain.

Pulsatilla should be considered when the sinus pain is worse at night, in a warm room, or on standing, stooping, or raising the eyes. The pains lessen in the morning and with pressure. Digestive symptoms such as nausea or indigestion may accompany the sinus pains.

People who need *Silica* have sinus pains distinctively improved with pressure, and such people may want to keep the head wrapped up tightly. They feel better also after warm applications. Their pains are worse with cold, mental exertion, noise, motion, stooping, talking, and light touch.

Spigelia should be considered when sinus pain begins after exposure to cold or cold wet weather, or when pain is much worse on stooping or bending the head forward. The head symptoms are relieved by cold applications or washing with cold water, and warmth is aggravating. The pains are made worse also by motion, jarring, noise, and light, whereas lying down with the head propped up improves them.

If the pain is made much worse by cold or touch, *Hepar sulph.* is probably the remedy. *Hepar* is particularly indicated for pain concentrated at the root of the nose that is worse in the morning. The scalp and whole head may feel bruised and sensitive to touch or to simple movements of the head or eyes.

BEYOND HOME CARE

GET MEDICAL CARE TODAY:

- if there is marked fever, severe pain, or foul-smelling discharge;
- if there is evidence of mild sinus infection (tenderness, thick yellow or green discharge) with no improvement after 48 hours.

CONJUNCTIVITIS

The conjunctivae are the thin transparent linings that cover the surface of the eyes and the inner eyelids. Infection, allergy, or exposure to irritating chemicals can cause inflammation and swelling of the conjunctivae, and the affected eye tears and looks bloodshot. This condition is known as conjunctivitis, or "pinkeye."

Both cold viruses and various bacteria can infect the conjunctivae. When the conjunctivae are infected with viruses, the discharge from the eye is clear and watery. Bacterial infections result in a thick yellow to green discharge.

Usually the symptoms begin in one eye and spread to the other within a few days. The affected eye is bloodshot, and the lids may be puffy and a bit red. The eyes may feel tired or as though sand has gotten in them. The eyelids often stick together as the discharge dries, especially during sleep. Vision is not affected, except by the discharge that covers the surface of the eye.

These infections are not dangerous so long as they do not move into deeper layers of the eye, an uncommon occurrence. Even without treatment, they clear up within ten days or so. Conventional practitioners give antibiotic eyedrops when bacteria is thought to be responsible for the infection, but there are no effective drugs for ordinary viral conjunctivitis.

Allergic reactions and irritation from smoke, smog, or other chemicals can cause similar symptoms of redness and tearing. You can readily distinguish these conditions from infectious conjunctivitis in most cases. Generally the infectious types are accompanied by cold symptoms or occur after exposure to someone else with the infection. When the conjunctivitis is caused by allergies or chemical irritation, usually you can remember the exposure to pollens, dust, fumes, or the like that led to it. Allergies and irritation usually begin by affecting both eyes and typically cause a watery or slightly mucous discharge. Allergic conjunctivitis is the only type frequently accompanied by much itching.

GENERAL HOME CARE

Avoid rubbing the affected eye(s), for this can injure the inflamed, weakened tissues and drive any infection into deeper layers of the eye. Touching the eye also spreads the infecting germs to your other eye and to other people. Periodically cleanse the eye with warm water to remove discharge and crusts. Be careful not to touch the unaffected eye, and be sure to wash your hands well every time you do touch your eyes or the surrounding area. If the conjunctivitis is caused by an allergy or irritant, rinse the eyes with artificial tears, sterile normal saline solution, or over-the-counter eyedrops, all available at a pharmacy.

HOMEOPATHIC MEDICINES

Give a dose of the indicated remedy three or four times a day for up to three days. Stop as soon as symptoms definitely improve.

Belladonna can be given at the earliest stage of conjunctivitis, when the main symptom is sudden onset of bright red, bloodshot inflammation of the membranes. The eye feels hot and may throb. Clear tears flow copiously. Light bothers the eyes (if this symptom is at all severe, see your practitioner).

Euphrasia (eyebright) has a well-deserved reputation in both home-opathic and herbal traditions for helping people with eye troubles. *Euphrasia* conjunctivitis is characterized by the copious flow of acrid, watery tears that burn the face. With time the discharge may become thick and mucous but never opaque or yellow-green. Often the eyes feel dry or as though there is dust or sand in them. The eyes and often the lids (especially the margins) are very red. There may be accompanying nasal drainage (see "Colds and Coughs").

Use *Apis* when swelling of the conjunctivae is extreme, especially if there is marked aggravation from heat. The conjunctival lining of the inner eyelid may be so swollen that it protrudes from behind the lid. The conjunctivae on the eyeball itself may be so swollen that the iris looks like it is sitting in a shallow depression (see your practitioner if swelling is this severe). The lids themselves and the areas above and below the lids may be puffy and swollen as if they are full of water. The eyes and often the lids are quite red. There are gushing, hot tears. The eyes may sting or burn, and the discomfort is worse in a warm room. Cold bathing of the eyes brings relief.

Pulsatilla is curative during infections characterized by discharge of much thick yellow-to-greenish matter from the eyes. The discharge generally does not irritate the skin, but the eyes may itch and burn, especially in the evening. The lids, especially the margins, also may itch intolerably. Going out in the open air as well as bathing the eyes in cold water afford relief. These eye symptoms may accompany a typical *Pulsatilla* cold, and the general symptoms of the medicine may be present.

Mercurius should be considered also when the discharge is yellow-green, but in this case the liquid is often irritating to the skin and may be less thick than the *Pulsatilla* discharge. Nighttime, warmth of the bed, and the glare of firelight may worsen symptoms of discharge and smarting of the eyes. There are likely to be eruptions of whiteheads or scales around the eyes and on the lids.

Consider *Hepar sulph.* if there is a thick puslike discharge, if eye discomfort is aggravated by cold and relieved by warmth, and if the general symptoms of the medicine are present (see the *materia medica* section).

BEYOND HOME CARE

GET MEDICAL CARE IMMEDIATELY:

- for severe eye pain;
- for any loss of vision;
- if there is an injury to the eye or a foreign body or chemical in the eye.

GET MEDICAL CARE TODAY:

- if there is any significant eye pain;
- if light causes pain in the eye;
- if the pupil is shaped irregularly or does not react to changes in light;
- if the worst redness is definitely in a circular pattern around the iris;
- if the area over the inner eye's tear duct is swollen or red.

CALL YOUR PRACTITIONER TODAY:

- if there is a thick yellow or greenish puslike discharge dripping from the eye.

BLOCKED TEAR DUCT

The tear ducts at the inner corners of the eyes allow the tears, which are forming constantly, to drain. Some newborn babies' ducts are too small or fail to open, causing the tears to back up into the eye and nourish bacterial growth. The child has a constant, thick yellow or green discharge of pus dripping from the eye. The eye itself is usually not involved and doesn't look badly bloodshot or swollen. This condition may last for a few months before the passageway of the tear duct opens fully.

Constitutional homeopathic treatment is generally the best way to help the child with this condition, unless the tear duct is completely absent and must be opened surgically. If you cannot obtain constitutional care from a homeopathic professional, you can try giving the child *Silica* 6x once or twice a day for ten to fourteen days. Conventional practitioners use antibiotic drops or attempt to dilate the tear duct with an instrument.

CHAPTER 5

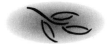

CHILDHOOD MALADIES

IN THIS CHAPTER we cover colic, teething difficulties, and bed-wetting, all very common childhood problems. We also address the infectious illnesses that typically affect children: measles, German measles, mumps, and chicken pox.

Of course, adults can get these infectious diseases, too. This is especially true today, since immunizations and better hygiene kept many grown-ups from being exposed when they were young. The symptoms of these illnesses are essentially the same during adulthood and childhood, so the information in these sections applies to adults as well.

GIVING HOMEOPATHIC MEDICINES TO CHILDREN

Giving a homeopathic remedy to an infant or young child can be a little tricky, depending on the form of medicine you have. It helps to keep in mind that the child doesn't have to swallow the medicine—it has its effect as soon as it contacts the inner surfaces of the mouth.

If the medicine is in liquid form, a small drop is plenty for each dose and won't cause choking. You need not give a whole medicine-dropperful. The tiny granules that look like cake sprinkles are almost as easy to use. Just pour several of them on the child's tongue—they'll stick there and dissolve almost instantly. If the remedy comes in a larger form, however, you should crush one of the pills or tablets into a powder between two pieces of clean paper using a heavy object. Alternatively, you can dissolve them in a spoonful of water and then give a small drop.

Older children love to take homeopathic remedies. Remind them to let the pills dissolve in the mouth, but don't worry if they chew them up.

COLIC

All babies cry a lot, but 10 to 20 percent have extended crying spells for no clear reason. Because these babies look like they have abdominal pain—they typically draw their legs up, harden the abdomen, and may pass gas—such crying spells are known as colic, a word implying cramping in the intestines.

Actually, the cause of colic remains a mystery. Abdominal pain resulting from trapped gas may in fact contribute in some cases, but other possibilities include oversensitivity of the tiny baby's nervous system, or simply a failure of the infant to have its needs understood and met quickly enough. At any rate, since nothing seems to console an infant with colic, you may worry that something is seriously wrong with the child, and you'll certainly feel extremely frustrated.

GENERAL HOME CARE

It should help to know that your child will definitely grow out of the problem, almost always by three months of age. Before the inevitable improvement, though, there are several steps you can try at home to ease the child's discomfort and reduce your own anxiety. First, however, you should take the baby to your health practitioner for a checkup. Other illnesses are unlikely if the child has no other symptoms, but you should be sure that such problems as ear infections and hernias are ruled out.

Colic seems to be more common in bottle-fed rather than breast-fed babies, perhaps because of air swallowing. If you bottle-feed your baby, hold the bottle upside down and check to see that a drop of milk drips out of the nipple each second. If not, enlarge the nipple hole. Also, some babies have sensitivities to milk protein. Switching from a cow's-milk formula to a soy- or casein-based formula may help.

In breast-fed babies, colic may be aggravated by foods the mother eats and passes to the baby in her milk. Cow's milk, citrus fruits, and cabbage are the most likely culprits. It can't hurt to experiment with eliminating these foods from your diet temporarily, as long as you make sure to replace them with other foods or supplements containing the missing nutrients. If you're breast-feeding, you should definitely avoid stimulants, including coffee, tea, and caffeinated soft drinks.

Babies cry for different reasons at different times. If you listen to your child closely, you may be able to distinguish a "hungry" cry from a "tired" cry. As soon as your baby starts crying, try to figure out what she's trying to tell you.

- She may be hungry. Remember that babies don't get hungry on schedule. If she wants food, feed her. Don't be concerned about overfeeding—she'll stop eating when she's had enough.
- She may want to suck, even though she's not hungry. If that's the case, she'll prefer a pacifier to the breast or a bottle.
- She may be bored. Even little babies have a great need for stimulation from the environment. She may want to be played with or propped up in a room where there's a lot going on. Sometimes rhythmic stimulation such as a rocking cradle or windup swing is just what she wants.
- She may be sleepy. If she is, picking her up or otherwise fussing over her may just make her cry more. Try putting her down alone in a dark, quiet room and letting her cry for a few minutes. If the crying quickly becomes a softer whimper, you're probably on the right track.
- She may need to be held. Babies crave physical contact, and they should get it. Don't worry about spoiling the child.
- She may be cold, hot, wet, or in pain. Always check to make sure that her diapers don't need changing, that she's properly dressed, and that nothing is jabbing or poking her under her clothes or under the blankets.

If crying persists after you've tried one response, just try another. By quickly identifying the reason for your baby's crying and responding appropriately, you may be able to keep the child from getting so frustrated and "wound up" that the crying becomes self-perpetuating.

Finally, be sure that you're getting enough rest yourself. A colicky baby can be physically and emotionally exhausting. If you can, arrange for a relative or friend to care for the child for an hour or two a day so you can get a break. You'll be better able to withstand the stress and, in turn, to communicate love and reassurance to your baby.

CASETAKING QUESTIONS FOR COLIC

Character of the symptoms:
• Does the child seem angry, or simply uncomfortable?
• Is the child restless, or does she lie still?

Modalities:
• Are the symptoms relieved by gentle, firm pressure on the abdomen?
• Does warmth relieve the symptoms or make them worse?
• How does motion affect the child? How about physical contact?
• Are the symptoms worse at a specific time of day?

HOMEOPATHIC MEDICINES

Infants with colic respond well to homeopathic treatment. You should notice improvement within an hour (often within ten minutes) when you give the correct medicine.

Colicky infants who need *Chamomilla* are extremely irritable, scream loudly, and appear to be in unbearable pain. Although nothing seems to please them, they may find temporary relief by being carried or rocked, but resume crying and screaming once they are put down. Typically, they toss about frequently. The pains are aggravated at night and by warm applications.

Give *Colocynthis* if the symptoms are relieved by firm pressure on the stomach or abdomen. Warmth may bring relief as well. The infant cannot keep still, and seems to be angry, screams loudly, and has an anxious and angry-looking face, though the irritability isn't as extreme as in the *Chamomilla* child. She tends to hold on to things or to people tightly.

Magnesia phosphorica is similar to *Colocynthis,* but you should use *Mag. phos.* first if symptoms seem primarily relieved by warmth. Gentle pressure also helps, and again, the infant often curls up with his knees against his chest. Hiccups may occur concurrently. *Mag. phos.* children usually aren't as persistently irritable as *Chamomilla, Colocynthis,* or *Nux vomica* infants.

Nux vomica is the choice for the infant who has colic after she or her nursing mother eats rich food, or when the nursing mother is taking any medicines, drugs, or alcohol. The child is irritable, but again, isn't typically as out of control as the *Chamomilla* infant.

The infant who needs *Bryonia* also is very irritable, but in this case the screaming is noticeably worse from the slightest motion. He is sensitive also to touching and heat. The infant lies motionless, often with his knees drawn up.

Like *Nux vomica, Pulsatilla* is indicated when the infant or nursing mother has eaten rich foods; like *Chamomilla* babies, the *Pulsatilla* child wants to be carried. The difference is subtle: *Pulsatilla* children have mild dispositions, and though they can be quite irritable, their cries are weaker and fundamentally less angry. Another point: the child may find relief in gentle motion; he wants to be carried primarily because he craves physical contact.

When a breast-feeding mother experiences grief or other strong emotions, her infant may "pick up" her feelings. Use *Ignatia* if colic occurs in such circumstances.

If the infant frequently spits up, drools, and is generally restless, consider *Ipecacuanha.*

Finally, *Jalapa* is another medicine to try when others haven't helped.

REMEDY SUMMARY FOR COLIC

Give the medicine: Up to every hour while the symptoms are worse, less frequently as the irritability or discomfort diminishes, for up to 2 days.

When to try another medicine: If there is no significant improvement after 12 hours.

CHAMOMILLA ★

Essentials
- Extreme irritability
- Loud, nearly constant screaming

Confirmatory symptoms
- Worse at night
- Relieved by being carried or rocked
- One cheek flushed, the other pale
- Worse from warmth

COLOCYNTHIS

Essentials
- Irritability and colic relieved by pressure on the abdomen; child pulls knees up to chest

Confirmatory symptoms
- Better from warmth
- Child holds on tightly to people and objects

MAG. PHOS.

Essentials
- Colicky symptoms relieved especially by warmth but also by gentle pressure on the abdomen

Confirmatory symptoms
- Infant lies with knees bent up to chest
- Angry irritability, but not typical

NUX VOMICA

Essentials
- Symptoms begin after the baby or mother eats rich food, or after the mother takes alcohol, drugs, or medicines

Confirmatory symptoms
- Angry irritability

PULSATILLA

Essentials
- General *Pulsatilla* symptoms—usual mild disposition, but irritable in a fussy rather than extremely angry way (see *materia medica* section)

Confirmatory symptoms
- Child wants to be carried and held; craves physical contact and affection as much as or more than the motion itself
- Symptoms may have started after eating rich food

BRYONIA

Essentials
- Worse from motion—the child lies still as it cries or screams, rather than thrashing about

IPECACUANHA

Essentials
- Frequent spitting up or vomiting

Confirmatory symptoms
- Excessive drooling

IGNATIA

Essentials
- Begins after emotional upset or stress experienced by mother or baby

JALAPA
- Helpful in some cases of colic when other medicines haven't been effective

---

BEYOND HOME CARE

GET MEDICAL CARE IMMEDIATELY:

- if there are black or bloody stools;
- if there is severe vomiting or diarrhea;
- if the child is pale, limp, lethargic, or feverish.

SEE YOUR PRACTITIONER TODAY:

- if the colicky symptoms are associated with vomiting or diarrhea;
- if the child is taking any medicines or has recently been immunized.

SEE YOUR PRACTITIONER SOON:
- for a thorough medical examination after the symptoms begin. This applies to *all* infants with colic.

TEETHING

Although the eruption of teeth through the gums is always uncomfortable, some children suffer terribly every time a new tooth comes in. In recent years, the success in treating teething children has convinced more people of the efficacy of homeopathy than anything else.

GENERAL HOME CARE

Rely on simple home-care measures for your teething child unless symptoms are severe. Offer her something soft but firm to gnaw on. Ice wrapped in a moist washcloth, or a commercial, frozen teething toy may help.

HOMEOPATHIC MEDICINES

Chamomilla is by far the medicine most likely to help the teething child. The gums are inflamed and the child can't keep her fingers out of her mouth. One cheek may be hot and red, while the other is pale. She screams with pain, and nothing can comfort her. She is terribly irritable. She demands things but rejects them as soon as she gets them, tossing them across the room if she's old enough. She may throw angry fits, screaming and hitting those around her. She is calm only if she is constantly carried about or rocked. During sleep she tosses about and cries out suddenly.

Ignatia may help if the child is extremely distressed by the pain but not so irritable. She sighs, sobs, and cries. She may tremble, and single parts of the body sometimes quiver or jerk. She may wake from sleep with piercing cries.

The *Kreosote* child suffers from extremely painful dentition. The gums are severely inflamed and red with a spongy consistency. The child is agitated and wakeful.

REMEDY SUMMARY FOR TEETHING

Give the medicine: Up to 3 times a day, repeating the medicine only when symptoms return.

When to try another medicine: If there is no significant improvement after 24 hours.

CHAMOMILLA ★

Essentials
- Screaming with severe pain; inconsolability
- Extreme irritability

Confirmatory symptoms
- Fingers constantly in the mouth
- Child is demanding but can't be satisfied; rejects things she has asked for
- Temper tantrums, striking out at others
- Relief from being carried or rocked
- One cheek flushed, the other pale

IGNATIA

Essentials
- Child is extremely distressed by the pain but not so irritable—sobbing, crying

Confirmatory symptoms
- Sighing
- Trembling; single parts of the body quiver or jerk
- Wakes from sleep with piercing cries

KREOSOTE

Essentials
- Much pain, but the child is not necessarily angrily irritable

Confirmatory symptoms
- Red, inflamed gums are swollen to the point that they appear "spongy"

BED-WETTING (ENURESIS)

Most children are ready for toilet training between the ages of two and three. Bowel control usually comes first, followed within six months or so by daytime control of the bladder. Staying dry at night is a little more difficult, though, and bed-wetting is considered normal until the child is six or so. After that age, your health practitioner may recommend tests to rule out infection or structural problems of the urinary system. These disorders are uncommon, however, and in all likelihood this problem will eventually clear up on its own.

Though it seems automatic, nighttime bladder control is a function of the higher brain, and it just takes time to learn this neurologically complex skill. How early a child learns to control his bladder does not reflect any other aspect of his psychological or physical development, so long as there are no other symptoms. Of course, concern about persistent bed-wetting is natural, and neither child nor parent likes the wet sheets and forced cleanup routine. Try to give your child acceptance and reassurance, however. Communicating anxiety or dissatisfaction with your child does not help him learn bladder control and may actually aggravate the problem.

There can be other causes of bed-wetting. Sometimes genetics is a factor, since the tendency to wet the bed runs in families. A child's food sensitivities or allergies also may play a role. Pediatrician Lendon Smith has estimated that reactions to such foods as milk, citrus fruits, chocolate, and sugar contribute to the problem in as many as one-tenth of all bed-wetting children.

Psychological factors can be responsible for bed-wetting. Stress can put demands on the child's psychological defenses, limiting the nervous system's capacity to learn new skills. Sometimes the child unconsciously uses bed-wetting as an easy way to get attention. In other cases wetting the bed may be an expression of bottled-up anger. Some children stop wetting the bed but then start again after facing a stressful situation or illness. The birth of a sibling, a move to a new home, or a serious illness may trigger the recurrence of bed-wetting.

On rare occasions, infection or structural abnormality of the urinary tract is responsible for bed-wetting.

GENERAL HOME CARE

The primary treatment for bed-wetting is "tincture of time," allowing the child to learn to control his bladder at his own pace. Helpful factors include providing a secure, guilt-free, loving home environment. Encourage his efforts to stay dry at night, just as you would encourage his efforts to draw or to ride a bicycle. You might also try gentle suggestions that allow his subconscious mind to associate urinating with being out of bed. For instance, every time he urinates, have him say something like, "My feet are on the floor. Now I'm going to the bathroom."

Limiting fluid intake during the latter part of the day and having the child urinate just before bedtime are traditional but generally unsuccessful measures for controlling bed-wetting. Some parents have a little better luck getting the child up to urinate during the night, especially if he wets the bed at a predictable time.

Since food sensitivities may be the reason for your child's bedwetting, consider eliminating possible offenders from your child's diet and see how it affects his bed-wetting. Remember, it's often the foods the child craves most that he is sensitive to.

Constitutional homeopathic treatment sometimes can be helpful to bed-wetters, but we are not tremendously impressed with the results. We have seen some children stop bed-wetting immediately after receiving a constitutional medicine, but more often there has been no apparent change in this symptom, even when the child improves in other ways.

The most helpful role your health practitioner is likely to play is in reassuring you that your child is healthy. If bed-wetting persists past the age of six or so, the practitioner will want to run tests on the urinary system to rule out infection or anatomical problems. He or she will consider also the role of stress and psychological factors. If problems are discovered in any of these areas, appropriate treatment can be given. Rarely is surgical or medicinal treatment necessary.

Some practitioners prescribe powerful drugs such as imipramine (an antidepressant), dilantin (an anticonvulsant), or dextroamphetamine (an amphetamine) for bed-wetting children. We are of course cautious about treatments that suppress symptoms without dealing with the underlying problem, especially when they involve powerful drugs with many potential adverse effects.

CASETAKING QUESTIONS FOR BED-WETTING

Character of the symptoms:
• Is the child especially hard to wake up?
• Does the child urinate while dreaming?

- Does the child lose urine during the day as well, such as when sneezing or laughing?

Modalities:
- Is there a time of night or season of the year when the bed-wetting is more frequent?
- Does the problem seem to be affected by weather?

Other symptoms:
- Is there any pain in the bladder?

HOMEOPATHIC MEDICINES

Generally, the best way to use homeopathy to help children who wet the bed is with constitutional treatment. Seek professional homeopathic care for this treatment. If this is unavailable, you may try one of the following medicines as long as there are no other health problems.

Kreosote is the medicine to start with when the only problem is bed-wetting and there are no striking symptoms to help you choose a different remedy. In the typical case, the child sleeps deeply and is very hard to awaken. He wets the bed while dreaming and may even tell you he was dreaming of urinating. As with several other medicines, including *Causticum* and *Sepia,* the child urinates shortly after falling asleep in the classic case.

In cases without specific symptoms, try *Causticum* if *Kreosote* doesn't help or isn't available. Of course, you can give *Causticum* also if its particular symptoms are present. Like *Kreosote,* this medicine is especially indicated when the child wets soon after falling asleep. The problem may be worse in the winter, on cold days or nights, and during changes in the weather, but is less frequent in the summer. The child may also dribble in his pants during the day while coughing or sneezing or after any excitement. He seems to pass the urine so easily that he is unaware of the stream.

Equisetum is another medicine to try when bed-wetting persists without many other symptoms. The old homeopathic textbooks say that *Equisetum* is indicated when the child still wets the bed out of habit. The child may experience a dull pain in the bladder and a sense of distention that is not relieved by urinating.

Sepia, like *Kreosote* and *Causticum,* can help when the child urinates shortly after going to sleep. You can consider this remedy also when the *Sepia* personality is evident: the child, usually a girl, is reserved, dislikes sympathy, and wants to be alone (see the *materia medica* section for more on the typical general symptoms of *Sepia*).

Belladonna is given to bed-wetting children who sleep restlessly, moaning and perhaps even screaming in their sleep. They are difficult to waken. They also may pass urine during the day, especially while standing.

Pulsatilla can be useful for bed-wetting children who are sensitive and gentle, weep easily, and crave affection. They may sleep on their back with hands above the head or on the abdomen.

REMEDY SUMMARY FOR BED-WETTING

Give the medicine: In just one dose in the thirtieth potency.

When to try another medicine: If there is no improvement after 3 to 4 weeks.

KREOSOTE ★

Essentials
• Child is very difficult to wake

Confirmatory symptoms
• Urinates early in the night
• Wets while dreaming; may dream of urinating

CAUSTICUM

Confirmatory symptoms
• Child wets the bed soon after falling asleep
• Wets more often in the winter, on cold days or nights, during changes in the weather; less often in the summer
• Dribbling of urine during the day while coughing, sneezing, or laughing, or after any excitement

EQUISETUM

Essentials
• Bed-wetting during dreams or without definite pattern

Confirmatory symptoms
- Passes large amounts of urine
- Dull pain in the bladder and a sense of distention unrelieved by urinating

SEPIA

Essentials
- Child urinates shortly after going to sleep

Confirmatory symptoms
- Loses urine during the day when laughing or coughing
- Mental and personality symptoms of *Sepia*—the child is reserved, dislikes sympathy, and wants to be alone (see *materia medica* section)

PULSATILLA

Essentials
- Child is gentle, sensitive, weeps easily, and craves affection

Confirmatory symptoms
- Sleeps on the back, perhaps with hands above the head or on the abdomen

BELLADONNA

Essentials
- Child sleeps restlessly, moaning or even screaming during sleep

Confirmatory symptoms
- Loses urine during the day, especially while standing

BEYOND HOME CARE

SEE YOUR HEALTH PRACTITIONER TODAY:

- if there are any other symptoms associated with the bed-wetting: frequent or painful urination, bloody urine, abdominal pain, or fever. Even if these symptoms are more mild, your child needs medical evaluation within a day or two.

SEE YOUR PRACTITIONER SOON:

- if your bed-wetting child is more than 6 years old;
- if your child has learned bladder control but has been wetting the bed again regularly for a month or so.

MEASLES

Measles is one of the most contagious diseases known. While uncommon in the United States, occasional outbreaks have occurred in recent years. The illness can be serious.

The symptoms of an early case of measles are identical to those of a bad cold. After an incubation period of ten to fourteen days, the symptoms begin with a hacking cough, nasal discharge, and a low-grade fever. Redness and watering of the eyes, along with sensitivity to light, are usually pronounced. After a few days, small white spots resembling salt crystals appear inside the mouth on the inner cheeks.

Within four or five days after the symptoms begin, there is a brief drop in fever, and then the classic measles rash develops as light-red spots on the face and neck. The spots come out in small, irregularly shaped blotches, which may be flat or slightly raised. As the rash rapidly spreads, the blotches run together, and new ones appear on the upper chest and arms. Over the next few days the rash spreads over the back, abdomen, and legs, eventually reaching the feet. By about this time the fever drops and the child starts to feel much better.

Serious complications, including pneumonia and inflammation of the heart, occur occasionally. Rarely—once in ten thousand cases or so—measles involves the brain and may result in permanent neurologic damage.

GENERAL HOME CARE

A child with measles usually has a diminished appetite. Don't try to force-feed him if he isn't hungry. His body is telling him that he doesn't need the food, or at least that he can't digest it efficiently.

With such a high fever, he is at risk of dehydration (see chapter 8), so make sure he receives enough liquids. The child's sore and inflamed eyes may be sensitive to light. Keep lights dimmed. Supplemental vitamin

A has been found in recent research to reduce the risk of serious complications; consult your health practitioner for advice.

CASETAKING QUESTIONS FOR MEASLES

Character of the symptoms:
- Have the symptoms come on suddenly, or gradually?
- Which are the more prominent symptoms: fever, general complaints such as restlessness or tiredness, eye irritation, runny nose?
- What is the color of any nasal discharge? Does it irritate the skin?

Modalities:
- How sensitive to light are the eyes?
- How does the child react to motion?

Other symptoms:
- Do the limbs or facial muscles jerk or twitch?
- Does the body feel especially heavy or tired?
- Does the patient have a cough or chest pains? Describe the cough.
- If there is a headache, where is the pain worse?
- Is the digestive tract affected with nausea, diarrhea, or constipation?

HOMEOPATHIC MEDICINES

According to Samuel Hahnemann, *Aconite* is "almost miraculous" in the treatment of measles; E. A. Farrington, a nineteenth-century American homeopathic authority, said it's "the best remedy for the beginning measles." *Aconite* is most useful early in the disease, especially if it has come on suddenly. At this point you won't know for certain that the illness is measles. There is fever, restlessness, nasal discharge, red eyes, sensitivity to light, dry croupy cough, chest stitches, restless sleep, and sometimes diarrhea.

Like *Aconite, Belladonna* is useful during the early stages of measles, but it can be used also after the rash has erupted. *Belladonna* is particularly indicated when predominant symptoms include a red face, throbbing headache, and moistened skin from the fever. These children are drowsy and at least a little delirious but may be unable to sleep. Their limbs may twitch or jerk. Light, noise, or the slightest jarring makes their symptoms worse.

Gelsemium is a third medicine possibly useful during the early stages of measles; like *Belladonna,* it also may be used during the rash stage. Unlike *Aconite* or *Belladonna,* the *Gelsemium* measles begins slowly. There is a gradual onset of fever and chilliness, and the child feels heavy and very tired. Sometimes raising the head or even keeping the eyes open is just too great an effort, and the child lies motionless. She is apathetic and doesn't want to be disturbed. The *Gelsemium* child usually is not very thirsty, and is apt to have a watery nasal discharge that burns the upper lip, a headache above the nape of the neck, and perhaps a harsh, croupy cough.

A prescription of *Euphrasia* is indicated during measles when the nasal discharge and the eye symptoms predominate. As distinct from that of *Gelsemium,* the *Euphrasia* type of nasal discharge is profuse and does not burn the upper lip. These children do, however, have acrid tears that stream out of their eyes. The eyes appear red or unusually bright. Sensitivity to light is especially intense. Their nasal and eye symptoms tend to improve in the open air. They have a dry cough and possibly hoarseness. They also tend to have throbbing headaches, which get better once the measles skin eruptions appear. (See also chapter 4 on colds and coughs.)

Bryonia is valuable for treating children with measles when the rash appears late and when the chest especially is affected. *Bryonia* children have a dry, painful cough, chest stitches, soreness of the limbs and body, and sometimes twitching muscles in the face, eyes, and mouth. The muscles ache badly, and the child lies still because it hurts to move, in contrast to the *Gelsemium* child, who is just too tired to move. The face is pale and the eyes are red. Constipation and frontal headaches can accompany the measles. As with all *Bryonia* fevers, dry mouth and an intense thirst for cold drinks are characteristic. The symptoms are made worse by motion and warmth and better by stillness and cold things.

Pulsatilla is primarily useful in the later stages of measles, when the fever has subsided or has completely gone. The nasal discharge is usually thick and yellowish, and profuse tearing comes from the eyes. The cough is typically dry at night and loose during the day. The *Pulsatilla* child desires cool air, is worse in the heat, and has little thirst. Feelings of queasiness or nausea accompanied by diarrhea may occur. Earaches commonly are experienced, too. *Pulsatilla* is useful also when eye problems linger after the measles.

Other medicines that can be helpful in treating children with measles are:

FERRUM PHOS.: Useful in the initial stages of measles if *Aconite* isn't working and if *Belladonna* doesn't seem indicated.

APIS: For high fever, much swollen skin, and greatly inflamed eyes and lips worsened by heat. The patient is thirstless, irritable, and may be delirious.

KALI BI.: Useful during the later stages of measles if earache occurs or swollen glands develop. Characteristically *Kali bi.* patients have a rattling cough, and the nose runs with thick, yellow, stringy mucus. There may be a sensation of pressure at the root of the nose and perhaps throbbing and burning in the nasal cartilage.

RHUS TOX.: For intensely itching rashes, worse at night and during rest; the patient is restless.

ARSENICUM: Indicated in severe cases of the measles with great restlessness, much weakness, delirium, and offensive and exhausting diarrhea.

REMEDY SUMMARY FOR MEASLES

See text for brief descriptions of other medicines that may be useful.
Give the medicine: Every 4 to 6 hours for up to 3 days.
When to try another medicine: If the symptoms haven't begun to improve after 3 days.

ACONITE ★

Essentials
- First stages of presumed measles with sudden onset
- Fever, restlessness, nasal discharge, red eyes, light sensitivity, dry croupy cough, stitching pains, restless sleep

BELLADONNA

Essentials
- Fever with red face, throbbing headache
- May be given in early stages of the illness or after rash has appeared

Confirmatory symptoms
- Drowsiness; delirium of any degree
- Limbs twitch or jerk
- Uncomfortably sensitive to light, noise, or slightest jarring

GELSEMIUM

Essentials
- Slow onset of symptoms with gradually increasing fever and chilliness
- Child feels heavy, tired
- Suitable before or after the rash appears

Confirmatory symptoms
- Little thirst
- Headache at base of skull
- Watery nasal discharge burning the upper lip
- Child apathetic, lies motionless, doesn't want to be disturbed

EUPHRASIA

Essentials
- Nasal discharge and eye irritation are predominant
- Eyes appear red or bright; painfully sensitive to light

Confirmatory symptoms
- Profuse watery nasal discharge that does not irritate the skin
- Nasal and eye symptoms relieved in open air
- Dry cough, hoarseness
- Throbbing headache which improves after the rash appears

PULSATILLA

Essentials
- Used in later stages of measles after fever has subsided
- Thick yellowish nasal discharge
- May be given at any stage if general symptoms of *Pulsatilla* are prominent (see *materia medica* section)

Confirmatory symptoms
- Cough; may be dry at night and loose during the day
- Queasiness, nausea, or diarrhea
- Earaches
- Eye problems that linger after the measles

BRYONIA

Essentials
• Late-appearing rash
• Marked chest symptoms: dry painful cough, stitching pains

Confirmatory symptoms
• Aching or soreness of the limbs and body, worse from motion
• Twitching of the face or around the eyes or mouth
• Constipation
• Frontal headaches
• Dry mouth; intense thirst for cold drinks

BEYOND HOME CARE

GET MEDICAL CARE IMMEDIATELY:

• if your child has a severe headache, excessive lethargy, vomiting, or drowsiness;
• if there is spontaneous bruising or ruptured blood vessels under the skin;
• if there is unexplained bleeding from the rectum, nose, or mouth;
• if there is difficult or rapid breathing.

GET MEDICAL CARE TODAY:

• if any infant less than 6 months old gets the measles;
• if there is earache;
• if significant coughing lasts more than 4 days.

SEE YOUR PRACTITIONER SOON:

• if the fever and cough do not subside as the rash peaks.

GERMAN MEASLES

German measles, or rubella, is a harmless disease to children. It is, however, a potential threat to pregnant women since those who contract it during the first three months of pregnancy have a fifty-fifty chance of delivering an infant who has serious birth defects, including blindness, deafness, heart condition, cleft palate, and mental problems. German measles is sometimes called the three-day measles. It is shorter and less severe in its symptoms than the "regular" measles, which typically lasts seven to ten days. The incubation period ranges from fourteen to twenty-one days. Even though symptoms are apparent for only three days, children with German measles are contagious to others from seven days prior to eruption of the rash and usually for five days after this time.

In a typical case of the German measles, the child becomes mildly ill with a low-grade fever and some nasal discharge about twenty-four to thirty-six hours before the rash develops. There is then painful swelling of the lymph nodes at the back of the head and neck and behind the ears. This swelling may last six or seven days, even beyond the disappearance of the rash. The rash consists of very small, slightly raised spots which begin on the face and spread over the rest of the body within twenty-four hours. Sometimes large areas of the body become flushed and red. The rash reaches the lower legs on the third day as the rash on the face begins to fade.

The above description of symptoms represents the classic form of German measles. Many children, however, have much milder cases. There is often no rash, and their symptoms may be impossible to distinguish from those of colds or other viral infections. Joint pains sometimes occur, though this happens more commonly in adults.

GENERAL HOME CARE

Children with the German measles are rarely very sick. They do not need to stay in bed and should be allowed to get up and even go outside on nice days. They should of course stay away from pregnant women.

HOMEOPATHIC MEDICINES

The following homeopathic medicines have been found to be most effective in treating children with German measles: *Aconite, Belladonna, Ferrum phos.,* and *Pulsatilla.* Read the chapters on measles, fevers, influenza, and the *materia medica* section for specific information on each medicine's symptoms.

BEYOND HOME CARE

Except for problems resulting from pregnant women getting German measles, there is no evidence that German measles causes significant complications.

MUMPS

No longer very common, mumps is a moderately contagious viral disease with an incubation period lasting fourteen to twenty-one days. The typical symptoms include the characteristic swelling of the parotid salivary glands, which lie just below and in front of the earlobe, along with fever ranging from 101°F to as high as 105°F, loss of appetite, and headache. Other salivary glands under the jaw sometimes are affected. Children are contagious from one day prior to onset of symptoms until the swelling of the salivary glands is completely gone. In adults, mumps may affect other glands such as the ovaries, testes, or pancreas, but sterility rarely occurs.

Nearly half of all children with mumps experience subclinical infections with either no symptoms or only mild symptoms appearing. Measurement of antibodies in the blood can determine if subclinical infections have already established immunity.

Encephalitis, a viral infection of the brain, is an occasional complication of the mumps. Since this condition can be serious, it is especially important to note the symptoms listed in "Beyond Home Care."

GENERAL HOME CARE

Bed rest isn't essential since mumps is a mild disease. The ill person should keep away from adults who have never had mumps, however. Acid liquids (such as lemonade, orange juice, or ginger ale) and spices should be avoided because they stimulate salivation and increase pain.

CASETAKING QUESTIONS FOR MUMPS

Character of the symptoms:
- Which glands are affected (parotid glands only, submaxillary glands under the jaw, testes or ovaries)?
- Do the affected glands feel very hard, almost rocklike?
- Are the affected glands visibly red and inflamed?

• What is the character of the pain? Does it extend into the ears or throat?

Other symptoms:
• Is the face red?
• Is there excessive salivation, bad breath, or a bad taste in the mouth?
• Is perspiration markedly increased?

HOMEOPATHIC MEDICINES

Belladonna is the most commonly prescribed medicine for the mumps. As with so many of *Belladonna*'s symptoms, the illness comes on rapidly and violently. The parotid glands are hot and red (they may, in fact, become scarlet red), and are sensitive to touch. Typical are burning pain in the throat and shooting pains in the glands, which come and go suddenly. Some spasmodic constriction of the throat may occur, especially when the child is drinking or swallowing. The face shows a glowing redness, and the child may appear dazed or a little delirious. In some cases the parotid gland swelling suddenly lessens, but a throbbing headache and increased delirium ensue.

Phytolacca is one of the remedies to consider when mumps involve the submaxillary glands, which lie under the jaw, as well as the parotids. Whichever glands are involved, they typically are quite firm, even stony hard, and the child experiences an uncomfortable sense of pressure and tension in them. Swallowing is difficult, especially anything hot, and may cause pain that shoots into the ear. The throat feels dry and rough. The face and skin tend to be pale, not *Belladonna*'s distinctively red color. The symptoms are worse in cold and wet weather, at night, and with the heat from the bed.

Pulsatilla is more valuable during the later stages of mumps. *Pulsatilla* children usually have a dry mouth and thickly coated tongue. *Pulsatilla* is also one of the prime medicines for adults when the mumps involve the breasts, ovaries, or testicles. As with other illnesses, the choice of this remedy is confirmed if the patient is weepy, whiny, craves affection, is thirstless, desires open air, and is worse when warm. The symptoms may be worse at night and after lying down.

Mercurius is another medicine to consider when mumps causes swelling of the submaxillary glands. The affected glands may feel hard to the touch, and are tender. Other distinct symptoms of this medicine include offensive sweat, foul taste on the tongue, foul breath, and excessive salivation. The *Mercurius* child often sweats a lot, especially at night. Although it isn't as readily available as the medicines we've mentioned so far, *Pilocarpinum* has a good reputation for treating mumps. Drs. Tyler and Burnett, two leading British homeopaths of the past, considered it a "near specific" for people with mumps (there is never just one specific medicine for a disease). Characteristic symptoms of *Pilocarpinum* are few; they include profuse sweat followed by great thirst, much salivation, and general weakness.

Other homeopathic medicines to consider in treating children with mumps include:

ACONITE: Useful during the earliest stages if there is a sudden onset of fever, great restlessness, and much thirst. The symptoms are worse in warm rooms and better in the open air.

RHUS TOX.: Appropriate when there is more swelling on the left side; aching in the limbs that is worse at night, during rest, and when first moving, but better during continued motion; extreme chilliness and sensitivity to cold; and dry, burning thirst. Cold sores on the lips may accompany the other symptoms.

BRYONIA: The patient is very irritable; the slightest motion causes pain—even the turning of the head hurts. She has dry lips and is quite thirsty for cold water.

ARSENICUM: When the patient has severe weakness, chilliness, clammy sweats, anxiety, and marked thirst, especially for sips of water. *Arsenicum* is good also if the symptoms have progressed to the breasts, ovaries, or testicles. The symptoms are worse after midnight.

CARBO VEG.: Used when the symptoms have progressed to the breasts, ovaries, or testicles. Other symptoms include chilliness, bluish skin, sluggishness, difficulty getting enough air, and lingering fever. Some digestive symptoms, such as gas and bloating, occasionally occur.

KALI BI.: Good for fleshy, light-complexioned children or those who have a thick, sticky, stringy nasal discharge accompanying the swollen glands.

REMEDY SUMMARY FOR MUMPS

See text for descriptions of other remedies that may be useful.
Give the medicine: Every 4 to 6 hours for up to 3 days.

When to try another medicine: If the symptoms haven't begun to improve after 2 days.

BELLADONNA ★

Essentials
- Illness begins suddenly
- Parotid glands hot and red

Confirmatory symptoms
- Child appears dazed, may be delirious
- Glowing redness of the face
- Shooting pains in the glands; burning in the throat

PHYTOLACCA

Essentials
- Very firm or rocklike swelling of affected salivary glands

Confirmatory symptoms
- Submaxillary glands involved
- Sensation of pressure or tension in the glands
- Pain shooting into the ear upon swallowing
- Pale face and skin

PULSATILLA

Essentials
- Especially useful during later stages of mumps, or when mumps involve the breasts, ovaries, or testicles
  or
- General symptoms of *Pulsatilla* are present (child is gentle, sensitive, weeps easily, craves affection, is thirstless, desires open air)

Confirmatory symptoms
- Dry mouth, thickly coated tongue

MERCURIUS

Essentials
- Foul taste on the tongue, foul breath, excessive salivation
- Increased and offensive perspiration, especially at night

Confirmatory symptoms
- Submaxillary glands involved

PILOCARPINUM

Essentials
- Alternative to *Belladonna* when no other remedy seems clearly indicated

Confirmatory symptoms
- Profuse sweat followed by great thirst, salivation, and general weakness

BEYOND HOME CARE

GET MEDICAL CARE IMMEDIATELY:

- if there are convulsions, stiffness of the neck, severe headache, or marked weakness.

GET MEDICAL CARE TODAY:

- if pain and swelling of the breast, ovaries, or testicles occur;
- if the child has difficulty hearing;
- if the patient has abdominal pains or begins vomiting.

SEE YOUR PRACTITIONER SOON:

- if you have any uncertainty about your child's illness;
- if your child has recurrent swelling of the parotid gland.

CHICKEN POX

Chicken pox is an infectious viral disease with an incubation period of ten to twenty-one days. It usually begins with a low-grade fever and a cold. Unlike the flat, barely raised spots typical of measles, chicken pox rashes are individual red spots that appear on the child's face, scalp, and torso. At first, these spots look like insect bites, but within hours they develop a small, clear blister in the center. These blisters eventually break and are replaced with a brownish scab. Sometimes the eruptions become infected with bacteria and develop into raw ulcers with pus. Consider your child contagious until all the pox have fully scabbed over.

Children experience chicken pox in different degrees of severity. Some children get only a few spots, and others are literally covered with them. Some may have intense itching; others barely complain. Most children fall somewhere in between these extreme cases. Infrequent complications of chicken pox include encephalitis and pneumonia. Reye's syndrome (see chapter 3 on fever and influenza) may follow chicken pox.

GENERAL HOME CARE

Bed rest is not required, but you should keep the child away from others since chicken pox is highly contagious. The child should be encouraged not to scratch at the eruptions, for this can cause infection and scarring. Trimming the fingernails is generally a good idea. When bathing children with chicken pox, pat them dry carefully to avoid breaking the blisters or disturbing the scabs. An oatmeal bath sometimes reduces some of the itching. Since a child's appetite is usually diminished during this illness, it is generally considered best to prepare small amounts of simple and nourishing foods.

Never give aspirin to a child with chicken pox. Aspirin is believed to help trigger Reye's syndrome, a life-threatening illness, in some children who have had chicken pox.

HOMEOPATHIC MEDICINES

Many homeopathic authorities have stated that *Rhus tox.* is the most effective medicine for people with chicken pox. British homeopath Margaret Tyler referred to it as "the only remedy required," and nineteenth-century American homeopath E. Harris Ruddock said *Rhus tox.* "should be given unless some other remedy is strongly indicated." Despite these declarations, other medicines also should be considered, since the exception to this valuable rule for chicken pox may be your child.

The *Rhus tox.* symptoms include intense itching that grows worse from scratching, at night, and at rest. The eruptions can be large and contain much pus. *Rhus tox.* children are very restless and often have great difficulty going to sleep and staying asleep.

Pulsatilla is indicated for children who have its general and mental characteristics. They weep easily but are not very irritable. They have little thirst despite the fever. They are worse in heat and at night, and are better in the open air.

The symptom that most clearly indicates *Antimonium tart.* is that the skin eruptions come out very slowly. In the classic case, each pock is quite large. Sometimes the rash is accompanied by a rattling cough and bronchitis.

Other medicines to consider for children with chicken pox include:

ANTIMONIUM CRUDUM: For both the physically and the emotionally irritable child who cries if washed, touched, or even looked at. Shooting pains occur when pressure is placed on the eruptions.

ARSENICUM: For large eruptions with much pus. The eruptions can become open sores. Burning pains accompany extreme chilliness. Pain and itching get worse just prior to and after midnight and in cold weather.

BELLADONNA: For chicken pox accompanied by severe headache, flushed face, hot skin, drowsiness, and inability to sleep.

MERCURIUS: For offensive and profuse sweat, and for large eruptions with much pus that sometimes become open sores. The lymph nodes in the neck may get swollen. Symptoms are worse at night and when the patient is hot or cold.

REMEDY SUMMARY FOR CHICKEN POX

See text for brief descriptions of other medicines that may be useful.

Give the medicine: Every 4 to 6 hours for up to 3 days.

When to try another medicine: If the symptoms haven't begun to improve after 2 days.

RHUS TOX. ★

Essentials
• Intense itching, worse from scratching, at night, and at rest

Confirmatory symptoms
• Child restless, unable to sleep
• Eruptions large, contain much pus

PULSATILLA

Essentials
• Child is gentle, sensitive, weeps easily, and craves affection

Confirmatory symptoms
- Little thirst, even with fever
- Child feels worse in warm rooms and at night, better in the open air

ANTIMONIUM TART.

Essentials
- Rash appears slowly

Confirmatory symptoms
- Large chicken pox blisters
- Rattling cough

BEYOND HOME CARE

GET MEDICAL CARE IMMEDIATELY:

- if there is severe headache, extreme weakness, convulsions, and stiffness of the neck;
- if there is any vomiting, or if respiration is rapid and shallow (Reye's syndrome must be ruled out);
- if spontaneous bruising or ruptured blood vessels appear under the skin.

GET MEDICAL CARE TODAY:

- if the skin eruptions become seriously infected;
- if an infant less than one year old gets chicken pox.

SEE YOUR PRACTITIONER SOON:

- if symptoms linger;
- if the child is breathing much more rapidly than normal.

Note: See also "Beyond Home Care" in chapter 4 on colds and coughs for more information.

CHAPTER 6

E A R A C H E S

E AR INFECTION IS the most common childhood illness other than simple runny nose. Almost every child has had at least one ear infection by the time he or she is six, and for many children and their parents, frequent recurrences of these infections is a major problem. Further, there's always the worry that the complications of ear infections can impair the child's hearing and even delay learning to speak. Adults sometimes get ear infections, too.

There are two main types of ear infections. Infection of the middle ear and eardrum is called otitis media. It is the more serious illness and is the type more often meant when a health professional diagnoses an ear infection. Otitis externa, as its name implies, is infection of the outer ear or of the canal that leads to the eardrum. It is actually a skin infection similar to those occurring elsewhere on the body, but it can cause a great deal of ear pain and discharge. We'll discuss each type of ear infection separately.

Not all earaches result from infections. During a cold, many people complain that their ears feel stopped up or that they experience twinges of sharp, brief pains. These symptoms are generally mild. They are due to pressure differences on either side of the eardrum caused by the inflammation and fluid secretion that accompany a cold. Pressure changes also account for earaches that happen in airplanes or in cars driving up or down a mountain. Some people get earaches whenever they are out in a cold wind or swim in cool water.

Otitis Media (Middle-Ear Infection)

The middle ear, the space behind the eardrum, becomes infected during an episode of otitis media. The eustachian tube leads from the middle ear forward and downward, connecting the middle ear to the cavity behind the nose. Normally, the tube opens to allow fluids secreted by mucous cells in the ear to drain into the throat, and to allow pressure in the middle ear to become equalized with the pressure of the atmosphere. At other times, the eustachian tube should be closed to prevent fluids in the nose, which are full of microorganisms, from reaching the middle ear.

Ear infections develop when the eustachian tube opens and closes improperly, allowing germ-laden fluids from the nose and throat to enter but not depart from the middle ear. Inflammation resulting from a cold or allergy may cause this improper function, but in young children sometimes the tube is just too small and short to work properly.

As a middle-ear infection progresses, white blood cells and antibodies are secreted into the tissues and the middle-ear area, where they attack and kill infecting bacteria. As dead bacteria and white blood cells accumulate, pus forms and puts pressure on the eardrum. The thin eardrum membrane bulges outward, and pain increases as it is stretched. Eventually it may tear, allowing pus to drain to the external auditory canal. Don't be alarmed if this happens (you'll see pus or blood dripping out of the ear)—this is the way the body expels the infected material, and a torn eardrum usually heals rapidly.

The symptoms of acute middle-ear infection are variable. A young child may seem to be in pain, often playing with or pulling at the ears. Older children or adults usually know if something is wrong with the ear, but sometimes even during a severe infection the ear just feels stuffed up. If the eardrum is ruptured, a discharge from the ear may be obvious, or the hair around the affected ear may be sticky or crusty.

Many children with recurrent ear infections have their own characteristic symptom patterns that parents learn to recognize early in the illness. Unusual irritability, emotional sensitivity, or clinginess may accompany ear infection, and sometimes a child's mood changes are the only evidence of the problem. There may be a high fever, but ear infections often occur without any fever at all. Sometimes the child vomits or has diarrhea because of an ear infection, with no sign that something is wrong with the ears. In most cases, if nothing else is responsible, these digestive symptoms clear up rapidly.

The diagnosis of an ear infection depends on accurate visual examination of the eardrum performed with an otoscope, a magnifying lens and light that illuminates the drum and external canal through a small speculum that fits into the canal. A normal eardrum has a pearly gray, slightly shiny appearance, and looks delicate and translucent. During an infection the most characteristic change is outward bulging of the eardrum from the buildup of pus inside. The eardrum becomes thickened and more opaque and often looks quite red. Redness of the drum, however, may be caused by fever, crying, or cold, and a diagnosis of otitis media should never be made on the basis of a red eardrum alone.

Traditionally, physicians have held that antibiotics effectively treat ear infections and prevent complications. However, many scientific studies over the past twenty-five years contradict such beliefs. In one large study of children with acute otitis media, those treated with antibiotics actually recovered at a slightly slower rate than those who were not.[1] Another found that children with chronic otitis maintained on prophylactic (preventative) antibiotics were two to six times more likely to have recurrent acute infections than those on placebos.[2] Recently, John Bailar, M.D., a Harvard professor and editorial board member at the *New England Journal of Medicine,* comprehensively reviewed the scientific literature on the treatment of otitis with antibiotics. He concluded that the available research "seems to demolish the conclusion that antibiotics improve the outcome [in otitis media]."[3]

In any case, be watchful if otitis media is diagnosed. Serious acute complications of middle-ear infection are rare but do occur. These include mastoiditis, infection of the bony area just behind the ear. Be alert for any redness, tenderness, pain, or swelling in this area, and report these symptoms immediately to your health practitioner. Mastoiditis can become a chronic problem and result in hearing loss and erosion of the bone.

Meningitis and other infections of the central nervous system may result from acute otitis media if the infection spreads through the bloodstream to bony structures. Symptoms of these problems include severe or persistent headache, stiff neck, persistent vomiting, and marked change in mood or alertness.

1. J. Froom, et al., "Diagnosis and Antibiotic Treatment of Acute Otitis Media: Report from the International Primary Care Network," *British Medical Journal* 300 (1990): 582–86.

2. E. I. Cantekin, T. W. McGuire, and T. L. Griffith, "Antimicrobial Therapy for Otitis Media with Effusion (Secretory Otitis Media)," *Journal of the American Medical Association* 266 (23): 3309–17.

3. J. Bailar, "The Practice of Meta-Analysis," *Clinical Epidemiology* 48 (1995): 149–57.

The most common complications of middle-ear infections are the chronic ear problems that often follow. Serous otitis media, accumulation of a translucent noninfectious fluid in the middle ear, interferes with normal motion of the eardrum and the tiny middle-ear bones so that hearing is reduced. Homeopathic constitutional treatment often is effective with chronic serous otitis. Antihistamines and decongestants are worthless, though they are often prescribed. Conventional treatment for persistent hearing loss due to serous otitis involves surgical insertion of polyethylene tubes into the eardrum to allow drainage of middle-ear fluid. These tubes seem to improve treated ears' hearing for a few months, and this may be very important to the child who is at a crucial stage of language development. Research has shown, however, that there is no long-term improvement in hearing when tubes are inserted, and eardrums in which tubes have been placed tend to become scarred. We believe that the tubes should be inserted for serous otitis only when there is a significant, documented hearing problem, when the risks of the surgery are clearly understood, and when the goal of treatment is improved hearing within a short period.

GENERAL HOME CARE

General recommendations for any infectious illness apply to people with acute middle-ear infections; they should rest, have plenty of liquids, and be comforted. A heating pad or hot washcloth applied to the ear may help reduce pain.

To help prevent ear infection, avoid nursing or bottle-feeding children when they are in a lying position; gravity may allow milk or juice to run into the eustachian tubes, encouraging infection. Allergies may predispose an individual to ear infection by causing inflammation and fluid buildup; identification of the substances that trigger allergic reactions for that person can be helpful.

BEYOND HOME CARE

See "Beyond Home Care" following "Otitis Externa."

OTITIS EXTERNA (OUTER-EAR INFECTION)

Outer-ear infections essentially are skin infections involving the canal that leads from the outer ear to the eardrum. The symptoms of external-ear infections often include much ear pain and throbbing due to inflammation. The pain is characteristically aggravated by moving the outer ear, so a helpful way to differentiate between middle-ear and external-ear infections is to pull on the earlobe. Both types of ear infections can be present at the same time, so you still should use the guidelines in "Beyond Home Care" to decide if medical consultation is needed. Often the ear canal is quite itchy during an external ear infection. If you look into the canal, you can see that it is red and scaly or wet, and a thick discharge may be present. Usually there is no fever or general symptoms of illness.

External-ear infections do not endanger the organs of hearing, although the discharge and swelling may reduce hearing for a time. As with all skin infections, there is some small danger that the infection will spread aggressively. Rapidly spreading redness or swelling of the outer ear or nearby skin is a danger sign, as is onset of fever.

GENERAL HOME CARE

Gently wash out the accumulated scaling and discharge by placing a piece of cotton soaked in dilute vinegar (half water/half vinegar) or Burow's solution (available at drugstores) in the ear canal, leaving it there for eight to twelve hours. Make sure you can pull out the cotton easily. Then briefly rinse the canal with warm water, using a bulb syringe. Let the ear drain after this, but put in a drop or two of the vinegar solution every eight hours or so.

CASETAKING QUESTIONS FOR EARACHES

Character of the symptoms:
- Does the pain extend into the throat, neck, or behind the ear?
- Describe the color and consistency of any discharge from the ear.

Modalities:
- At which time of day is the pain worse?
- Is the ear tender or sensitive to touch?
- How do heat and cold affect the pain?
- How is the pain affected by stooping or bending over, motion in general, and lying down? Does it help to lie on the affected ear?
- Does swallowing make the pain worse?

Other symptoms:
- What is the color and consistency of any nasal discharge?
- Is perspiration or salivation increased?

Note: See the appropriate chapters if the earache is accompanied by runny nose, cough, sore throat, or any other symptoms.

HOMEOPATHIC MEDICINES FOR ALL EARACHES

These descriptions apply to children with ear infections, but the indications for adults are the same. Most of the descriptions of physical-exam findings (color and shape of the eardrum) apply to otitis media, but all the other symptoms are applicable to those with both middle-ear infections and otitis externa. You can use these descriptions also to treat the person with an earache resulting from something other than infection.

Many of these medicines share similar symptoms. For example, *Silica, Hepar sulph.,* and *Mercurius* all are equally indicated by the presence of painfully swollen lymph nodes in the head and neck that commonly occur with ear infections. If no medicine is strongly indicated, start with either *Pulsatilla,* if the child is more clingy than usual, or *Hepar,* if the child is somewhat irritable or severe pain is the predominant feature of the illness.

Belladonna is the most commonly indicated homeopathic medicine during the early stages of an ear infection or earache, especially when the illness begins suddenly with few prior cold symptoms. Within an hour or two, the child is in intense pain. He may have had a watery runny nose for a short while, but the mucus isn't cloudy, colored, or thick. The outer ear, ear canal, or eardrum may be bright red, but pus hasn't formed and the eardrum is still normally shaped. A sudden high fever (see the description of *Belladonna* fevers in chapter 3) often begins about the same time as the earache. The ear pain may extend down into the neck, and there may be associated sore-throat or facial pain.

Ferrum phos. is used in much the same way as *Belladonna,* in the early stages of suddenly occurring earaches not yet accompanied by pus formation. The onset is not quite as sudden, the fever is not so high, and the overall condition of the child is a little less intense. You can give *Ferrum phos.* also if you've already tried *Belladonna* and it still seems indicated, but hasn't worked.

Chamomilla is indicated chiefly by the effects of the illness on the child's mood, and less so by particular symptoms. Children for whom

Chamomilla is indicated are extremely irritable. They scream and cry angrily, do not want to be touched, and can't be comforted. They may ask for things which they then reject, and they are likely to hit you for crossing them at all or for no apparent reason. Sometimes the child can be calmed by being carried. The earache generally doesn't come on as quickly as in the *Belladonna* case, but the pain is severe and the child may scream. The symptoms may be made worse by stooping or bending over, and improved by warmth or being wrapped in warm covers. A discharge from the ear is less typical of *Chamomilla* than of other medicines discussed later. Usually there is a watery runny nose and, less often, a very thick discharge. As with *Belladonna,* the nasal mucus usually is not colored. Whatever the particular symptoms, though, be sure to consider *Chamomilla* for the child who is in severe pain, especially if he is extremely irritable.

Another commonly effective medicine is *Pulsatilla.* In contrast to *Chamomilla,* it is indicated for children who are sweet, placid, loving, and mild during the earache. The *Pulsatilla* child may be irritable, but the irritability is weak and whiny, not violent as is the *Chamomilla* or *Hepar* child. *Pulsatilla* children want to be held and cuddled and are comforted when given affection. They too may scream with the pain but are just as likely to weep piteously. *Pulsatilla* is more frequently indicated for ear infections that develop after cold symptoms have been persistent for a few days. The nasal discharge has become thick and yellow to green in color. Though pain may be fairly severe, sometimes there seems to be no pain at all. Examination often shows a red, swollen eardrum and a buildup of pus in the middle ear. A thick yellow-green discharge may be seen at the external canal. The pain is typically worse at night and in a warm room. There may be a sensation of pressure in the ear. The child may or may not be feverish, but tends to feel uncomfortably warm and wants fresh air. She is noticeably less thirsty than usual, even with a high fever. In any case, the strongest indication for *Pulsatilla* is the characteristic mildness and clinginess of the child.

Silica also is indicated for the middle and later stages of a cold accompanied by an ear infection. The child who needs *Silica* also is mild and whimpering, but is less loving and less interested in affection than the *Pulsatilla* child. Also characteristic of children for whom *Silica* is indicated are marked physical weakness and tiredness. The illness seems really to have worn them out. They are definitely chilly and want warm covering. They may have sweat about the head or on the hands or feet. If there is pain in the ear, it may be intense, but usually not as severe as the pain of some of the other medicines. It tends to occur at night and is made worse by cold applications, moving, sitting for a long time, and noise. *Silica* is the remedy most prominently indicated for pain behind the ear in the region of the mastoid, though many other medicines also cover this complaint. There may be itching in the ear (also symptoms of *Hepar sulph.* and *Mercurius*) or a stopped-up sensation. The examination may show inflammation and pus formation, and there may be drainage of pus or watery fluid from the ear. A nasal discharge, of any character, often accompanies the infection.

The physical symptoms indicating *Hepar sulph.* are similar to those of *Silica* but more intense. Again, this is a remedy best given during the middle and late stages of colds and ear infections, when a thick, colored nasal discharge often precedes or accompanies the earache and when inflammation in the middle ear has progressed to the point that pus has formed. You should think of *Hepar* when the child is intensely, even violently, irritable about everything. Although this emotional state is similar to that described for *Chamomilla,* the child is a little less expressive, is less prone to scream constantly or hit, doesn't have such a strong aversion to being held, and is less likely to throw away things she asked for. But the *Hepar* child lets you know, in no uncertain terms, that she is angry. *Hepar* is indicated for children who are very chilly—cold air or coldness of any sort makes them uncomfortable and provokes symptoms. The child wants the heat turned up, and she wants lots of blankets. The earache is usually severe and is worse at night. It is made worse also by cold air, open air, and cold applications, and is improved by warmth and bundling up.

Mercurius also is indicated for earaches after pus formation has occurred. The child needing *Mercurius* is somewhat irritable and may act impulsively or hastily, or he may be less alert than normal. He may be generally bothered by heat or cold or both, but this particular earache is typically made worse by warmth, especially the warmth of the bed. Pain is worse at night. Characteristic *Mercurius* symptoms also include profuse and offensive perspiration, head sweats, increased salivation, bad breath, puffiness of the tongue, and trembling or twitching.

REMEDY SUMMARY FOR EARACHES

Give the medicine: Every 3 to 6 hours for 2 to 3 days, stopping when there is definite improvement; repeat when symptoms begin to get worse again, or if no further improvement has occurred after 12 hours.

When to try another medicine: If there is no significant improvement after 12 to 24 hours.

BELLADONNA ★

Essentials
- Earache begins suddenly with intense pain and few prior symptoms of a cold (no thick or colored nasal discharge)

Confirmatory symptoms
- Bright-red outer ear, ear canal, or eardrum without pus formation
- Accompanied by sudden high fever (see chapter 3)
- Ear pain extends down into the neck, or accompanied by sore throat or facial pain

FERRUM PHOS.

Essentials
- Early stages of earaches before pus has formed; symptoms similar to *Belladonna* but not as sudden or severe
- Give if *Belladonna* seems indicated but hasn't helped

HEPAR SULPH. ★

Essentials
- Sharp, severe earache
- Earache accompanied by thick, colored discharge from nose or ears
- Irritability

Confirmatory symptoms
- Chilliness and aversion to the cold or uncovering; desire for warmth
- Earache worse in cold, open air, from cold applications, or at night; better from warmth

PULSATILLA ★

Essentials
- Mild disposition; craves affection and physical contact
- Yellow to green thick discharge from the nose or ears

Confirmatory symptoms
- Ear pain worse at night and in a warm room
- Worse in general from warmth; wants fresh air
- Little or no thirst

CHAMOMILLA

Essentials
- Extreme irritability; child screams and cries angrily, doesn't want to be touched or comforted, and may strike out
- Severe ear pain

Confirmatory symptoms
- Child calms down when carried
- Earaches during teething
- Symptoms worse when stooping or bending over, and improved by warmth or being wrapped in warm covers
- Clear nasal discharge, usually of watery consistency

MERCURIUS

Essentials
- Another common earache remedy after pus has formed in the middle ear

Confirmatory symptoms
- Earache worse from warmth and at night
- Profuse, bad-smelling perspiration; head sweats
- Increased salivation, bad breath, puffiness of the tongue
- Symptoms worse when stooping or bending over, and improved by warmth or being wrapped in warm covers

SILICA

Essentials
- Later stages of an earache
- Physical weakness and tiredness
- Chilliness, desire for warm covering

Confirmatory symptoms
- Mild and whimpering disposition, but less interested in affection than the *Pulsatilla* patient

- Pain behind the ear in the region of the mastoid
- Sweating about the head or on the hands or feet

BEYOND HOME CARE

GET MEDICAL CARE IMMEDIATELY:

- if earache is accompanied by severe weakness, loss of alertness, severe headache, or stiffness of the neck.

GET MEDICAL CARE TODAY:

- if a baby begins to pull or rub her ears;
- for any definite earache or any ear discharge in a child under 7 years old;
- for anyone with severe earache, especially if it's accompanied by fever or ear discharge;
- if there is tenderness or redness in the bony area behind the ear;
- if there is sudden, significant decrease in hearing, with or without pain.

SEE YOUR PRACTITIONER SOON:

- if an older child or adult has had mild ear pain or discharge lasting longer than 1 or 2 weeks;
- if mild hearing loss lasts longer than 2 weeks

CHAPTER 7

SORE THROATS

A SORE THROAT MAY be the sign of a viral or bacterial infection, but just as commonly it results from a postnasal drip or simply from dryness of the throat. Most sore throats, even when they result from infections, are self-limited symptoms that the body can heal on its own. Medical practitioners use laboratory tests to determine whether the *Streptococcus* bacteria is involved. The most accurate test is still a throat culture, but you must wait up to two days for the results. In many offices, swab tests that give almost instant results are used instead. Usually, no attempt to identify other germs other than strep is made.

NONINFECTIOUS SORE THROATS

Mucus trickling down the back of the nose and into the throat often causes enough irritation to produce pain. Postnasal drip can be a problem for those with acute colds or acute attacks of allergies like hay fever or reactions to cat fur. It can trouble also those who have chronic nasal congestion due to allergy. People with acute symptoms can be treated at home according to the guidelines in chapters 4 and 12 on colds and allergies, but those with chronic or recurrent symptoms should be treated by a professional homeopath.

Sore throats commonly are also the result of dryness caused by open-mouthed breathing or artificially heated air.

VIRAL AND NON-STREP BACTERIAL INFECTIONS OF THE THROAT

A substantial number of infectious sore throats are precipitated by the same viruses that cause the common cold. Bacteria other than *Streptococcus* also are frequently involved in sore throats. Symptoms accompanying viral or non-strep bacterial throat infections are various. Pain may be minimal or intense; fever, swollen lymph nodes, and pus in the throat may or may not be present. Cold symptoms often occur.

Less commonly, other germs infect the throat with more severe symptoms. Both herpangina and true herpes viral throat infections may cause marked general symptoms and small blisters or sores on the throat tissues. Mononucleosis, another viral infection, may cause severe sore throats. We discuss mononucleosis in more detail later in this chapter. Gonorrhea, covered in the chapters on women's and men's health concerns, also can infect the throat.

Most sore throats that result from infections caused by viruses or non-strep bacteria are not very serious. They clear up on their own, though the patient with mononucleosis may be sick for quite a while. Other kinds of bacteria that infect the throat produce self-limited illnesses and rarely lead to serious complications.

Conventional medicine offers no treatment for viral infections associated with sore throat—antibiotics are useless and can be risky. At this time there are no simple tests to detect non-strep bacterial sore throats (with the exception of gonorrhea). Since such infections don't cause serious problems, and since they clear up by themselves, antibiotic treatment is unnecessary.

STREP THROAT

"Strep" refers to a particular type of bacteria, the group A beta-hemolytic *Streptococcus*. Although a person with a strep throat is often sicker and has a higher fever and more pain than one with a viral sore throat, the disease itself is not serious; the symptoms clear up within a few days. Cold symptoms and coughs are less likely to accompany a strep throat than a viral sore throat. Scarlet fever may occur, but this is simply strep throat accompanied by a rash, and the treatment of a person with scarlet fever is no different from one with simple strep throat.

The main reason for the concern about strep throats is that they can—only rarely—lead to serious illnesses, including kidney inflammation and rheumatic fever. The person with a kidney disease resulting from a prior strep infection becomes quite ill, but usually recovers without any permanent ill effects. On the other hand, rheumatic fever can lead to permanent heart damage to one or more of the valves of the heart. Rheumatic fever has become quite rare, but still it is important to take it seriously.

Rheumatic fever can be prevented if all the strep germs are killed within the first ten to twelve days of the infection. Often, the body's own defenses have eradicated the strep within that time. Still, to be safe and to prevent the spread of the infection to others, when the lab test is positive for strep infection, pediatric authorities recommend that children with strep throat receive penicillin or another appropriate antibiotic treatment. In order to prevent rheumatic fever, antibiotic treatment must be begun within the first week or so after the symptoms begin.

Antibiotics also relieve discomfort and shorten the course of the symptoms, especially when treatment is begun during the first day or two of the illness. However, this period often has passed by the time a strep infection is diagnosed. Also, various studies have shown that even the proper use of orally administered penicillin fails to eradicate strep bacteria in up to 30 percent of those treated.

Taking these complexities into account, you should start with homeopathic treatment. Homeopathy often is very effective in helping the person with strep heal the illness. And if you do decide to use antibiotics, there's nothing wrong with continuing the homeopathic treatment concurrently.

Regarding the use of antibiotics, sometimes the decision is easy. Any child with a family history of rheumatic fever definitely should receive antibiotics. People of any age who have already had rheumatic fever must take antibiotics preventively from the onset of any significant sore throat, even before the type of infection is known.

If there is no history of rheumatic fever, the choice can be a little more difficult. On balance, we feel it's reasonable to forego antibiotics even for children, since rheumatic fever is so rare today. But because these rare cases do occur mainly in kids, we wouldn't argue with a decision to opt for antibiotics. Adults in generally good health need not take antibiotics, but might consider doing so if they will be exposing others to the disease.

MONONUCLEOSIS

"Mono" is a viral infection of the whole system and is most common in people ten to thirty-five years old. Symptoms often include a very painful sore throat, red swollen tonsils (sometimes spotted with white material), exhaustion, aches, and fever. The lymph nodes, especially in the neck, are always swollen. Mono is like the flu, but mono lasts longer than the flu, and the sore throat is worse. Mono also may be accompanied by cough, hepatitis (liver inflammation), swelling of the spleen, or symptoms affecting the nervous system. A blood test is required to confirm mono. Mono has no orthodox medical treatment, and it usually resolves itself in two to four weeks, though it may last up to three months. Homeopathic treatment may reduce the length of the illness.

EPIGLOTTITIS

The epiglottis is the flap of tissue that covers the entrance to the larynx; when one swallows, it prevents food from getting into the tube leading to the lungs. Rarely, the epiglottis becomes infected by bacteria, resulting in a serious medical emergency, since swelling of the epiglottis may totally block the windpipe. The symptoms—severe sore throat, sense of constriction, and marked fever—begin suddenly. As the swelling worsens, swallowing becomes so difficult that drooling occurs. Struggling to breathe, the patient often sits leaning forward and open-mouthed. Epiglottitis occurs most often in children under six, but older children and adults also can get it. It requires immediate emergency treatment in a hospital.

GENERAL HOME CARE

Sore throats caused or aggravated by dryness are often relieved simply by reducing room heat, running a humidifier, and remembering to take frequent sips of liquid. Gargling with warm salt water, lemon juice and honey in warm water, or dilute apple cider vinegar temporarily relieves sore throat pain. Throat lozenges may help, too. Sucking on a 100 mg or 500 mg tablet of vitamin C may be soothing, but be careful not to irritate the tongue or throat. If you are being treated with homeopathic medicine, however, do not take lozenges containing menthol or eucalyptus, since these substances may interfere with the action of the medicine.

Home treatment for mononucleosis is the same as for other sore throats or for flus. Vigorous activity must be avoided, since the spleen is vulnerable to rupture.

CASETAKING QUESTIONS FOR SORE THROATS

Character of the symptoms:
- How would you describe the throat pain (for example, raw, burning, or stinging)?
- What other sensations are present? Does the throat feel swollen, or do you feel as though there is a splinter or a lump in the throat?
- On which side, if any, is the pain worse? Did it start on one side and move to the other?
- Are there patches of white material or pus on the tonsils or throat?
- Does the pain extend to the ear?
- Is the external throat sensitive to touch?

Modalities:
- How does swallowing warm or cold drinks affect the pain? How is the pain affected by empty swallowing or swallowing only saliva?
- Is the pain affected by warm or cold weather or rooms?
- Is the pain worse at a particular time of day?

Associated symptoms:
- How does the tongue look—is it red with raised "bumps" or coated yellow? Is the tongue painful?
- Is salivation increased? If drooling isn't obvious, check if the pillow is wet or if the mouth simply feels full of saliva.

HOMEOPATHIC MEDICINES

When a person has a sore throat, *Belladonna* is the first medicine to think of. During the first twenty-four hours, if the pain has come on suddenly, particularly if it is accompanied by fever and flushed skin, *Belladonna* is the likely medicine. The throat is very red and may be quite swollen, but little or no pus is evident. The tongue may have a "strawberry" appearance, as with scarlet fever. Swallowing, especially liquids, makes the throat pain worse, and the patient may have an aversion to drinking. There also may be a great sense of dryness in the throat.

Consider *Aconite* when the sore throat is accompanied by high fever, and thirst comes on suddenly (the *Belladonna* patient is not so thirsty and may actually be averse to liquids). The condition may have begun after exposure to cold or drafts. *Aconite's* other characteristic mental symptoms may be present (see the *materia medica* section).

Arsenicum should be considered when the general symptoms of the medicine are evident: chilliness even during fever, thirst, and restlessness combined with fatigue. Most typically, the throat pain is burning in character. Warm drinks relieve the pain, whereas swallowing, cold drinks, or exposure to the cold make it worse.

The *Rhus tox.* person has a painfully sore throat that is made better by warm drinks and warmth in general. The pain in the throat is usually worse in the morning. The pain often begins after straining the throat while speaking or singing or after exposure to cold, wet weather. Sometimes the pain is worse when first swallowing but gets better after repeated swallowing. The *Rhus tox.* patient is very restless but is less tired and more achy than the *Arsenicum* patient. He may be anxious, irritable, and weepy.

Lycopodium sore throats are typically worse on the right side or begin on the right side and spread to the left. The pain may be relieved by either warm or cold drinks, whereas being in cold air may make it worse. There may be pain extending up into the ears. In general, the illness doesn't begin particularly suddenly, and usually the patient isn't terribly sick. She typically wants fresh air. The symptoms in general, sometimes including the sore throat, may be worse in the late afternoon, between 4 and 8 P.M. in classic cases.

When the sore throat is severe and is accompanied by fever and weakness, *Mercurius* may be indicated. The throat is red and swollen, and pus or other white or yellow material may be seen on the tonsils or walls of the throat. Generally the *Mercurius* patient can be sensitive to both heat and cold. Becoming cold aggravates the throat pain, but a warm bed also may make it worse. Liquids of any temperature aren't known to influence the symptoms particularly. The sore throat tends to be more painful at night. A classic *Mercurius* sore throat symptom is the tendency to salivate and drool. The pillow may be wet, or more frequent swallowing may be noticeable. The tongue often looks or feels swollen or puffy, and at times the teeth make imprints on the tongue. The breath may smell bad. There may be cold symptoms such as thick greenish or yellow mucus draining from the nose.

Hepar sulph. is similar to *Mercurius* in severity of infection. Pus has formed, and the throat and tonsils are very swollen. Often the person says he feels something stuck in his throat like a splinter (*Lachesis* and *Apis* also may have this symptom, though less characteristically). The patient is irritable and easily angered. Chilliness is a predominant symptom, and both the general condition and the sore throat are definitely aggravated by exposure to cold. Warm drinks and warmth in general soothe the sore throat. The pain may extend to the ears.

Lachesis is particularly useful when the throat pain is worse on the left side or begins there and spreads to the right. Drinking, especially drinking warm liquids, makes the pain worse (sometimes cold drinks bring some relief). Swallowing can be difficult, with solid foods being harder to swallow than liquids. Typically the symptoms are made worse from warmth in general, and the pain often is worse in the morning, especially upon waking, and during the day. The throat is sensitive to touch, and clothing around the neck may cause pain or a choking sensation. A sensation of swelling in the throat is a strong symptom of *Lachesis* (as well as *Hepar, Rhus tox.,* and *Sulphur*).

When the pain of a sore throat is stinging in character, *Apis* may be the medicine, particularly if the pain is made better from cold drinks or a cool environment, and worse from warm drinks or warmth. The throat, tonsils, and tongue are swollen and characteristically appear as though they are filled with water. Absence of thirst is typical.

Phytolacca should be given when there is much aching in the body along with the fever, and when the sore throat is worse from warm drinks. The appearance of the throat may be dark red or even purplish or bluish, and the glands are swollen. The pain may shoot up to the ears, particularly during swallowing. People who need *Phytolacca* tend to have an incessant desire to swallow, despite the fact that it is painful to do so. They are cold and like to be covered, but still they may feel chilly. Their body aches may cause them to be restless, but these pains are worse during motion. One rare but distinctive feature of people who need *Phytolacca* is an acute pain felt at the base of the tongue when protruded.

Sulphur should be considered when a sore throat lingers or when the indicated medicine is not working, as long as some of the general and particular symptoms of *Sulphur* match the person's own. There is much burning pain in the throat, with dryness of the mucous membranes, diminished appetite, and increased thirst. Despite the burning, the pain is better when the patient drinks warm liquids. The pain in the throat also can be stitching, pressing, or cutting. A sensation like a lump, splinter, or hair in the throat may be felt. The general symptoms of *Sulphur*—particularly discomfort from warmth; general lethargy; and offensive breath, sweat, and discharges—are important for determining when to use it.

REMEDY SUMMARY FOR SORE THROATS

Give the medicine: Every 6 to 8 hours for 2 to 3 days, stopping when there is definite improvement.

When to try another medicine: If there is no significant improvement after 24 hours.

Note: All medicines below cover swollen lymph nodes in the neck and scarlet fever rash.

BELLADONNA ★

Essentials
- During the first 24 hours when the pain has come on suddenly and is accompanied by fever and flushed skin
- Redness of the throat or tonsils, often with swelling, but no pus is present

Confirmatory symptoms
- "Strawberry" appearance of the tongue, as with scarlet fever
- Throat pain worse from swallowing, especially liquids
- Sensation of dryness in the throat

PHYTOLACCA ★

Essentials
- Sore throat with body aches and fever
- Throat appears dark red or even purplish or bluish
- Pain worse from warm drinks

Confirmatory symptoms
- Pain shooting up to the ears during swallowing
- Incessant desire to swallow
- Chilliness
- Pain at the base of the tongue when protruded

MERCURIUS

Essentials
- Pus or white/yellow material in the throat
- Excessive salivation, drooling

Confirmatory symptoms
- Sensitivity to both heat and cold
- Throat pain worse at night
- Thirst
- Swollen or puffy tongue, bad breath

LYCOPODIUM

Essentials
- Sore throat worse on the right side or beginning on the right and spreading to the left
- Pain relieved by warm drinks and warm food (see text)

Confirmatory symptoms
- Feels worse in general in the late afternoon, between 4 and 8 P.M.

LACHESIS

Essentials
- Pain worse on the left side or spreading from left to right
- Pain worse from drinking liquids

Confirmatory symptoms
- Sore throat worse in the morning, especially on waking
- Throat sensitive to touch; clothing around the neck causes discomfort or choking sensation
- Person feels worse in general from warmth

HEPAR SULPH.

Essentials
- Pus has formed, and the throat and tonsils are very swollen
- Irritability
- Chills

Confirmatory symptoms
- Sensation of a splinter or something stuck in the throat
- Throat pain worse from cold and better from warm drinks and external warmth

ARSENICUM

Essentials
- Sore throat accompanied by chilliness, thirst, and restlessness combined with fatigue
- Throat pain relieved by warm drinks

Confirmatory symptoms
- Throat pain burning in character
- Pain worse from swallowing in general, cold drinks, or exposure to the cold

RHUS TOX.

Essentials
- Throat pain better from warm drinks and warmth in general
- Restlessness

Confirmatory symptoms
- Symptoms begin after straining the voice or exposure to cold, wet weather
- Thirsty for sips of water
- Dry mouth, dry sore throat
- Aches and pains while lying still; worse when first starting to move but get better with continued motion

APIS

Essentials
- Stinging sore throat pain
- Marked swelling of the throat or tonsils

Confirmatory symptoms
- Throat pain better from cold drinks and worse from warm drinks and external heat
- Swollen parts of the throat appear as though filled with water
- Absence of thirst

SULPHUR

Essentials

- Lingering sore throats
- One or more of the following general symptoms: discomfort from warmth; general lethargy; and offensive breath, sweat, and discharges

Confirmatory symptoms

- Burning throat pain with dryness of the mucous membranes; better from drinking warm liquids
- Sensation of a lump, splinter, or hair in the throat

BEYOND HOME CARE

GET MEDICAL CARE IMMEDIATELY:

- if there is a severe sore throat and great difficulty swallowing, or if there is much drooling or difficulty breathing.

GET MEDICAL CARE TODAY:

- if there is swelling of the region around the tonsils to the extent that it is bulging or pushing the uvula to one side;
- if a sore throat is accompanied by a fever and a red rash that feels like sandpaper;
- if a child has a significant sore throat, or a sore throat and fever, for more than a day or two (adults can wait safely a few days longer);
- if there is white or yellowish material on the tonsils or throat;
- if a person who previously had rheumatic fever gets a sore throat.

CHAPTER 8

DIGESTIVE PROBLEMS

FOR MANY PEOPLE, the gastrointestinal tract is the first system of the body to develop symptoms when stress levels rise. Many less serious digestive conditions can be cared for at home with homeopathic medicine or other home treatment measures. These include the common causes of vomiting, diarrhea, and abdominal pain. Appropriate homeopathic medicines for all of these conditions are listed together. Vomiting and diarrhea are the more common causes of dehydration, although it can occur during any acute illness. Therefore, we include a section on the prevention and recognition of dehydration in this chapter. We have a few comments about the frequently troublesome indigestion and constipation complaints, for which we think simple home-care measures usually suffice.

Along with playing many other physiological roles, the liver is an important digestive organ. Hepatitis, acute liver disease, always requires professional medical attention, but still you may want to use home treatment with homeopathic medicines to speed the healing process. We also cover the homeopathic treatment of hemorrhoids and motion sickness in this chapter.

GASTROENTERITIS AND OTHER CAUSES
OF VOMITING AND DIARRHEA

Often called stomach flu, acute gastroenteritis is the generic medical term for the common infectious illness of the gastrointestinal tract. The symptoms include some combination of vomiting, diarrhea, and abdominal cramping. Acute gastroenteritis is usually virus related, but you can contract bacterial gastroenteritis also by eating spoiled food (food poisoning). Both types of gastroenteritis are short-term, self-limited illnesses that get better once the body neutralizes the infecting germs or bacterial toxins. They can, however, make you feel very sick, often with fever and general achiness in addition to the digestive symptoms.

The main risk with these illnesses is that prolonged vomiting or diarrhea may exhaust reserves of body fluid before healing takes place. Children and especially babies are at much greater risk of serious fluid loss than adults. Today worldwide, more infant deaths result from dehydration caused by diarrhea than from any other condition.

The chief digestive symptoms of gastroenteritis—vomiting and diarrhea—can be caused by other conditions as well. Some of these can be treated at home, but others require medical assistance.

VOMITING

Although it is decidedly an uncomfortable experience, vomiting is an important and effective defense mechanism. It allows the body to rid itself of poisons and germs, and it can remove food that the gastrointestinal tract is not digesting and absorbing properly. Nausea usually precedes vomiting and serves as a useful warning that all is not well with the digestive system and that eating would not be a good idea.

The most common cause of vomiting in any age group is gastroenteritis. Vomiting, especially children's, may be caused also by infection elsewhere in the body. Conditions like ear infections, colds and flus, urinary infections, and more serious illnesses all can lead to vomiting, sometimes before the symptoms of the "real" illness are apparent. Usually vomiting associated with other infections is mild and happens only once or twice, but if the vomiting itself requires treatment, the advice in the "General Home Care" section should be followed. Homeopathic treatment should be based on the overall symptom picture no matter what the name of the disease. If a cold or ear infection is accompanied by significant vomiting, try to find the one remedy that best covers all of the person's symptoms.

Children vomit easily. Their digestive tracts generally are more sensitive than adults'. Psychological upset as well as eating too much food or too many sweets may make a child vomit once or twice, whereas an adult might just feel queasy.

Many babies spit up frequently after nursing or bottle-feeding. The milk comes up because the muscular valve that should close off the bottom of the esophagus is not yet fully developed. Babies can spit up what seems to be quite a lot of their food and still grow and gain weight adequately. So long as the vomited material is simply burped up and doesn't come up forcefully, and so long as the child seems comfortable and is gaining enough weight, there is no cause for concern; the condition eventually corrects itself.

Other uncommon conditions associated with vomiting in both children and adults may be serious or even life-threatening. We will indicate these in "Beyond Home Care."

DIARRHEA

Diarrhea is defined as an increase in both the frequency and looseness of stools. Frequency is important because even a very loose bowel movement is of little immediate significance if it occurs only once or twice a day. Diarrhea, like vomiting, is another way the body can quickly eliminate germs, toxins, and irritants from the gastrointestinal tract. When the intestinal linings are infected, or when poisons or irritants are present, absorption of fluids and nutrients is reduced, and the muscular walls of the intestine contract more vigorously and more rapidly. The result that you are aware of is a loose or liquid stool, but the body has accomplished the disposal of harmful materials.

Acute diarrhea, like vomiting, occurs more often with gastroenteritis or along with other infectious illnesses such as ear infection or flu; again, this is more common in children. The main concern with diarrhea caused by these conditions is excessive loss of body fluids, especially in children (see the following section on dehydration for more information about this problem). Otherwise, home treatment and careful observation usually are all that's necessary.

Breast-fed babies normally have very loose stools as frequently as eight times a day or so. Once the child is fed formulas or solids, the stools generally get firmer and come less often. Children have more sensitive digestive tracts than adults, and may have diarrhea after fairly minor psychological or dietary upsets. No treatment other than avoidance of irritating foods and relief of stress is necessary in these cases.

Diarrhea caused by one-celled, microscopic animals (*Giardia lamblia* and *Entomeba histolytica* in the majority of these cases) is becoming increasingly common in the United States. Sexual contact with an infected person, drinking contaminated water (*Giardia* can be found in many streams and lakes), and poor hygiene among infected children or during their diaper changes spread these infections. Travelers to foreign countries are especially vulnerable to these infections. Symptoms vary from none at all to severe and debilitating diarrhea. When a family member has a suspected or confirmed infection, professional medical care is essential, but you may use homeopathic medicines in addition to other prescribed treatments to help restore health to the intestinal tract.

Other causes of acute and chronic diarrhea may be serious and should not be treated at home. Again, check the "Beyond Home Care" section.

GENERAL HOME CARE

When acute vomiting or diarrhea occurs, the best way to help the body heal is to carefully limit what you eat and drink. Food and even liquids irritate the inflamed linings of the stomach and intestines, attracting more fluid from the bloodstream and touching off renewed bouts. Adults and children should begin home care by spending six to twelve hours without food or drink of any kind.

When the symptoms have calmed down a bit, try taking clear liquids in sips or teaspoonfuls to replace the water and minerals the body has lost and to provide some simple sugars for energy. Fruit juice or flat soft drinks diluted to half water, vegetable broth (simmer mixed vegetables in water for ten or fifteen minutes, then strain), or rice water (use an excess of water to cook rice) all are good choices. Broth or soup stock made with oil or animal fat should be avoided, as should milk. Gradually increase the amount of clear liquids over a day or two, and then begin trying low-fiber foods such as white rice or toast, low-fat yogurt or cottage cheese, or bananas.

Younger children and babies do not have the fluid reserves of adults, so begin replacing their fluid losses at once. The breast-fed baby should continue its nursing, but all other liquids and solids should be discontinued. If a baby has been vomiting, you should try to reduce the breast milk taken per feeding to avoid touching off more vomiting. If diarrhea is present without vomiting, offer the breast frequently and allow the baby to drink as much as she wants.

Babies on formula, and young children who have been weaned should receive clear liquids only (as outlined above) from the time the symptoms become apparent. Discontinue formula and milk products. If the child has been vomiting, it is vital that you get her to hold down some fluids to replace those lost. You may have to start with tiny amounts of liquids, perhaps only a teaspoonful every fifteen minutes. Children who have diarrhea can drink fluids only when they feel they want them. Be sure to offer them frequently, even when the child doesn't ask. If the child refuses to drink, you'll have to watch carefully for signs of dehydration.

Begin reintroducing the child's normal diet as the symptoms improve, usually a day or two after they began.

DEHYDRATION

The body is composed mostly of water; the brain, the kidneys, various hormones, and other systems all work together in intricate harmony to maintain the body's vital fluid balance. Water is constantly lost in the urine, in perspiration, in the stool, and in water vapor that leaves the lungs when we breathe. In healthy people with an average activity level, about half the body's water loss occurs through the skin and lungs. Illness increases these losses since perspiration and deep, rapid breathing accompany fevers, respiratory illnesses, vomiting and diarrhea, and any type of stress.

Although there are powerful regulatory mechanisms that conserve fluids and minerals if intake is low or losses are high, and although there are sizable reserves of fluid in the body, the body is not always able to cope with low intake or excessive loss of fluids. Once fluid levels drop below the necessary minimum, function of many crucial systems of the body becomes impaired. This is dehydration. Mineral losses that occur when large amounts of fluids are lost through vomiting, diarrhea, and such also may cause serious problems, since minerals play necessary roles in such vital physiological functions as contraction of muscles, transmission of nerve impulses, and regulation of heartbeat.

Babies less than six months old are at the greatest risk of dehydrating and suffering its severe consequences. Their metabolic rate is high, their kidneys don't retain water well, and they lose greater proportions of water per pound than adults do. The risk of dehydration decreases with age, but it can happen to anyone if fluid losses are great enough. Older people, who may have impaired kidney function and reduced fluid reserves, also are at increased risk.

GENERAL HOME CARE

Anyone with an acute illness should drink some extra liquid. If there is little fever and no respiratory symptoms, the increase need not be large—a couple of extra glasses of water or juice a day is fine. If fever, congestion of the nose, or cough are present, another couple of glasses should be taken. Instructions for making sure the person with vomiting or diarrhea gets enough fluid are given in this section under "Gastroenteritis." Anyone who is sick, but particularly children and elderly people, should be offered liquids every hour or two, since they may be just too tired or woozy to respond to thirst.

Anyone with severe vomiting or diarrhea, and babies with any degree of these symptoms or decreased thirst with their illness, should be watched closely for signs of dehydration. The first indication that fluid losses are too great is dryness of the mouth and eyes—so long as the person still has tears and saliva, he is not yet markedly dehydrated. As dehydration worsens, later signs are (1) loss of the normal texture of the skin (if you pinch up some skin it does not immediately snap back into place); (2) sunken eyes; and (3) in babies, a sunken "soft spot" at the top of the head. A definite reduction in the quantity of urine also is a bad sign. Immediate medical attention should be obtained as soon as you notice dry mouth or lack of tears.

BEYOND HOME CARE

GET MEDICAL CARE IMMEDIATELY:

- if the eyes or mouth is truly dry (no saliva or tears);
- if there is loss of normal skin texture: if skin is pinched up and does not immediately snap back into place;
- if the eyes appear sunken;
- in babies, if the soft spot at the top of the head is sunken;
- if the quantity of urine is markedly reduced (in babies, you should count how many times the child wets the diapers and notice how wet they are compared to normal).

ABDOMINAL PAIN AND INDIGESTION

Abdominal pain can be caused by acute gastroenteritis, but it is more often a symptom of indigestion. Indigestion is a vague term we use to refer to minor disruptions of the function of the esophagus, stomach, and intestines, causing symptoms such as heartburn, queasiness, burping, and gas.

Acute bouts of such symptoms usually are the result of bad diet or psychological stress. Eating too much, too rapidly, or too many foods at one meal may cause as much trouble as particular problem foods or beverages. The pain accompanying indigestion normally is just a nuisance, but at times it can be intense.

There are many serious causes of acute abdominal pain also, including appendicitis, inflammation of the gall bladder or pancreas, intestinal obstruction, and diverticular disease (diverticuli are small intestinal out-pouchings). In women, abdominal pain may be caused by infections in the reproductive organs, or pregnancies that lodge in the ovarian tubes. Even experienced surgeons can have trouble diagnosing the problem, so don't hesitate to consult your health practitioner (see "Beyond Home Care" on pp. 160–61 for specific recommendations). If the pain is not extreme, and so long as there are no worrisome accompanying symptoms, you can treat the person at home for a few hours.

If mild abdominal pain or other symptoms recur or become chronic, it should prompt you to see your health practitioner. Once a diagnosis is made, professional homeopathic treatment can be helpful.

APPENDICITIS

Long thought to have no function in the body, the appendix is known now to contain lymphatic tissue and to play a role in the immune system of the gastrointestinal tract. It may be a kind of filter that helps protect the large intestine from harmful microbes. This makes questionable the common practice of removing the appendix "preventively" during abdominal surgery for other reasons.

Of course, the appendix can become diseased. When it gets clogged with fecal material, it may become inflamed and swollen and a bacterial infection may develop in its walls. As the swelling stretches the walls, pain becomes severe. Eventually the appendix bursts, and inflammation and infection spread throughout the abdomen. This complication, called peritonitis, is extremely dangerous. Therefore, it's very important to diagnose appendicitis before the appendix bursts. As with other causes of abdominal pain, appendicitis is hard to diagnose. The most typical pattern of symptoms runs as follows: After a short period of disinterest in food, and perhaps a mild episode of vomiting, the person with appendicitis begins to feel pain in the area of the navel. Within another few hours the pain moves from the center of the abdomen and becomes localized in the right lower section of the abdomen. Touching the painful area increases the pain, and as inflammation progresses, the muscles of the abdomen become tense and hard. There may be a fever of a degree or two above normal, and the person may be constipated.

There are other conditions that mimic this pattern of symptoms, but still you should be extremely wary of appendicitis if you see this pattern. When the classic symptom pattern is apparent, it is not such a problem as when appendicitis causes different symptoms, however. Some authorities estimate that the "typical" pattern occurs in only one-fifth of the cases. Young children and older people especially are likely to have confusing symptoms. The diagnosis of appendicitis can be made more definite by careful examination of the abdomen and rectum and with blood tests, but the diagnosis cannot be confirmed until during surgery.

GENERAL HOME CARE

The milder symptoms of indigestion are best treated at home by letting them pass and refraining from doing anything that might aggravate the system further. You may do well to put off eating altogether, but certainly avoid spices, coffee, alcohol, and fatty or oily foods. Herb teas such as peppermint or raspberry leaf are good for helping relieve gas. Changing position frequently or walking slowly may help gas move more freely.

Relaxation exercises and other ways of effectively dealing with stress are briefly discussed in chapter 11 on headaches. They are a good idea if your symptoms were brought on by stress, and even when this isn't the case, they sometimes help relieve indigestion or abdominal pain.

If you have definite abdominal pain, avoid solid foods and take only clear liquids. So long as you don't have diarrhea or vomiting, plain water is best. Some people get relief using a hot water bottle or heating pad, applying slight pressure, or bending double.

For cases of mild to moderate abdominal pain, we think that it makes sense to watch and wait for a few hours before seeking medical care. Most often the pain will pass, and in those few cases where there are serious problems, the wait won't hurt. Don't hesitate to try an appropriate homeopathic medicine while waiting for the seriousness of the problem to become clear. Even if you eventually need more extreme medical measures, the correct medicine may well help your body heal more rapidly.

CASETAKING QUESTIONS FOR DIGESTIVE PROBLEMS

Character of the symptoms:
- What are the symptoms—queasiness, nausea, vomiting, diarrhea, or pain—and which are worse?
- How would you describe the pain—sharp, burning, pressing, or some other sensation?
- Where exactly is the discomfort felt? Does it radiate or extend elsewhere?
- What is the color and appearance of the vomited material? The stool?

Associated symptoms:
- Is the tongue coated?
- Has the complexion changed?

Modalities:
- How are the symptoms affected by drinking or eating? Are there any specific foods or drinks that affect the symptoms? Does the temperature of food or drink make a difference?
- How are the symptoms affected by hot or cold applications, hot or cold rooms, motion, standing, or lying down? What affect does pressure or bending double have on the pain?
- At what time of day are the symptoms worse?
- In what way, if any, is the person sensitive to the smell of food?
- Does vomiting relieve the nausea? How does a bowel movement affect the symptoms?

HOMEOPATHIC MEDICINES

The symptoms of *Arsenicum* match those of many acute gastrointestinal affections. The classic patient has violent vomiting and diarrhea that can be accompanied by a great deal of pain in the stomach or intestines. The presence of *Arsenicum*'s general characteristics determine the choice of this medicine: The patient is quickly exhausted by the illness, greatly weakened yet extremely restless; she constantly changes position until the weakness becomes completely debilitating; she may be very fearful and specifically afraid to be alone; the *Arsenicum* adult or older child often fears she has a serious illness and may die; usually there is a marked thirst—sometimes she repeatedly wants to drink small amounts of water; and there may be a high fever, though the *Arsenicum* patient is typically very chilly and wants to stay under the blankets. When this combination of restlessness, exhaustion, fear, chilliness, and thirst is present during an acute digestive illness, you should give *Arsenicum* no matter what the specific digestive symptoms.

The gastrointestinal symptoms of *Arsenicum* include severe nausea, vomiting, diarrhea, and abdominal pain. The symptoms come on or are worse at night, often after midnight. Vomiting is made worse from eating and drinking, and drinking even very little may cause immediate vomiting. Moving around or drinking milk also may result in renewed vomiting. Typically there is burning or cramping in the stomach or abdomen. In spite of the terrible burning, cold drinks aggravate the pain and warm drinks help. External warmth also is likely to help relieve the pain, whereas the patient's becoming chilled makes it worse. The diarrhea also is made worse from eating or drinking, particularly eating cold foods like ice cream, or drinking cold liquids. Burning may be felt in the rectum during or after the bowel movement. Great exhaustion follows. *Arsenicum* is the most commonly indicated medicine for food-poisoning illnesses.

Ipecac. is indicated chiefly by persistent and extreme nausea, whether or not other symptoms such as vomiting or diarrhea are present. Even after vomiting, when most people would get at least temporary relief, the *Ipecac.* patient may continue to feel sick to his stomach. The patient usually is not so severely ill in general as the *Arsenicum* patient, though certainly he can have a fever and feel weak. The nausea is made worse from the smell of food, and the condition sometimes can be traced to having eaten too much rich or fatty food. Most often there is a great deal of vomiting, sometimes becoming nearly continuous. Vomiting is worse after eating or drinking. Usually the person has little thirst and is not particularly anxious or chilly. The vomited material often contains much mucus. Pinching, cutting pains may be felt in the abdomen, and often the person must pass much gas. Diarrhea accompanied by nausea also is a symptom of *Ipecac.* Stools are green, sometimes as green as grass, or frothy like yeast; often they are mucous. Usually the tongue is clean and uncoated, and often there is increased salivation and drooling.

Colocynthis is indicated when the person complains of cramping, clutching abdominal pains that can be relieved with pressure and warmth.

The patient may double up with the pain, press his fist into the painful area, or lie over a hard object to get relief. Infants with *Colocynthis* colic are better when lying on the stomach, but worse again if they are moved from that position. Warmth brings relief as well. The pain is made worse from eating and particularly drinking. When the pain becomes severe enough, vomiting may occur; often it seems related to the intensity of the pain. Diarrhea may occur, preceded by the cramping pains described above. The bowel movement usually relieves the pain, at least for a time. Whatever the combination, the symptoms may have been brought on by the person's anger or suffering of an insult to his sense of justice.

Similarly, *Magnesia phos.* is useful to those with abdominal pain made better from warmth and pressure. If the two medicines can be distinguished, the *Magnesia phos.* patient finds greater relief in warmth and doesn't seek pressure so insistently. Vomiting and diarrhea are rare.

As always, *Belladonna* is indicated in the early stages of the illness if the symptoms came on suddenly. The accompanying general symptoms—fever, flushed face, and dullness—are as prominent as the nausea, vomiting, or diarrhea. Vomiting is not clearly related to eating or drinking; the vomited material contains mucus or partly digested food. *Belladonna* is likely to be helpful when infection elsewhere in the body comes on with vomiting or diarrhea in addition to the fever. There may be diarrhea with mucous stools. *Belladonna* also covers abdominal pains that are sharp and come on in spells, appearing and disappearing suddenly. The pains are worse after drinking and from motion, being jarred, walking, or standing. Gentle pressure aggravates it, whereas firm pressure brings relief.

Bryonia often is the remedy for acute gastroenteritis. The general characteristic of this medicine, aggravation caused by motion, applies to all the digestive symptoms—nausea, vomiting, diarrhea, and abdominal pain all may be touched off by the slightest motion. Sometimes moving even a single part of the body is enough to bring on the symptoms. Vomiting comes on after eating or drinking. The smallest quantity of liquid may cause vomiting, though in some cases nausea is relieved by drinking. Abdominal pain often is relieved by pressure or by lying on the painful area, and it may improve after a bowel movement. Diarrhea is worse in the morning, after the patient gets up and moves around, and sometimes during hot weather. The stool is most often pasty or mushy. In general, the person feels warm, is irritable, and wants to be left alone to lie still.

Phosphorus also covers certain symptoms of acute gastroenteritis. The symptoms are similar to those of *Arsenicum*: much vomiting and diarrhea, burning pains, weakness, anxiety and restlessness, and thirst for cold drinks. Usually, *Arsenicum* is a better first choice when these are the main symptoms, unless specific *Phosphorus* symptoms are present. Nausea is worse after warm drinks or even after putting the hands in warm water. Vomiting after eating or drinking is typical, but more specifically, the *Phosphorus* patient may vomit as soon as water becomes warm in the stomach or after drinking the smallest quantity of liquid. Warm water aggravates the vomiting immediately, and looking at water may cause renewed vomiting. Cold water momentarily relieves nausea and pain, but within a few moments it becomes heated and the symptoms begin again. Often there is a general sense of emptiness and weakness in the stomach or entire abdomen, and an empty, hungry feeling may keep the person awake at night. The *Phosphorus* patient may experience diarrhea with involuntary stools. Sometimes the anus will not close and stool oozes out uncontrollably, or there may be only a sensation of an open anus.

Violent diarrhea, usually accompanied by vomiting, may best be covered by *Veratrum album*. The stools may look like water used to cook rice, or they may look watery and greenish, containing small green flakes. The stool is ejected forcefully from the body (more so than in the *Arsenicum* case) in great quantity. These symptoms are always accompanied by colicky cramps in the abdomen, which are temporarily relieved by the diarrhea. Violent vomiting often is associated with the diarrhea, and the person may purge from both the mouth and the rectum at the same time. Motion brings on renewed diarrhea and vomiting. The general symptoms of this medicine are marked and include severe chilliness, cold perspiration (especially on the forehead), and great weakness. The body is cold, and even the breath may be cold. There is much thirst for large quantities of cold water.

Podophyllum is one of the more commonly indicated medicines for those with acute diarrhea. Profuse, offensive-smelling stools are characteristic. You may wonder where it all comes from since so much passes with each bowel movement and the movements are so frequent. The stools may be yellowish or greenish and often are completely liquid. The diarrhea is made worse from eating, drinking, and moving around, and it sometimes alternates with a headache. This medicine is well suited to the person with common diarrhea when he is a bit less energetic but not terribly sick; diarrhea seems to be the main symptom. Eventually, after frequent, profuse stools, he does become exhausted. *Podophyllum* diarrhea may be completely painless, or there may be abdominal pain that is worse before or during the bowel movement. Sometimes cramps in the muscles of the feet, calves, and thighs accompany the diarrhea, or yawning and stretching may be noticeable. Vomiting is rare, but dry heaves or gagging do occur at times.

When the symptoms have been brought on by mental exertion, overeating, or use of alcohol, coffee, or other drugs, *Nux vomica* can be a good medicine. Heartburn, nausea, empty retching, and sour burps are manifestations of a general disorder of the stomach. Headache, irritability, drowsiness, and dullness are typical of the *Nux* patient with digestive upset. The symptoms are worse in the morning and are aggravated also by eating; uncomfortable queasiness, bloating, and gas accumulation occur after meals. The patient often feels that this discomfort would be relieved if he could vomit, and vomiting after eating is common. This may take the form of retching up only small amounts of food. Vomiting or retching may follow his attempts to bring up phlegm from the throat. Diarrhea with brown liquid or mucous stools that come frequently in small amounts is characteristic. There may be a strong, sometimes constant urge to move the bowels, but little or no stool passes. A bad backache often precedes or accompanies the bowel movement. *Nux* matches the symptoms of many hangovers.

Pulsatilla also covers the digestive symptoms resulting from improper diet, in this case especially from rich foods, fats, or particularly ice cream. But *Pulsatilla* may benefit anyone with a gastrointestinal condition if the general symptoms of the medicine are pronounced. Usually nausea, vomiting, and diarrhea are not too severe. There is heartburn, queasiness, a bad taste in the mouth, and a sense of heaviness after eating. The tongue may be coated thickly with white or yellow material. The person experiences nausea after drinking, especially warm liquids, and cold drinks may relieve the nausea. Food eaten long before may be vomited up only partly digested. *Pulsatilla* also covers diarrhea with green or mucous stools, or stools that constantly change in character or color. The diarrhea is likely to be worse at night, in a warm room, or when the patient gets warm.

REMEDY SUMMARY FOR DIGESTIVE PROBLEMS

Most of the medicines listed here may be useful for people with any combination of digestive symptoms, including vomiting, diarrhea, or abdominal pain.
Give the medicine: Every hour (during intense pain or incessant retching) to every 12 hours (if vomiting or diarrhea is mild).
When to try another medicine: Severe symptoms should improve rapidly, and you need allow only an hour or two before switching

to another medicine if there is no change. Wait 12 to 24 hours if symptoms are mild.

ARSENICUM ★

Essentials

- Violent vomiting and/or diarrhea accompanied by much pain in the stomach or intestines
- Any digestive symptoms accompanied by restlessness, exhaustion, fear, chilliness, and thirst
- Most commonly indicated medicine for food poisoning; give if no other remedy is better indicated

Confirmatory symptoms

- Burning pains relieved with warmth, worse from cold; burning in the rectum during or after bowel movement
- Thirst for small amounts of cold water
- Symptoms come on or are worse at night, often after midnight
- Vomiting worse from eating and drinking, especially cold things; drinking small amounts causes immediate vomiting

IPECAC.

Essentials

- Persistent, extreme nausea with any digestive symptoms; nausea persists after vomiting

Confirmatory symptoms

- Vomiting can be severe, worse after eating or drinking
- Nausea worse from smell of food
- Little thirst
- Pinching, cutting pains in abdomen
- Green stools
- Tongue not coated, but increased salivation and drooling

COLOCYNTHIS

Essentials

- Cramping, clutching abdominal pains relieved with pressure and warmth

Confirmatory symptoms
- Pain worse from drinking or eating
- Vomiting as pain becomes more severe
- Diarrhea preceded by cramping pains; bowel movement relieves the pain, at least for a time
- Symptoms follow anger or being insulted

MAGNESIA PHOSPHORICA

Essentials
- Abdominal pain better with warmth and/or pressure; vomiting or diarrhea less prominent than in *Colocynthis*

BELLADONNA

Essentials
- Early stages of the illness when symptoms come on suddenly
- Prominent general symptoms such as fever, flushed face, and dullness
- Also helpful when other illnesses begin with vomiting or diarrhea in addition to the fever

Confirmatory symptoms
- Sharp pains come and go suddenly
- Pains worse after drinking, from motion, being jarred, and gentle pressure; better from firm pressure
- Vomited material or diarrhea contains mucus

BRYONIA

Essentials
- Any digestive symptom decidedly aggravated by motion

Confirmatory symptoms
- Person irritable, wants to be left alone to lie still
- Moving a single body part brings on symptoms
- Vomiting after eating or drinking, even tiny amounts of liquid
- Abdominal pain relieved by pressure or after a bowel movement
- Diarrhea worse in the morning, after getting up; stool pasty or mushy

NUX VOMICA

Essentials
- Digestive problems brought on by mental exertion or tension, overeating, or use of alcohol, coffee, or other drugs; primary hangover medicine
- Heartburn, nausea, empty retching, and sour burps
- Irritability

Confirmatory symptoms
- Worse in the morning
- Eating causes queasiness, bloating, gas, or vomiting
- Diarrhea with brown liquid or mucous stools that come frequently in small amounts
- Strong urge to move the bowels but little or no stool
- Backache before or during bowel movement

PULSATILLA

Essentials
- Digestive symptoms after eating rich foods, fats, or particularly ice cream
  or
- In any digestive condition, if the general symptoms of *Pulsatilla* are pronounced (see *materia medica* section)

Confirmatory symptoms
- Heartburn, queasiness, bad taste in the mouth, and a sense of heaviness after eating
- Tongue coated thickly with white or yellow material
- Nausea after drinking, especially warm liquids; relieved by cold drinks
- Vomiting of partly digested food
- Diarrhea with green or mucous stools or stools that constantly change in character or color

PHOSPHORUS

Essentials
- Symptoms are similar to *Arsenicum*: much vomiting and diarrhea, burning pains, weakness, anxiety and restlessness, and thirst for

cold drinks (try *Arsenicum* first unless patient has symptoms listed below)

Confirmatory symptoms
- Nausea and vomiting worse after warm drinks; vomiting as soon as water becomes warm in the stomach
- Vomiting after eating or drinking even very small amounts
- Diarrhea with involuntary stools; stool oozes out uncontrollably, or sensation of an open anus
- General sense of emptiness and weakness in the stomach or entire abdomen; empty, hungry feeling may keep the person awake at night

VERATRUM ALBUM

Essentials
- Violent diarrhea ejected forcefully accompanied by colicky cramps in the abdomen; the diarrhea temporarily relieves the cramps
- Stools look like water used to cook rice, or watery and greenish, containing small green flakes
- Violent vomiting commonly accompanies the diarrhea; simultaneous vomiting and diarrhea

Confirmatory symptoms
- Motion causes diarrhea and vomiting
- Severe chilliness, cold perspiration (especially on the forehead)
- Great weakness
- Thirst for large quantities of cold water

BEYOND HOME CARE

These indications are for vomiting, diarrhea, indigestion, and abdominal pain.

GET MEDICAL CARE IMMEDIATELY:
- for any severe abdominal pain;
- if there is incessant vomiting;

- if there is evidence of dehydration: lack of tears, truly dry mouth, loss of normal skin texture, sunken eyes, sunken soft spot in baby's head;
- if there is a possibility of poisoning or drug use;
- if stools or vomited material is bloody, black, red, tarlike, or resembles coffee grounds;
- if there is vomiting, diarrhea, or pain after an abdominal or head injury;
- if a child's vomiting is accompanied by marked irritability, inconsolable screaming, or marked lethargy;
- if vomiting begins unexpectedly during the course of a viral respiratory illness.

GET MEDICAL CARE TODAY:

- if there is significant vomiting or pain and no bowel movement for 24 hours;
- if the patient is or could possibly be pregnant;
- if the patient is diabetic;
- if there is yellowing of the skin or eyes, if the urine is very dark, or if the stools are gray or nearly white;
- if there is swelling or pain in the groin or where the lower abdomen meets the thighs.

CALL YOUR PRACTITIONER TODAY:

- if you are taking any medications.

SEE YOUR PRACTITIONER IN THE NEXT FEW DAYS:

- for recurrent abdominal pain, vomiting, or diarrhea, even if the symptoms are mild, or for any definite change in bowel habits lasting longer than 2 weeks.

CONSTIPATION

To stay in good health, it is not necessary to have a bowel movement every day, and no immediate health problems will result even if you go for a long time without one. Still, infrequent, difficult bowel movements are symptomatic of sluggishness of the intestines, which can contribute to cancer, diverticular disease, and a variety of other degenerative diseases of the intestine and possibly of the whole system.

GENERAL HOME CARE

The best way to alleviate constipation and maintain active bowel function is to drink adequate liquids and eat a diet rich in fiber. All plant foods contain a certain amount of indigestible "roughage." Since this material is not absorbed by the body, and in fact attracts and holds water, the stool is larger and stretches the intestinal walls. This stretching stimulates a reflex that speeds the movement of the stool through the intestine smoothly.

The foods richer in fiber content are whole grains and fresh vegetables; most fruits have less. You don't need to eat bran, the indigestible outer layer of grain, or to take any sort of laxative, as long as your diet includes plenty of whole grains and vegetables. It may help to avoid milk and other dairy products.

Sometimes these dietary measures fail to relieve constipation. At times, an important factor may be stress of one kind or another, since the nervous system regulates the contraction of the intestinal muscles. Travelers commonly become constipated for this reason. A lack of exercise also may contribute to the problem.

Sometimes an internal imbalance is the real trouble, and no amount of dietary adjustment or stress reduction helps. Homeopathic treatment for people with chronic constipation can be helpful, but you should consult a professional. Avoid laxatives and enemas.

BEYOND HOME CARE

Anytime there is a marked change in bowel movement pattern that lasts more than a week or two, whether the new pattern develops slowly or gradually, you should consult your medical practitioner, especially if you are older than thirty-five.

HEMORRHOIDS

Hemorrhoids are one of the more common afflictions of people who live in the developed countries of North America and Europe. Fifty percent or more of the population of the United States experience this undignified and often painful malady at some time in their lives.

Although hemorrhoids are still not completely understood, they are known to be swollen blood vessels in the anal area. You could think of them as anal varicose veins, though this description probably isn't precisely correct in scientific terms. At any rate, if the blood vessels involved originate from the outer portion of the anus, you can see and feel the hemorrhoid as a soft bluish-purple lump. On the other hand, you probably won't notice simple hemorrhoids that occur inside the anus, since usually they are painless.

Wherever they develop, hemorrhoids commonly cause painless rectal bleeding. You may notice a little blood on the toilet paper, a few drops in the bowl, or some streaking of blood on the outside of the stool. There may be mild soreness or burning, and you may experience itching also, since the irregularly swollen tissues are difficult to keep clean.

You'll become much more uncomfortable if an ordinary hemorrhoid becomes clotted or thrombosed. The resulting inflammation and additional swelling can lead to increased bleeding and acute pain. Interior thrombosed hemorrhoids often protrude from the anus, while those that formed on the outside become larger and exquisitely tender.

In conventional medical practice, intractable, severely inflamed thrombosed hemorrhoids may be removed by constricting them with rubber bands or by excising them surgically. Most hemorrhoids eventually resolve on their own without treatment. After healing is complete, you may notice a small projection of skinlike tissue at the hemorrhoid site. These skin tags are painless and need no treatment.

GENERAL HOME CARE

As always, prevention is the best treatment. Hemorrhoids are rare in cultures with high-fiber diets—yet another argument for eating plenty of fiber yourself. Avoid straining while on the toilet, since it puts pressure on the abdominal blood vessels and in turn on those in the anal area (see the previous section on constipation).

If you're prone to hemorrhoids, limiting yourself to about a minute on the toilet helps to ensure that you don't strain too much. Regular exercise speeds circulation of the blood and thus helps prevent hemorrhoids; conversely, sitting allows blood to pool in the lower body, where it may overload the veins. If your job requires you to sit for long periods, be sure to get up and walk around for a few minutes every hour or two. And be sure to minimize pressure on the blood vessels by maintaining weight at a near-ideal level.

If you do develop hemorrhoids, the first symptom you might notice is painless bleeding from the rectum. Even though hemorrhoids themselves are no threat to your general health, you should be checked by your health practitioner for any new rectal bleeding; even if you do have hemorrhoids, the bleeding may come from another site, and cancer *must* be ruled out. At a minimum, your stool should be tested for the presence of blood, and the rectum and last part of the large intestine should be examined.

Once you've had the proper examination, home care of hemorrhoids is simple. Hemorrhoids on the outer part of the anus can be difficult to clean, but there are alternatives to toilet paper that work better. Obviously, soaking in a warm bath is a great way to get clean, and many find the warmth soothing. Sitz baths, in which you squat in a few inches of warm water, are recommended often since the squatting position spreads the anal tissues and makes cleaning easier.

Drugstores sell pads soaked in witch hazel solution; the wet pad provides gentler, more thorough cleansing, and witch hazel is a mild astringent that may slightly reduce hemorrhoidal swelling. Witch hazel, made from the bark of a shrub native to the southern U.S., is used in homeopathy under its botanical name, *Hamamelis*. Though this medicine often is given orally for hemorrhoids, homeopathic pharmacies also sell topical preparations of *Hamamelis* either alone or in combination with other plant-based hemorrhoid remedies.

If you're unfortunate enough to develop a thrombosed hemorrhoid, you should lie down whenever possible—the force of gravity when standing simply adds to the inflammation. Hot or cold applications may help reduce the pain a bit. Again, use warm baths to keep the area clean.

CASETAKING QUESTIONS FOR HEMORRHOIDS

Character of the symptoms:
- How severe is the pain, and how would you describe it? Are the hemorrhoids tender?
- Is there itching or any other sensation in the rectal area (such as pressure or pulsation)?
- How much bleeding is there? What is the color of the blood?

Associated symptoms:
- Is there constipation or diarrhea?
- Is there any back pain?

Modalities:
- At what time of day are the symptoms worse?
- How are they affected by warm or cold applications, motion (passive or active), or having a bowel movement?

HOMEOPATHIC MEDICINES

Aesculus is one of the more commonly useful homeopathic medicines for hemorrhoids and may be given if you can't find a better-fitting remedy for the symptoms below. It is definitely indicated when the hemorrhoids are accompanied by aching in the lower back and at the base of the spine. There may be a sensation in the rectum like splinters or sticks, or a sensation of heaviness or pressure in the rectum as if it would protrude. *Aesculus* is a good choice when there isn't much bleeding.

Nux vomica is useful for many people with simple hemorrhoids. There may be stinging pains, constricted sensations, and a constant uneasy feeling in the anal area, but severe tenderness isn't too common. Pain or discomfort is worse usually in the early morning, in cold or open air, when uncovered, and in tight-fitting clothing, especially pants. Although bleeding may be present, *Nux* is one of the better medicines when there is no bleeding (a characteristic it holds in common with *Aesculus*). Itching may be troublesome, but will likely be relieved by cold water. Chronic constipation often contributes to the problem, and there may be an ineffective urge to defecate. *Nux* is a good choice also for people who are sedentary or who overuse laxatives, coffee, medications, or drugs.

When itching is the predominant symptom, *Aloe,* made from the aloe vera plant, is likely to be the right medicine. There may be significant burning or soreness, described as feeling as if the rectum has been scraped. Cold water provides relief. Diarrhea rather than constipation may be present, and some people who need *Aloe* have a feeling of weakness in the rectum, as if they won't be able to hold in the stool when passing gas or urinating. Most typically their symptoms are worse in the morning, and they may even be awakened by discomfort.

Belladonna is ideal during the first day or two of acute inflammation around the hemorrhoids, when there is much redness and swelling and great pain and tenderness. There may be a lot of bright-red blood.

The key symptom indicating *Muriatic acid* is tremendous tenderness. Perhaps even more than with *Belladonna,* the sufferer can barely stand even a very light touch on the inflamed hemorrhoid. The pain is increased significantly by walking or riding, but warm water makes it better. Bleeding is common. The hemorrhoids may protrude only during a bowel movement or when urinating, and there may be an involuntary stool when passing gas or urinating.

Pulsatilla may be the correct remedy if cold applications relieve the discomfort and the general symptoms of the medicine listed in the *materia medica* section are present (thirstless, moody, weepy, and "warm blooded"—that is, they are sensitive to or are aggravated by heat, and require fewer clothes than others). One distinguishing symptom of people who need *Pulsatilla* is a tendency to have changing stools; no two stools are alike in color or consistency. *Pulsatilla* is a common remedy for hemorrhoids during puberty and pregnancy.

Hamamelis should help when significant amounts of dark, thick blood flow from the hemorrhoids. Though often very sore or even raw, the hemorrhoids aren't necessarily extremely tender to touch. Pulsations may be felt in the rectum.

REMEDY SUMMARY FOR HEMORRHOIDS

Give the medicine: Two to 3 times a day for up to 3 days.
When to try another medicine: If there is no improvement after the third day.

AESCULUS ★

Essentials
- Aching in lower back and base of spine

Confirmatory symptoms
- Sensation in rectum like splinters or sticks, or of heaviness or pressure, as if rectum will protrude
- Little or no bleeding

NUX VOMICA

Essentials
- Relatively mild discomfort: stinging pains, tight sensation, or vague uneasy feeling
  or

- General symptoms of *Nux* are present (see *materia medica* section), or the problem appeared after overuse of laxatives, coffee, medications, or drugs

Confirmatory symptoms
- Discomfort worse in early morning, in cold or open air, when uncovered, and in tight-fitting clothing
- Little or no bleeding
- Itching; relief from cold water
- Chronic constipation; ineffective urging to defecate is typical

BELLADONNA

Essentials
- Early, acute inflammation around the hemorrhoids, with much redness, swelling, pain, and tenderness

Confirmatory symptoms
- Bright-red blood

HAMAMELIS

Essentials
- Dark, thick blood

Confirmatory symptoms
- Though sore and painful, the hemorrhoids are relatively non-tender
- Pulsations in the rectum

ALOE

Essentials
- Much itching

or
- Burning or sore pains, as if the rectum has been scraped

Confirmatory symptoms
- Relief from cold water
- Diarrhea; feeling of weakness in the rectum, as if stool will pass when passing gas or urinating
- Pain worse in the morning; may awaken the patient

MURIATIC ACID

Essentials
- Great tenderness; even very light touch provokes much pain

Confirmatory symptoms
- Pain worse while walking or riding, better from warm water
- Bleeding
- Hemorrhoids protrude only during a bowel movement or when urinating
- Involuntary stool when passing gas or urinating

PULSATILLA

Essentials
- Relief from cold applications
  or
- General symptoms of *Pulsatilla* are present (see *materia medica* section)

Confirmatory symptoms
- No two stools are alike in color or consistency
- Hemorrhoids during puberty and pregnancy

BEYOND HOME CARE

GET MEDICAL CARE IMMEDIATELY:

- for profuse rectal bleeding.

SEE YOUR PRACTITIONER SOON:

- for any new-onset rectal bleeding;
- for any new lumps or swellings in the anal area.

HEPATITIS

Hepatitis, or inflammation of the liver, is caused most often by a viral infection. The more common hepatitis infections are hepatitis A, usually passed in the stool, and hepatitis B, passed mostly through blood or during sexual contact. Hepatitis B is more dangerous because a substantial proportion of those who come down with the disease develop chronic hepatitis, a serious illness. Other viruses can cause hepatitis, too, including mononucleosis. Sometimes poisons or drugs cause noninfectious hepatitis. The symptoms of hepatitis include extreme fatigue, low-grade fever, disinterest in food, and queasiness. The liver (located in the upper right part of the abdomen, under the ribs) may feel heavy, painful, and tender. Jaundice, a yellowing of the skin and eyes, sometimes but not always accompanies hepatitis. Likewise, very light-colored stools and very dark urine may or may not be noticed.

GENERAL HOME CARE

Hepatitis is a serious illness, and you should have professional medical help to diagnose it and to follow its course. There are, however, no effective conventional medicines for hepatitis. Various preventive medications are available for people who have been or may in the future be exposed to hepatitis, and you should speak to your practitioner about them if you think you might be exposed.

If you have hepatitis, get as much rest as you feel you need, and eat a well-balanced diet of moderate protein and low fat content. Try to eat well even if you aren't very hungry. Avoid irritating spices, oily food, coffee, and drugs. You should abstain entirely from alcohol.

CASETAKING QUESTIONS FOR HEPATITIS

Character of the symptoms:
- How would you describe the liver discomfort—soreness, or sharp pain?
- Does the discomfort or pain extend elsewhere? Exactly where?

Associated symptoms:
- Is the mouth affected—is there bad breath or a bad taste, a swollen or coated tongue, or increased salivation?
- How is digestion affected—is there gas, bloating, fullness, diarrhea, or constipation?

Modalities:
- How is the discomfort affected by eating, motion, being jarred, breathing, or lying on the right side?
- Is the liver area tender to touch or pressure?

HOMEOPATHIC MEDICINES

Treatment with homeopathic medicines often has been successful in shortening the course of the illness and helping the person recover vitality. We have observed dramatic improvement in many cases. It is best to receive treatment from an experienced professional. If none is available, however, we think that you should treat yourself and your family. You should be receiving professional medical care whether or not you are using homeopathy at home.

The earliest stage of acute liver disease sometimes calls for *Aconite* if the general symptoms of the remedy also are present—high fever, moaning, restlessness, and fearful anguish. Shooting pains in the region of the liver may be felt.

Belladonna also may be indicated for the person with hepatitis in the early stages, again, if the general characteristics of this medicine are evident. The pains in the liver come and go suddenly, and breathing, jarring motion, and lying on the right side worsen them.

Hepatitis with pain extending from the liver into the back and just below the right shoulder blade often indicates *Chelidonium*. The pains are sore or sticking in character, and eating may bring relief. From the region of the liver, they may radiate in any direction, rather than just to the back. There is diarrhea with gray or yellow stools. The person feels heavy-headed and chilly, and there may be fever, jaundice, and a bitter taste in the mouth. The tongue may be coated yellow. There may be a craving for milk.

Lycopodium is an important medicine for people with hepatitis. The pains may extend into the back (as with *Chelidonium),* but they don't tend to be as sharp. There is likely to be a sense of being too full after only a few mouthfuls of food. Gas, bloating, and general abdominal discomfort develop immediately after eating, and often there is rumbling in the upper abdomen. The liver area can be sore to the touch and painful when lay upon, and the abdomen in general may be sensitive to the pressure of clothing.

The *Mercurius* hepatitis patient suffers from distressing symptoms of the upper digestive tract. The tongue may be coated a dirty yellow color, and it is likely to be swollen and puffy, taking the imprint of the teeth. The gums become swollen and weak and bleed easily. The liver is swollen and tender, and lying on the right side is painful. Stools may be light gray or yellowish green. Often the skin and eyes are yellowed. There may be pronounced, clammy perspiration. A general sensitivity to both heat and cold is typical.

Nux vomica may be useful for the person with hepatitis, especially if she is a heavy alcohol or drug user. The accompanying digestive symptoms may include those described for *Nux* earlier in this chapter. The liver may be swollen or sensitive to touch, and the pain is sometimes worse after mental work.

China suits the person with hepatitis when the liver is markedly sensitive to pressure and to touch. The patient is chilly and sensitive to open air. Like the *Nux* and *Lycopodium* patient, he may have a sense of heaviness or fullness in the stomach and abdomen, especially after eating. He may burp frequently, but this gives no relief. Burps taste bitter or like the food he has eaten. He may have cravings for cold drinks, sweets, or coffee.

REMEDY SUMMARY FOR HEPATITIS

Give the medicine: Every 6 to 12 hours for up to 6 doses, stopping as soon as you notice any real change in the quality or intensity of the symptoms.

When to try another medicine: If there has been no change within 3 or 4 days; sooner if symptoms are worsening.

ACONITE

Essentials
- Earliest stage of acute liver disease if the general symptoms of the remedy are also present—high fever, moaning, restlessness, and fearful anguish

Confirmatory symptoms
- Shooting pains in the region of the liver

BELLADONNA

Essentials
- Early stages of hepatitis if the general characteristics of *Belladonna* are present (see chapter 3 on fever)

Confirmatory symptoms
- Liver pains come and go suddenly
- Pains worse from breathing, jarring motion, lying on the right side

CHELIDONIUM ★

Essentials
- Pain extending from the liver into the back and just below the right shoulder blade (or radiating from the liver in any direction)

Confirmatory symptoms
- Sore or sticking pains; relieved by eating
- Diarrhea with gray or yellow stools
- Person feels heavy-headed and chilly
- Bitter taste in the mouth
- Tongue coated yellow
- Craving for milk

MERCURIUS

Essentials
- Several of the following typical *Mercurius* symptoms:
  — tongue swollen, takes imprint of the teeth, and is coated a dirty yellow color
  — bad breath
  — gums swollen and weak, bleed easily
  — liver swollen and tender; painful lying on right side
  — stools light gray or yellowish green
  — clammy perspiration
  — sensitivity to both heat and cold

LYCOPODIUM

Essentials
- Pain extending from liver into the back, typically duller than with *Chelidonium*
  or
- Characteristic general symptoms of *Lycopodium* are present (see *materia medica* section)

Confirmatory symptoms
- Liver area sore to touch and painful when lay upon; abdomen sensitive to the pressure of clothing
- Sensation of fullness after only a few mouthfuls of food
- Gas, bloating, and abdominal discomfort after eating; rumbling in the upper abdomen

NUX VOMICA

Essentials
- Hepatitis in those who abuse alcohol or other drugs, especially if general symptoms of *Nux* are present (see *materia medica* section)

Confirmatory symptoms
- Liver swollen and tender
- Liver pain worse after mental work
- Other digestive symptoms of *Nux* (see section on digestive complaints earlier in this chapter)

CHINA

Essentials
- Liver is markedly sensitive to pressure and touch

Confirmatory symptoms
- Sense of heaviness or fullness in abdomen, especially after eating
- Frequent burping, but not relieved by it
- Cravings for cold drinks, sweets, or coffee

BEYOND HOME CARE

GET MEDICAL CARE TODAY:

- if there is yellowing of the skin or eyes, if the urine is very dark, or if the stools are gray or whitish.

SEE YOUR PRACTITIONER SOON:

- if you think you have been exposed to hepatitis;
- if you have been experiencing unusual, unexplained fatigue or discomfort in the upper right part of the abdomen for more than a few days.

Note: Consult "Beyond Home Care" for abdominal pain earlier in this chapter if the pain in the upper right of the abdomen is significant.

MOTION SICKNESS

Most people have been carsick or seasick at one time or another and know what an unpleasant experience it can be. If you are frequently bothered with the affliction of motion sickness, try homeopathic medicines to prevent or treat the discomfort. Give a dose as often as every twenty to thirty minutes up to three times when nausea is severe. If the medicine seems to help, repeat it thereafter only when the symptoms return. Try a new medicine if there is no relief within fifteen minutes after the third dose.

HOMEOPATHIC MEDICINES

Cocculus covers the severe nausea, vomiting, and dizziness characteristic of motion sickness. Nausea and dizziness force the person to lie down; rising up, especially out of bed, and noise make them worse. The sight, smell, or even thought of food brings on new waves of severe nausea. The symptoms are worse also when the throat is dry or when the patient gets cold. *Cocculus* is the first medicine to try for motion sickness if the symptoms don't point you to any one remedy.

The *Petroleum* patient gets dizzy and nauseated when riding in a car or boat. He becomes faint and pale and breaks out in a cold sweat. There may be pain in the back or the head, or there may be an empty, even painful sensation in the stomach that eating can relieve. He salivates excessively.

Tabacum symptoms include deathly nausea, possibly even worse than that of the other two medicines. The patient is cold and pale, and his body is bathed in cold perspiration. He suffers from violent vomiting with renewed retching every time he moves. His symptoms are particularly worse in warmth and are better in the open air, when the eyes are closed, and in a quiet, dark environment. Occasionally he'll feel better after he uncovers the abdomen.

All of the above medicines are lesser-known homeopathic remedies and may be hard to come by. *Nux vomica* is a more commonly used medicine that also fits many of the symptoms of motion sickness. There is constant nausea, a splitting headache, and buzzing in the ears. More information on *Nux* appears earlier in this chapter and in the *materia medica* section toward the end of the book.

CHAPTER 9

WOMEN'S HEALTH PROBLEMS

H OMEOPATHIC MEDICINE COMPLEMENTS other self-care measures for women's health needs. Self-care with homeopathy can be very effective for some simple women's problems, and in this chapter we will cover three particularly common conditions: vaginal inflammation, menstrual cramps, and cystitis. Women with many other gynecological problems also can be helped with homeopathy, but those with more complex conditions such as irregular periods, abnormal menstrual bleeding, ovarian cysts, uterine fibroids, breast conditions, sexual difficulties, and so on should receive treatment from a professional homeopathic practitioner.

The homeopath values the symptoms of the reproductive system as some of the more important clues about the well-being of the whole person. The health of the reproductive system is a direct reflection of the delicate balance and dynamic interplay between two of the more central regulatory mechanisms of the body, the hormonal and nervous systems.

The drugs and surgery used in conventional medicine to treat women's problems can alleviate symptoms, but they do not remedy the underlying disharmony. Conventional treatment of some women's disorders, especially serious infections and cancerous conditions, clearly is sometimes necessary. Nevertheless, we believe it is preferable whenever possible to seek homeopathic care that encourages true healing before resorting to suppressive treatments.

Commonly given hormonal medications—estrogens and progestins—deserve special comment. These are given for a variety of conditions, including menstrual irregularity and abnormal bleeding. Homeopaths are wary of such treatments that simply mask symptoms without restoring health. When the symptoms are no longer clearly apparent, it can be much harder to choose the correct homeopathic medicine. In addition, the body must compensate for the presence of the medicine in the system and for the changes in body chemistry it causes.

Hormone treatment makes most sense when given to replace natural hormones the body can no longer make following menopause, or after surgery that removes the ovaries. Even then, of course, these medications work only for as long as they are taken—they don't cure the underlying cause of the deficiency. Still, many women find them extremely helpful in mitigating the symptoms that result from reduced levels of hormones, such as hot flashes and irritability. And there is increasing evidence suggesting that following menopause, replacement estrogen can be helpful in preventing osteoporosis and heart disease. A decision to take replacement hormones may make sense for many women and does not usually interfere with homeopathic treatment.

VAGINITIS

The lining of the vagina is a mucous membrane similar to the inside of the mouth. It is kept moist by secretions from cells in the membrane. The amount of fluid secreted by these cells changes in relation to the phase of the menstrual cycle and in response to sexual excitement. In addition, the cervix secretes liquid material that varies also in quantity and consistency during the menstrual cycle. Thus, the vagina normally contains small to moderate amounts of liquid. At certain times of the month, the accumulation can be great enough to be noticed as a discharge, even when there is no infection or other problem with the vagina.

Abnormal discharge with vaginal inflammation or infection is termed vaginitis. There may be a substantial increase in the discharge; a change in its color, consistency, or odor; or accompanying symptoms such as itching or soreness. Sometimes the latter symptoms occur even though there is no appreciable discharge.

Prior to menopause, the more common causes of vaginal inflammation are infections. Like the mouth and skin, the vagina is normally populated by a variety of microorganisms that serve to discourage infection. These "good" organisms control infectious germs by competing with them for food, by maintaining a chemical environment that inhibits their growth, and by forming a protective physical barrier. The vaginal lining also has a variety of immune defenses to further defend against infection. Women who have passed menopause or whose ovaries have been removed often experience vaginitis because of the reduced supply of hormones needed to maintain the vaginal tissues.

Vaginal infections begin when these normal protective mechanisms are disrupted. Contributing causes can include physiological imbalance, friction (as in vigorous sexual activity), antibiotics that kill the good organisms, medications that alter hormone balance, or chemical irritation caused by diaphragm jelly or other products. Even wearing restrictive clothing or underwear made of synthetic materials may alter the vaginal environment enough to allow infection.

Of course, the infecting organism is part of the process too. Most types of vaginal infections are sexually transmitted diseases, although the *Candida* fungus normally is present in the vagina in small numbers. Short of abstinence, the best way to avoid sexually transmitted diseases is by practicing safer sex, which includes limiting the number of sexual partners, selecting them carefully, and using condoms correctly until you've been in a long-term, strictly monogamous relationship with no evidence of STDs in either partner. These measures do not guarnatee you will escape infection, but they will improve your chances dramatically. At any rate, if you do have a vaginal infection, simultaneous treatment of your sexual partner may be necessary.

There are several common types of vaginal infections. Yeast, or monilial, infections are caused by the same fungal organism, *Candida albicans,* responsible for thrush in the mouth and for yeast rashes on the skin. This organism is actually a normal inhabitant of the human body and ordinarily lives in harmony with other microbes of the vagina. But when an imbalance occurs, the yeast invades the vaginal lining and reproduces rapidly. The infection, coupled with the body's reaction, produces the familiar symptoms of yeast vaginitis: thick, creamy or curdy, whitish discharge, often accompanied by itching or redness and rawness of the external genitals.

Bacterial infections of the vaginal lining also are common. The type of bacteria most frequently found in association with vaginal infections has been given various names (including *Hemophilus*), but is now called *Gardnerella.* Various other bacteria are sometimes found in association with vaginitis.

The third common cause of vaginal infection is the *Trichomonas* organism, an amoebalike microbe much larger than bacteria. *Trichomonas* infections typically result in a yellowish or greenish, sometimes frothy vaginal discharge. Often the cervix is involved in the infection and appears irregularly raw and reddened.

More serious infections of the female reproductive organs do occur, and they are not at all rare. When bacteria such as *Gonococcus* (which causes gonorrhea) or *Chlamydia* infect the cervix, uterus, or fallopian tubes, symptoms range from none at all or mild vaginal discharge to pelvic inflammation and pain, severe infection with pus cavities, and symptoms of general illness. If untreated, these infections can result in infertility due to scarring within the fallopian tubes, and they can be passed on to your sexual partner.

Vaginal inflammation and discharge can occur also without an infection, or when infection plays only a minor role in causing the symptoms. Mechanical or chemical irritation brings the body's local defenses into play to protect the tissues. Specific causes of such irritation include vigorous sexual activity, substances in products such as diaphragm jelly, feminine hygiene products, or tampons and foreign objects in the vagina. Vaginal discharges that result from forgetting to remove a tampon also are fairly common. In such cases, the vaginal lining becomes red and swollen with extra blood, and secretions increase as an effort is made to flush the irritation away. Infection may result if the irritation allows germs to enter the tissues, but discomfort and a discharge don't necessarily mean an infection is present.

GENERAL HOME CARE

If you're experiencing the early stages of mild vaginitis, you can certainly begin treatment at home. You don't have to know exactly what's causing the symptoms as long as you observe the guidelines in "Beyond Home Care." Even if you end up seeing your practitioner and perhaps receiving treatment, many of these self-care guidelines probably will apply.

First, consider whether or not there is something responsible for the vaginal-tissue irritation. Be sure you haven't left a tampon in place. If you've recently begun using a spermicidal jelly, contraceptive device, or vaginal deodorant, you may want to experiment with different brands or just avoid these things for a while to see if the irritation stops.

Remember to avoid synthetic fabrics in underwear, since these materials don't allow enough air to circulate. Loose-fitting clothing is preferable when possible.

Getting plenty of rest, limiting stress, and eating right often make the difference in how quickly and completely vaginitis resolves. Diet has proven especially important to many women who have found that eating well-balanced meals and avoiding sweets in particular were helpful in preventing vaginal infections.

One of the specific measures more effective in helping heal vaginitis is using a vinegar douche, prepared by diluting two tablespoons of either white or apple cider vinegar in a pint of warm water, twice a day at first and then once a day as the symptoms improve. The healthy vagina is slightly acidic, and maintaining an acid pH by using vinegar helps promote the growth of the normal microorganisms that protect the lining and inhibit the growth of bacteria and *Trichomonas*. Yeast organisms prefer a more acidic environment, but vinegar has the specific ability to inhibit their growth. In addition, the douche cleanses the vagina of the overgrowth of infectious organisms. Douche only when you already have vaginitis; avoid routine douching when you don't have symptoms, since it may cause irritation leading to vaginitis.

Another treatment for vaginitis some women have found effective involves garlic. You can use garlic as a vaginal suppository by peeling off the clove's outer skin (while leaving the last thin layer of the skin intact) and inserting the clove into the vagina for twelve hours. Alternatively, you can place a crushed clove of garlic in vinegar and then, after straining the vinegar to remove the bits of garlic, use this liquid for a douche.

Trichomonas infections are particularly resistant to self-care measures. Some women have tried douching with strong chaparral tea *(Larrea divaricata),* though results have been inconsistent.

Medical treatments for common vaginal infections vary with the infectious organisms. Fungal infections are treated with antifungal vaginal suppositories and creams; oral medications are now being used as well. Metronidazole (Flagyl) is given orally for both *Trichomonas* and *Gardnerella* bacterial infections. Generally, oral tetracycline-type drugs are used to treat *Chlamydia* infection.

CASETAKING QUESTIONS FOR VAGINITIS

Character of the symptoms:
- What is the color and consistency of the vaginal discharge?
- Are the tissues irritated, red, or swollen?
- Is there much itching or a strong odor?
- Is the woman pregnant?

Modalities:
- At what time of day is the discharge heaviest?
- How do walking and lying down affect the discharge?
- In relation to the menstrual cycle, when is the discharge worse (just before, just after, or between the periods)?

Other symptoms:
- Is there pain or other discomfort in the pelvic area? In the back?

Home treatment with homeopathy is indicated if you have no major health conditions and if your symptoms are not recurrent. During a vaginal infection, pay close attention to your symptoms before you use any douche or other treatment, since the original symptoms determine the choice of the correct medicine.

Kreosote is the first medicine to consider when the discharge causes or is associated with great irritation and rawness of the vagina and external genitals, though other remedies also cover this symptom. There is much soreness, smarting, burning, and itching in the tissues, and they become noticeably red and swollen with the inflammation. *Kreosote* discharges generally have a very foul smell. The discharge may be increased in the morning and upon standing, and less severe when the patient is sitting or lying down. In some cases it is intermittent, returning again as bad as ever after nearly ceasing.

Pulsatilla is useful to women with white vaginal discharges that have a consistency like milk or cream. Yellow discharges also are covered if the general symptoms suggest this medicine. The discharge may be either bland or irritating. It is one of the medicines appropriate for women with vaginitis during pregnancy (as are *Kreosote* and *Sepia*) or for pubescent girls with this problem (as are *Calcarea* and *Sepia*). Lying down may cause an increase in the discharge.

Calcarea carb. suits women with thick discharges that are either white or yellow. The discharge is likely to cause intense itching of the genitals. The flow of the discharge may come in sporadic gushes (as with *Graphites* and *Sepia*). This medicine may be indicated for young girls with vaginitis. Usually the choice of this medicine is confirmed by its general symptoms.

Graphites is indicated for the woman with a thin, white, and burning discharge, especially when it occurs in large, periodic gushes. Weakness of the back or tension in the abdomen may accompany the vaginitis. Walking may increase the discharge, and also it may be worse in the morning (as with *Sepia* and *Kreosote*).

Sepia's most striking characteristic is a flow that is yellowish or greenish, but *Sepia* may suit women with almost any kind of flow. Offensive odor is typical of *Sepia* cases. The symptoms usually become worse shortly before the menstrual periods or midway between them. As with *Graphites,* the *Sepia* discharge is likely to be more profuse in the morning and during walking. Sensations of uncomfortable pressure and weight ("bearing-down" pains) in the pelvic organs and lower abdomen are common in women who need *Sepia*. If no other symptoms suggest another medicine, give *Sepia* first when treating a child with vaginitis.

Another important medicine indicated when the discharge is acrid, irritating, and offensive-smelling is *Nitric acid*. The *Nitric acid*-type discharge is greenish, brownish, tan-colored, or sometimes like transparent, stringy mucus. Aggravation soon after the menstrual period is characteristic.

Borax is indicated when the vaginal discharge is clear and thick, like the white of an egg, or is thick and white, like liquid starch or sometimes even like white paste. The discharge may be bland or may irritate the genitals. A sensation of warmth may accompany the discharge, perhaps as if warm water is flowing over the organs. Sometimes the discharge is worse midway between the menstrual periods (as with *Calcarea, Kreosote,* and *Sepia*). General symptoms of this medicine include a dread of downward motion and a marked sensitivity to sudden noises; however, these symptoms need not be present in every case.

REMEDY SUMMARY FOR VAGINITIS

Give the medicine: One to 3 times a day, depending on severity of the symptoms, for up to 3 days. Stop as soon as the symptoms seem to be improving or changing substantially.

When to try another medicine: Allow 2 to 3 days without medicine before going on to another one if the first remedy doesn't seem to help.

KREOSOTE ★

Essentials
- Great irritation and rawness of the vagina and external genitals; tissues are sore, smarting, burning, and/or itching, and are red and swollen
- Offensive odor

Confirmatory symptoms
- Discharge increased in the morning and upon standing; much decreased when sitting or lying down
- Intermittent discharge

SEPIA

Essentials
- Yellowish or greenish discharge
- Offensive odor
- When treating a child with vaginitis if symptoms aren't decisive for another medicine

Confirmatory symptoms
- Discharge worse shortly before or midway between the periods
- Discharge more profuse in the morning and during walking
- Sensation of uncomfortable pressure and weight ("bearing-down" pains) in the pelvic organs and lower abdomen

CALCAREA CARBONICA

Essentials
- Thick discharge, either white or yellow
- Intense itching of the genitals (may be worse after urinating)
- Women with the general symptoms of *Calcarea* (see *materia medica* section)

Confirmatory symptoms
- Flow of the discharge comes in gushes
- Vaginitis in young girls

GRAPHITES

Essentials
- Thin, white, burning discharge

- Discharge comes in large gushes

Confirmatory symptoms
- Discharge increased from walking
- Discharge worse in the morning
- Weakness of the back or tension in the abdomen

BORAX

Essentials
- Discharge thick and clear, like the white of an egg, or thick and white, like liquid starch or white paste

Confirmatory symptoms
- Sensation of warmth, perhaps as if warm water is flowing over the genitals
- Discharge is worse midway between the menstrual periods
- Dread of downward motion
- Marked sensitivity to sudden noises

NITRIC ACID

Essentials
- Discharge is greenish, brownish, tan-colored, or of transparent, stringy mucus
- Discharge is acrid, irritating, and offensive smelling

Confirmatory symptoms
- Discharge worse after the menstrual period

PULSATILLA

Essentials
- White discharge with consistency of milk or cream
  or
- Any type of discharge if the typical general symptoms of this medicine are strongly present: weepy, clingy mood, craving affection; changeable moods; thirstless; worse in a warm room

Confirmatory symptoms
- Discharge increased from lying down
- Vaginitis during pregnancy
- Vaginitis in young girls

BEYOND HOME CARE

See "Beyond Home Care" following "Menstrual Cramps and Premenstrual Syndrome."

MENSTRUAL CRAMPS AND PREMENSTRUAL SYNDROME (PMS)

Many women experience discomfort of one sort or another in association with their menstrual periods. Cyclic recurrences of symptoms such as uterine cramping, leg or back pain, nausea or diarrhea, bloating, swelling and tenderness of the breasts, irritability and depression, fatigue and listlessness, dizziness, rashes or pimples, and headaches may come before, during, or after the period, usually following a characteristic pattern for each woman.

There are many possible contributing causes for menstrual discomfort. Regulation of the phases of the menstrual cycle involves an intricate balance of complex physiological functions. There are cyclic variations in hormone levels, blood flow, nervous system function, prostaglandin levels, and so forth. Any imbalance may result in disordered menstrual function.

Unresolved emotional conflict may predispose some women to menstrual difficulties, acute or chronic. In other women, structural changes in the reproductive tract such as development of uterine fibroids or endometriosis make the menstrual periods painful. Substances in the body called prostaglandins have been blamed for much of the trouble with difficult periods, but from the homeopathic viewpoint, the prostaglandin disorder is really a *symptom* of a deeper imbalance.

GENERAL HOME CARE

Reducing stress levels may help prevent menstrual discomfort. Once you have cramps or other symptoms, certainly you should rest and take it easy as much as possible. Heat may bring some relief. Many women find that exercise during menstrual cramping also helps. Attention to general good nutrition can help minimize menstrual problems. In addition, some women have found that specific dietary measures including limiting intake of salt and dairy products reduce symptoms. Calcium and magnesium supplements may help as well; recommended amounts and proportions of these two nutrients depend on the individual's symptoms.

CASETAKING QUESTIONS FOR MENSTRUAL CRAMPS

Character of the symptoms:
* How would you describe the pains?
* Where are the pains felt? Do they extend or radiate?
* Is there a feeling of weight or pressure in the pelvis or lower abdomen?

Modalities:
* In relation to the menstrual cycle, when is the pain worse (before or during the periods)? Is the pain relieved when the menstrual flow starts?
* How does motion, being jarred, bending over, or walking affect the pain?
* How is the pain affected by heat, coldness, or warm rooms?
* Does pressure on the abdomen relieve or worsen the symptoms? How about light touch?

Other symptoms:
* Is there lower back pain?
* What other symptoms accompany the cramping?

HOMEOPATHIC MEDICINES

Though symptoms may be relieved by taking conventional medicines that, for example, block the action of prostaglandin, menstrual problems are not caused by simply one chemical abnormality that can be "fine-tuned" at will with drugs. In contrast, homeopathic constitutional treatment can catalyze a response of the entire system so that a better overall balance is achieved.

Recurrent menstrual cramps and other chronic difficulties associated with periods are best treated constitutionally. In some cases, even symptoms that are blamed on structural abnormalities resolve with homeopathic treatment. If constitutional care is not available, it is certainly acceptable to use homeopathic self-care when symptoms are acute. If you are under constitutional treatment already, however, you should not take homeopathic medicines without first consulting your homeopath.

Belladonna is commonly indicated for women suffering acute pain with their periods. The pains tend to begin suddenly and end just as suddenly. They may take the form of cramps or something like labor pains. There also may be a feeling of intense weight and pressure in the lower abdomen and pelvis, sometimes as though the pelvic organs are about to fall out. *Belladonna* patients with these bearing-down pains get relief from applying pressure to the genitals or abdomen. No matter what type of pain the woman has, *Belladonna* is indicated when motion, walking, or being jarred worsen it. Sitting bent over aggravates the pain, whereas straightening up makes it better. Pain may extend from the region of the uterus to the back. Pain in the ovaries before or during the menstrual period (again, if it is made worse by motion or jarring) is also typical of *Belladonna*. Headaches before and during the menstrual periods are common (see chapter 11 on headaches).

If you have menstrual cramps that are unaccompanied by other symptoms and are relieved from pressure or warmth, either *Magnesia phosphorica* or *Colocynthis* is your choice. *Magnesia phos.* may bring relief if your menstrual pains are cramping in character or feel like the pains of childbirth, and if they are relieved by warmth, pressure, and bending forward. The pain centered in the uterus may radiate in all directions.

Colocynthis has nearly identical indications, with the pain being relieved by doubling up, pressure, and warmth. With *Colocynthis,* the relief from pressure and especially from doubling over tends to be more prominent, whereas relief from warmth is generally more obvious when the remedy is *Magnesia phos.* (since this can be a subtle distinction, you may need to switch from one of these medicines to the other). *Colocynthis* also covers sharp pains in the ovaries, especially when they occur shortly before the period. The *Colocynthis* patient is more likely to be irritable or angry than the woman who needs *Magnesia phos.* The cramps may have begun after the patient became angry or after she suppressed angry feelings (see also the paragraph on *Chamomilla* if irritability is prominent).

Cimicifuga covers menstrual cramps that make the patient double over with pain. The particular indications for this medicine are sharp pains that dart from side to side in the abdomen, and marked lower back pain during the flow. Motion aggravates the pain.

Chamomilla is selected during menstrual distress largely on the basis of the patient's mood. Marked irritability, such as faultfinding or snapping over little things, is typical, and the patient may become openly angry. Sometimes the pains seem to develop after the patient gets angry. If these emotional changes are the predominant symptoms, give *Chamomilla* first; *Colocynthis* is indicated when the irritability is present in addition to that remedy's other characteristic symptoms, or if *Chamomilla* doesn't help. *Chamomilla* menstrual pains may be felt so acutely that they cause the woman to cry out. They feel like cramps or labor pains. Many remedies cover menstrual cramps that feel like labor pains, but *Chamomilla* fits this symptom better than any other homeopathic medicine. Sensations of weight and bearing down also may occur in the pelvis. The pains are relieved by warmth.

The woman who needs *Pulsatilla* also may be irritable during her period, but not with the same angry intensity of the *Chamomilla* patient. She is sensitive, moody, weepy, or depressed, and perhaps a bit touchy, but she wants and appreciates gentle comforting. The menstrual pains may be of nearly any type and may be worse before or during the flow. They are sometimes bad enough to cause the woman to cry out or moan. Many other symptoms associated with periods may occur. Dizziness, fainting, nausea, vomiting, diarrhea, back pain, and headaches preceding or accompanying menstruation all are covered by *Pulsatilla*. Also, the woman has no thirst; heat worsens her condition, and open air makes it better.

The strongest indication for the self-care use of *Lachesis* is that the symptoms are relieved when the menstrual flow begins. This keynote characteristic pertains to any of the various symptoms that *Lachesis* suits: uterine pains, ovarian pain (especially on the left side), back pain, dizziness, headaches, and diarrhea. All of these may be severe before the period and then suddenly better once menstruation actually starts. Uterine cramps and soreness are likely to be made worse from the pressure of clothing on the abdomen, especially tight belts or elastic bands. The pains may extend into the upper abdomen or chest. Classic *Lachesis* symptoms begin or worsen during sleep or immediately upon wakening.

Caulophyllum should be considered when cramping pains are particularly bad before the period starts, though there is less immediate relief from the onset of the flow than with *Lachesis*. Pain in the small of the back or dizziness also may precede menstruation.

REMEDY SUMMARY FOR MENSTRUAL CRAMPS

Give the medicine: Up to every 4 hours or so during acute menstrual discomfort, repeating only when symptoms return.
When to try another medicine: If you find no relief after 6 to 8 hours.

BELLADONNA ★

Essentials
- Pains begin and end suddenly
- Cramping or laborlike pains
- Worse from motion, walking, or being jarred

Confirmatory symptoms
- Sensation of intense weight and pressure in the lower abdomen and pelvis, sometimes as though the pelvic organs are about to fall out; relieved by applying pressure to the genitals or abdomen
- Pain extends from the uterus to the back
- Pain in the ovaries before or during the menstrual period
- Pain aggravated by sitting bent over, better from straightening up
- Headaches before and during periods

MAGNESIA PHOS.

Essentials
- Relief from pressure or warmth
- Pains cramping in character or feel like the pains of childbirth

Confirmatory symptoms
- Relief from bending forward
- Pain centered in the uterus, radiating in all directions

COLOCYNTHIS

Essentials
- Relief from doubling up, pressure, and warmth
- Sharp pains in the ovarian region, especially occurring shortly before the period

Confirmatory symptoms
- Irritable or angry mood; cramps may begin after patient becomes angry or suppresses angry feelings

CIMICIFUGA

Essentials
- Sharp pains darting from side to side
  and/or
- Lower back pain during the flow

Confirmatory symptoms
- Pains force the woman to double over (but doubling over doesn't necessarily relieve the pain)
- Pain aggravated by motion

CHAMOMILLA

Essentials
- Intense pain causes crying out
- Marked irritability or anger

Confirmatory symptoms
- Best medicine for menstrual cramps that feel like labor pains
- Sensation of weight or bearing down
- Pains come on after getting angry
- Relief from warmth

LACHESIS

Essentials
- Pain and other premenstrual symptoms (see text) improve dramatically when the menstrual flow begins
- Symptoms worse from touch or pressure, even of clothing

Confirmatory symptoms
- Left-sided pain; pain in region of left ovary
- Pains extending into upper abdomen or chest
- Symptoms begin or worsen during sleep or immediately upon wakening

PULSATILLA

Essentials
- Weepy, clingy mood, craving affection; changeable moods; may be irritable, but not with angry intensity; thirstless; worse in a warm room

Confirmatory symptoms
- Pains worse before or during the flow
- Pains cause the woman to cry out or moan
- Other symptoms before or during the period, including dizziness, fainting, nausea, vomiting, diarrhea, back pain, or headaches

CAULOPHYLLUM

Essentials
- Cramping pains worse before the menstrual flow begins (better but not immediately relieved after the flow starts)

Confirmatory symptoms
- Pain in the small of the back
  and/or
- Dizziness before the period starts

BEYOND HOME CARE

GET MEDICAL CARE IMMEDIATELY:

- if there is severe pain (other than menstrual cramps) in the pelvic organs or abdomen.

GET MEDICAL CARE TODAY:

- if there is significant lower abdominal pain (not menstrual cramps), especially when accompanied by fever or vaginal discharge or bleeding. See the section on abdominal pain in chapter 8;
- if there is vaginal discharge with lower abdominal pain or fever, or if it comes after you or a partner have had recent new sexual contact;
- if a girl develops a significant vaginal discharge or irritation before puberty;
- if there are sores on or in the genitals or nearby areas, unless they are definitely recurrences of previously diagnosed herpes, or if there are any shallow open sores anywhere on the body that are not wounds;
- if you have had sexual contact with someone known to have or suspected of having gonorrhea, syphilis, a *Chlamydia* infection, AIDS, or any other major sexually transmitted disease;
- if there is heavy vaginal bleeding, even without pain, between the menstrual periods (see below for milder bleeding).

SEE YOUR PRACTITIONER SOON:

- if there has been persistent or recurrent painless vaginal bleeding between the periods. If the bleeding lasts longer than 10 days or recurs more than 3 months in a row, you need medical attention. If there is pain with the bleeding, seek care *now.* Very mild bleeding or "spotting" between the periods is common and is not a danger sign unless it is persistent or recurrent;
- in post-menopausal women, if there is *any* vaginal bleeding;
- if there has been heavy vaginal discharge or significant genital irritation, or if a mild vaginal discharge lasts longer than 2 weeks;
- if there has been unusually heavy menstrual bleeding every month, or if you have severe menstrual cramps recurrently.

CYSTITIS (BLADDER INFECTION)

Fifteen percent of all adult women get repeated cystitis, or bladder infections, and such infections are fairly common in girls as well. Symptoms include a burning pain during urination, a frequent and powerful urge to urinate though little urine may be passed, and cloudy or bloody urine. Pain or tenderness in the lower abdomen or the back, fever, and a general feeling of illness also may accompany cystitis, although symptoms may be completely absent.

The reasons females are so susceptible to urinary infections are that the urethra, the tube connecting the bladder to the outside of the body, is only a half-inch long and that the opening of the urethra is close to the anus. Bacteria from the intestinal tract can easily travel to the urethra and then into the bladder, where they can infect susceptible tissues. Bladder infections are more likely to occur after sexual activity or improper hygiene, which allows germs to spread to the urethra. Anything that irritates the urethral tissue, such as an improperly fitted diaphragm, spermicidal jelly, or tight-fitting clothing, may weaken resistance to infection. Urinary tract infections are more frequent also during pregnancy.

So long as the infection is confined to the urethra and bladder, cystitis may be uncomfortable but it's not dangerous. If the danger signs discussed in the "Beyond Home Care" section aren't present, you can use home treatment and homeopathy for a day or two before calling on your health-care provider.

Occasionally, however, the infection spreads into the kidneys or bloodstream. Kidney infection—with its high fever, marked weakness, and back pain—can be a serious illness. But of greater concern is that inflammation occurring during a kidney infection can result in permanent damage to the kidneys. Uncommonly, bacteria from a urinary infection spread into the blood, causing a serious generalized illness.

Conventional medical treatment for a urinary tract infection involves antibiotics. If antibiotics are prescribed, your health practitioner may recommend that you return for follow-up tests, since recurrences are fairly common and sometimes have no symptoms. Antibiotic treatment for acute infections does nothing to prevent future bouts.

Some women experience the symptoms of cystitis but do not have a bacterial infection. The symptoms may be related to viral infections, caffeine, chronic inflammation of unknown cause, or emotional stress. Antibiotics are not helpful in such cases. If symptoms are recurrent or severe, your health practitioner may recommend special tests to clarify the diagnosis.

GENERAL HOME CARE

Many urinary infections can be prevented by simple self-care measures. Hygiene is important. Always wipe from front to back after using the toilet, and be sure to change tampons or sanitary napkins frequently during menstruation. Drink lots of fluids, and urinate often, at least every two hours, to help wash germs out of the urethra. Urinating as soon as possible after lovemaking is especially important. Avoid potential irritants such as deodorant tampons, feminine hygiene products, and strong or perfumed soaps and bubble baths. Use cotton underwear. Avoid caffeine, which may irritate urinary tract tissues. Diaphragms should be fitted properly to prevent pressure on the urethra. If you use birth control pills, get a low- or no-estrogen kind.

If you do begin to notice symptoms, immediately begin drinking more liquids to dilute the bacteria in the bladder and flush them out. If your general health is good, you should drink *lots* of water or juice—get in a few gallons during the first day or so if you can (people with chronic illnesses such as heart or kidney problems should not increase their fluid intake except under medical supervision). Making the urine more acidic by drinking plenty of unsweetened cranberry juice or by taking vitamin C (the ascorbic acid form, not ascorbate) helps slow down the reproduction of the bacteria.

CASETAKING QUESTIONS FOR CYSTITIS

Character of the symptoms:
- Describe the urinary pains that are experienced.
- Where does it hurt (in the urethral opening, in the bladder)?
- Does the pain extend anywhere?
- How strong and frequent is the urge to urinate?
- Does the urine flow freely, or only in spurts or drops?
- Is a specific position necessary in order to urinate freely?
- Is there incontinence (involuntary urination)? When?

Modalities:
- At what time of day is the pain worse?
- In relation to urination, when is the pain most severe? At the beginning, during, or at the close of urination, or when not urinating?
- How does pressure, motion, lying down, or being jarred affect the symptoms?
- How does heat or cold affect the symptoms?

HOMEOPATHIC MEDICINES

As with many inflammatory conditions, *Aconite* should be considered during the earliest stages of a bladder infection. The patient may notice at first that it is difficult to pass urine, and then begins to experience burning pain during urination. At the same time, the general symptoms of *Aconite* may be developing (see the *materia medica* section).

Cantharis is the most commonly effective homeopathic medicine in treating those with urinary tract infections. Patients who need *Cantharis* have a frequent, strong urge to urinate, and a great deal of burning is felt during urination. The patient may be compelled to rush to the toilet, and the urgency may be such that she loses urine before she gets there. Despite the intolerable urging, however, urine may pass in drops only. Strong urging may be felt immediately after voiding or even while the patient is urinating. Tremendous burning, cutting, or stabbing pains are felt in the urethra and bladder before, during, and after urination, or along with the urge to urinate. The patient is restless, even frantic, with the severe pain. Sexual desire may be increased.

Nux vomica also fits well the typical symptoms of bladder infection.

Characteristic urinary symptoms of *Nux* include pain in the bladder or urethra before or during urination, and needlelike pains in the urethra extending back toward the bladder. Sometimes a strong urge to have a bowel movement accompanies the urinary urging and pain. *Nux* may be given also on the basis of its general characteristics (see the *materia medica* section). The woman may experience her urinary symptoms after excesses of food, alcohol, coffee, or drugs.

Mercurius may be indicated during a bladder infection if the symptoms are worse at night, or if the general symptoms of the medicine are clearly present. All the typical symptoms of cystitis are covered by *Mercurius,* including burning, uncontrollable urges, dark urine, and passage of urine in small amounts. *Mercurius* is one of the few medicines indicated when burning pain is worse when the patient is not urinating; burning may be severe also just before urination, upon beginning to urinate, or when the last drops are passed.

Sarsaparilla should be considered when the most severe pain in the urethra comes at the end of urination. It may not be burning in character. The bladder is less likely to be painful than it is in the *Cantharis* or *Nux* patient. Sometimes the patient can urinate only in dribbles while sitting down, and must stand up to get urine to flow freely.

Staphysagria is indicated when a woman experiences a bladder infection shortly after sexual activity, especially when no other remedy is clearly indicated. It is indicated also when a bladder infection is experienced soon after the woman is physically or emotionally abused, or after some type of serious embarrassment. A keynote physical symptom of women who need this remedy is the sensation that a drop of urine is continually rolling through the urethra.

Berberis should be considered when there are pains during or after urination, cutting or shooting either from the bladder to the urethra or from the urethra to the pelvis, thighs, or back. Motion may bring on pain. The patient may also experience pain in the back in the area of the kidneys or ureters (the tubes carrying urine from the kidneys to the bladder), pain that worsens with pressure, motion, or jarring.

Pulsatilla is used more often to treat women who have cystitis as well as the classic *Pulsatilla* disposition. Although the pain may not be quite as intense as that of the *Cantharis* patient, there is significant smarting and burning. Lying on the back may aggravate the urging enough to rouse the patient from sleep if she turns from her side onto her back. Urine may pass only in dribbles, and there may be involuntary dribbling at the slightest provocation, including coughing, sneezing, laughing, or being surprised.

Apis should be considered when treating people who have cystitis with severe pain and urging similar to those described for *Cantharis*. The burning and especially stinging pains are worse in the heat and at night, and better in cold. Though there is violent urging, the patient must strain to urinate, and the urine passes only in drops. The abdomen is sensitive to the slightest touch.

Though it has few distinguishing symptoms, *Equisetum* often is helpful during acute bladder infections. Bladder pain is prominent, especially after urinating.

REMEDY SUMMARY FOR CYSTITIS

Give the medicine: Every 6 to 8 hours for up to 3 days, stopping as soon as the symptoms significantly change.
When to try another medicine: If you find no relief after 24 hours.

CANTHARIS ★

Essentials
- Frequent, strong urge to urinate
- Great burning or cutting pains before, during, or after urination

Confirmatory symptoms
- Urine passes in drops only
- Strong urging during urination
- Severe pain making patient restless, frantic
- Increased sexual desire

ACONITE

Essentials
- Earliest stages of a bladder infection, with first signs of difficult or painful urination

Confirmatory symptoms
- General symptoms of *Aconite*: anxiety, fear, restlessness

SARSAPARILLA

Essentials
- Severe pain in the urethra at the end of urination

Confirmatory symptoms
- While sitting, patient can urinate only in dribbles; must stand up to urinate freely

MERCURIUS

Essentials
- General symptoms of *Mercurius* are present (see *materia medica* section)

Confirmatory symptoms
- Burning pain in the urethra worse when the patient is not urinating; just before urination, upon beginning to urinate, or when the last drops are passed
- Symptoms worse at night

NUX VOMICA

Essentials
- Symptoms begin after excesses of food, alcohol, coffee, or drugs, or other general symptoms of *Nux* are present (see *materia medica* section)
  or
- Pain in the urethra and/or bladder before or during urination, or during urge to urinate

Confirmatory symptoms
- Urge for bowel movement accompanies painful urge to urinate
- Needlelike pains in the urethra extending back toward the bladder

APIS

Essentials
- Stinging or burning pains, worse in the heat, better in cold
  or
- Severe pain and urging
- If *Cantharis* doesn't help and no other remedy is clearly indicated

Confirmatory symptoms
- Symptoms worse at night
- Abdomen sensitive to the slightest touch

STAPHYSAGRIA

Essentials
- Bladder infection that follows sexual activity if other remedies don't seem clearly indicated or haven't helped
- Bladder infection that follows physical or emotional abuse or some type of great embarrassment

Confirmatory symptoms
- Sensation that a drop of urine is continually rolling through the urethra

BERBERIS

Essentials
- Pain in the back in the area of the ureters or kidneys, worse with pressure, motion, or jarring
  or
- Pains during or after urination extending from the bladder to the urethra, or from the urethra to the pelvis, thighs, or back

PULSATILLA

Essentials
- General symptoms of *Pulsatilla* are prominent (see *materia medica* section)

Confirmatory symptoms
- Urging worse lying on the back or turning from side onto the back
- Involuntary dribbling from coughing, sneezing, laughing, or surprise

EQUISETUM

Essentials
- Bladder pain worse especially after urination

Confirmatory symptoms
- Involuntary urination (incontinence), perhaps at night

BEYOND HOME CARE

GET MEDICAL CARE TODAY:

- in general, whenever there is onset of acute urinary symptoms: burning pain in the urinary passageway, frequent or strong urges to urinate, or definitely cloudy urine. Adults may postpone medical care for 48 hours if pain is slight, frequency is mild, and there are no other symptoms;
- if the patient who has urinary pain or who must urinate frequently is a diabetic or has a history of high blood pressure or kidney disease;
- for a child who has urinary pain or urinates frequently;
- if there is blood in the urine (the urine may look smoky red or brown);
- if there is headache, vomiting, back pain, muscular twitching, convulsions, or chills along with urinary tract pain;
- if there are sharp pains in the kidney area, located in the back above the lower ribs;
- if a fever accompanies urinary pain;
- if there is any swelling of the face, ankles, or abdomen.

SEE YOUR PRACTITIONER SOON:

- if there are any recurrent urinary symptoms;
- if there is significant weight change.

Note: If there is a vaginal discharge, consult "Beyond Home Care" for vaginitis.

CHAPTER 10

MEN'S HEALTH PROBLEMS

THE HEALTH OF the male reproductive system is a reflection of overall well-being as well as sexual habits. We cover common men's health concerns, including sexually transmitted diseases, urethritis, prostate problems, irritation of the foreskin, and less common serious problems of the testicles.

SEXUALLY TRANSMITTED DISEASES

Sexually transmitted diseases, or STDs, include about fifteen infectious illnesses that may be transmitted during lovemaking. Symptoms of these infections can include discharge from the penis, various kinds of eruptions or sores on the genitals or surrounding skin, and swelling of the lymph nodes in the groin. Any such symptom requires medical evaluation and treatment. Two of the more common STDs are genital herpes simplex and venereal warts; homeopathic treatment can be helpful during either of these infections and is discussed in chapter 13.

Serious illnesses such as AIDS and some forms of hepatitis also can be transmitted during sex. They are beyond the scope of homeopathic self-care.

Short of abstinence, the best way to avoid sexually transmitted diseases is by practicing safer sex, which includes limiting the number of sexual partners, selecting them carefully, and using condoms correctly until you've been in a long-term, strictly monogamous relationship with no evidence of STDs in either partner. These measures do not guarantee you will escape infections, but they will improve your chances dramatically.

URETHRITIS

Urethritis is an infection and inflammation of the lining of the urethra, the tube that runs the length of the penis carrying urine and semen. Urethritis is most often associated with sexually transmitted infections, though sometimes no infection can be documented. A variety of germs can infect the urethra and trigger the body's inflammatory response, which can result in symptoms of burning and stinging as well as discharge of mucus or pus.

The *Chlamydia* bacteria is one of the germs more frequently associated with urethritis. Occasionally this infection leads to chronic symptoms of urethral irritation and discharge, and to infections of the prostate or testicles. Of more concern, *Chlamydia* often is passed on to women, where it may cause infections of the female reproductive tract that result in pain and sterility.

The most worrisome infection of the urethra is gonorrhea, since the *Gonococcus* bacteria can spread to other parts of the body, causing general illness and infections in the large joints, usually elbows and knees. It, too, can cause serious infections in women. A gonorrhea infection of the urethra usually causes the penis to discharge a copious, thick, yellowish pus, along with burning pain at the opening of the urethra felt during urination especially. In some cases, however, the discharge may be watery, scanty, or completely nonexistent, and there may be no pain. Gonorrhea also can infect other mucous membranes. Gonorrhea infections of the throat and rectum after oral or anal sex are not uncommon. Rectal gonorrhea may result in pain or discharge of pus, or there may be no symptoms at all.

There are many other kinds of germs associated with urethritis in men. Most of these are not considered causes of other health problems, but they have not been well studied. Urethritis can sometimes be caused by physical irritation—by soap, for example—or it may occur after taking antibiotics. Health practitioners may give the diagnosis of "nonspecific urethritis" if no infection with *Chlamydia* or *Gonococcus* is found.

We want to point out that the symptoms of all urethral infections, even when caused by gonorrhea, are largely evidence of the body's efforts to heal and remove the aggressive germs. Inflammation brings blood to the area so that more white blood cells, antibodies, and other components of the body's immune system are available to help destroy the bacteria. The extra blood also helps carry away dead cells and speeds the replacing of tissue damaged by the infection. The discharge flushes away debris and dead bacteria and blood cells, as well as infecting germs. Still, we strongly recommend antibiotic treatment, along with homeopathic treatment, for anyone with gonorrhea or *Chlamydia* urethral infections.

Discharges are uncommon in children but may develop if a child has put something in the urethra. A child with a penile discharge needs medical care.

BLADDER INFECTIONS

Unlike women, men rarely get bladder infections (cystitis), because the male urethra is longer and not so near the anus. A bladder infection in a boy or man often is evidence that something is structurally wrong with the urinary organs, and he must be evaluated by a urologist.

GENERAL HOME CARE

Home treatment of urethritis should be begun whether or not you ultimately take antibiotics. Drink extra fluids and urinate frequently to wash the germs out of the urethra. You should pay attention to the general health practices of resting, eating a simple and nutritious diet, and avoiding stress, for these enable the body's own defenses better to fight the germs and heal the inflamed tissue.

CASETAKING QUESTIONS FOR URETHRITIS

Character of the symptoms:
- What is the color and consistency of the discharge from the penis?
- If there is pain, what is its character—cutting (sharp), burning, or otherwise?

Modalities:
- At what time of day are the symptoms worse?
- Is ejaculation painful?

Other symptoms:
- Does the urine smell unusually strong?

HOMEOPATHIC MEDICINES

Natrum muriaticum is one of the primary medicines for men with urethritis. The discharge is usually thin and clear, mucous, or milky in color. Sometimes a greenish discharge occurs. The discharge may appear clear when it is wet but then leaves yellow spots on the underwear. There may be cutting or burning pains at the urethral opening during or after urination, or just as urination is finished.

Pulsatilla should help men with thick yellow or green urethral discharge that is bland and causes little pain. The medicine's general symptoms may indicate its use more than the specific symptoms of the discharge.

Mercurius is indicated when thick mucus or pus is accompanied by inflammation and burning pain of the urethra. The discharge may be white, yellow, or green. Often the symptoms are worse at night.

Sulphur should be considered for thin or mucous discharges when there is burning pain during ejaculation or when the general symptoms of the medicine are evident (see the *materia medica* section).

Nitric acid is another alternative when the discharge is accompanied by burning pain during ejaculation. In this case, the discharge is more likely to be thick and greenish or yellowish. The urine may smell very strong, and the patient is usually chilly in general (whereas the *Sulphur* patient is "warm blooded"—that is, he is sensitive to or aggravated by heat, and tends to wear fewer clothes than others).

REMEDY SUMMARY FOR URETHRITIS

Even if antibiotics are prescribed, homeopathic medicines also should be given, particularly if symptoms continue after completing antibiotic treatment.

Give the medicine: Twice a day for up to 5 days. As soon as the symptoms have improved significantly, repeat the dose only when they worsen again.

When to try another medicine: If there is no improvement after 2 days (wait until the third day to make this decision).

NATRUM MURIATICUM ★

Essentials
• Thin discharge that is clear, mucous, or milky in color

Confirmatory symptoms
• Discharge appears clear when it is wet but leaves yellow spots on the underwear
• Cutting or burning pains at the urethral opening during or after urination, or just as urination is finished
• Painless discharge

MERCURIUS

Essentials
• Thick mucus or pus accompanied by inflammation and burning pain of the urethra

Confirmatory symptoms
• Discharge white, yellow, or green
• Symptoms often worse at night

SULPHUR

Essentials
• Thin or mucous discharges with burning pain during ejaculation
or
• The general symptoms of the medicine are evident (see *materia medica* section)

NITRIC ACID

Essentials
• Burning pain during ejaculation
• Thick greenish or yellowish discharge

Confirmatory symptoms
- Strong-smelling urine
- General chilliness

PULSATILLA

Essentials
- Thick yellow or green urethral discharge that is bland, causing little pain or irritation
  and/or
- The general symptoms of *Pulsatilla* are present (see *materia medica* section)

PROSTATE PROBLEMS

The walnut-size prostate is located at the floor of the pelvis behind the base of the penis. During ejaculation, the prostate contributes a milky alkaline fluid to the semen to enhance the fertility of the sperm. Several maladies involving the prostate are fairly common in men, including prostatitis (prostate infections), benign prostatic hypertrophy (prostate enlargement), and prostate cancer.

BENIGN PROSTATIC HYPERTROPHY

The prostate grows larger with age. Once a man reaches middle age, problems with urinating often result as swelling of the prostate gland constricts the urinary passage. This is called prostatic hypertrophy. There may be trouble getting the urinary stream started, or the stream may be weak or interrupted. Frequent urging to urinate, together with passing of only small amounts, also is common. These symptoms should be evaluated medically.

Constitutional homeopathic treatment can be helpful during the early stage of prostatic hypertrophy. Conventional treatments include various recently introduced medicines as well as surgical procedures.

PROSTATE CANCER

The treatment of cancer is beyond the scope of this book, but we do have a few words of advice: Since prostate cancer is one of the more common malignancies in men, regular contact with your doctor after the age of forty is wise, even if you have no symptoms. Screening tests for cancer include physical exam of the prostate, and a blood test for the prostate specific antigen (PSA). Although the value of screening for prostate cancer is controversial (the benefits of treating cancer detected by screening tests aren't clear), your practitioner will have some recommendations and can keep you informed of medical progress in this area.

Prostate cancer often is very slow-growing, and your doctor may not recommend specific treatment. Constitutional homeopathic care would be appropriate under these circumstances.

PROSTATITIS

Because the urethra passes through the prostate on its way from the bladder, bacteria can travel through the urethra and settle in the prostate. The prostate gland is susceptible both to acute infection and to chronic infection or inflammation. An acute infection can cause severe pain and tenderness in the region of the prostate, sometimes extending up into the genitals, pelvis, or back. Other symptoms can include increased urge to urinate, burning during urination, difficulty starting urination, discharge from the penis, and general symptoms such as fever and weakness.

Chronic inflammation of the prostate can develop after an acute infection or on its own. Symptoms are similar to but milder than those of acute infection, and tend to come and go over long periods. Vague aching in the region of the prostate, dribbling of urine, trouble starting or maintaining a forceful stream of urine, and discharge of prostatic fluid from the penis after a bowel movement, for instance, are common symptoms. Often it is impossible to identify the bacteria involved in chronic prostatitis; it may well be a self-perpetuating problem that persists even after infecting bacteria have been eliminated.

GENERAL HOME CARE

Home treatment for acute prostatitis includes drinking plenty of fluids, urinating frequently to help wash out the infecting bacteria, resting, eating a simple and nutritious diet, and avoiding stress.

Chronic prostatitis is difficult to cure completely. Still, the measures used for acute prostatitis can be helpful. In addition, hot sitz baths may bring some relief. Also you can try Kegel exercises as a mild form of self-massage to express excess fluid from the prostate and thereby reduce symptoms: Firmly tighten the muscles you would use to interrupt the flow of urine, repeating 50 to 100 times per day. Some urologists advise their patients to ejaculate regularly to expel some of the prostatic fluid and reduce pressure in the gland.

CASETAKING QUESTIONS FOR PROSTATITIS

Character of the symptoms:
- What is the character of the pain or discomfort—is it an ache, a sensation of pressure, or sharp pain like a needle?

Modalities:
- How is the pain affected by sitting, standing, walking, and urinating?

Other symptoms:
- Describe the color and consistency of any discharge from the penis. Is there pain in the urethra or bladder?

HOMEOPATHIC MEDICINES

During either acute or chronic prostatitis, homeopathic care can complement conventional medical treatment. In acute cases, you can use homeopathic medicines to speed the healing process while you take antibiotics. If symptoms persist after antibiotic treatment, or in chronic cases that have developed with no acute onset, you may try homeopathy instead of antibiotics (after seeing a health practitioner to rule out dangerous infections such as gonorrhea or *Chlamydia*). We recommend you see a professional homeopath if one is available, but if not, go ahead and try homeopathy at home.

Unfortunately for the homeopath, the typical case of prostatic trouble gives rise to few distinguishing symptoms that help in remedy selection. If no remedy stands out as a good match for the affected person's symptoms, you can try the ones listed below one at a time.

Pulsatilla is a good medicine for the man who experiences aggravation of pain in the prostate after urination. There may be sharp pains or spasms in the region of the prostate that extend into the bladder and pelvis. A thick, bland discharge from the penis may be present. Men who show strong general symptoms of this medicine can be given *Pulsatilla* even when the specific symptoms don't clearly confirm it.

Chimaphilla umbellato is more difficult to find—even at some home-opathic pharmacies— than most of the medicines covered here, but it is well indicated for many men with prostatitis. Soreness in the region of the gland is worse from pressure, especially during sitting. There may be a sensation of sitting on a ball or simply of painful swelling. A discharge of mucus from the penis or the presence of stringy mucus in the urine may be noted.

The *Kali bichromium* patient's prostate pain is worsened by walking, and he must stand still for relief. The pain may be needlelike, or there may be drawing pains extending from the prostate into the penis. There may be burning in the urethra after urination. A discharge of particularly thick, sticky, or stringy material may be found at the urethral opening.

With *Causticum* there are pressure and pulsations in the prostate, with pain extending into the urethra and bladder after a few drops of urine have passed. In contrast, *Lycopodium* covers pressure in the gland that is worse during and after urination. Needlelike pains in the bladder and anus especially indicate this medicine.

Sabal serrulata also has been found effective during prostatic prob-lems. However, its indications are fairly general: enlargement of the prostate with difficulty passing urine, or burning while urinating.

REMEDY SUMMARY FOR PROSTATITIS

Give the medicine: During acute symptoms, one dose twice a day for up to 5 days, less frequently as the symptoms improve. For chronic cases, one dose of the thirtieth potency per day for 5 days, or a low potency twice daily for up to 2 weeks.

When to try another medicine: In acute cases, if there is no im-provement after 36 to 48 hours. In chronic cases, if the symptoms haven't improved within 10 to 14 days.

PULSATILLA ★

Essentials
- Pain in the prostate after urination
  or

- The general symptoms of *Pulsatilla* are present (see *materia medica* section)

Confirmatory symptoms
- Sharp pains or spasms in prostate area extending into the bladder and pelvis
- Thick, bland discharge from the penis

CHIMAPHILLA UMBELLATO

Essentials
- Soreness in the region of the gland is worse from pressure, especially during sitting

Confirmatory symptoms
- Sensation of sitting on a ball or of painful swelling
- Discharge of mucus from the penis or the presence of stringy mucus in the urine

KALI BICHROMIUM

Essentials
- Prostate pain aggravated by walking; must stand still for relief

Confirmatory symptoms
- Needlelike pain or drawing pains extending from the prostate into the penis
- Burning in the urethra after urination
- Discharge of very thick, sticky, or stringy material from the penis

CAUSTICUM

Essentials
- Pressure and pulsations in the prostate, with pain extending into the urethra and bladder after a few drops of urine have passed

SABAL SERRULATA

Essentials
- Chronic prostatic enlargement with difficult urination; there may be burning during urination as well

LYCOPODIUM

Essentials
• Pressure in the prostate aggravated during and after urination

Confirmatory symptoms
• Needlelike pains in the bladder and anus

FORESKIN IRRITATION

If a skin irritation on or under the foreskin develops, you can treat it at home by gently pulling the foreskin back, applying dilute *Calendula* tincture (see chapter 14), and allowing the area to dry before returning the foreskin to its normal position. If a sexually active adult has sores or a rash, or if pus has formed, see your practitioner.

Occasionally the foreskin may get stuck in a retracted position and become swollen or inflamed. Apply ice wrapped in a cloth to the area and gently try to work the foreskin back into its normal position. If you are not immediately successful, emergency care is required.

TESTICULAR PROBLEMS

Pain or swelling in the testicles or vicinity requires medical attention. A variety of problems may cause such symptoms.

Epididymitis is an infection of the epididymis, a compact, coiled tube attached to each testicle and in which newly formed sperm mature. Although epididymitis does not occur too often, it is more common than orchitis, infection of the testicles. Both of these infections cause pain and swelling in the testicular area.

Testicular pain also may be caused by twisting of the testicle and the structures within the scrotum that connect it to the body. Called testicular torsion, this is not only extremely painful but also dangerous, because if the blood supply is interrupted, the testicle may be lost in a few hours.

Testicular cancer is one of the more common cancers in men under thirty. You should get checked immediately if you notice a change in the size of or any lumps or nodules in a testicle. A cancerous testicle is typically painless. Usually testicular cancer is easy to treat when it is discovered early. Men should make it a habit to feel their testicles regularly (in the shower is a good time) to be sure that no changes have occurred.

BEYOND HOME CARE

GET MEDICAL CARE IMMEDIATELY:

- if there is significant pain in the testicles;
- if you pull the foreskin back and cannot return it to its normal position.

GET MEDICAL CARE TODAY:

- for babies, if the opening of the foreskin is too small to allow urine to pass freely;
- if there is swelling or lumps within a testicle;
- if there is a sore on the genitals or nearby areas, unless you are sure it is a recurrence of previously diagnosed herpes. Sores caused by syphilis in particular can appear elsewhere on the body, often on the hands or in or around the mouth. If you develop an unexplained, shallow, open sore, whether or not it is painful, and if you or a partner have had new sexual contacts within the previous two months, see your health practitioner right away;
- if there is significant pain in the prostate region, particularly if there is also a fever or back or pelvic pain;
- if there is a discharge from the penis, particularly if you or a partner have had new sexual contacts within the previous two weeks.

SEE YOUR HEALTH PRACTITIONER WITHIN THE NEXT FEW DAYS:

- if you have had sexual contact with someone known to have or suspected of having gonorrhea, syphilis, HIV, or *Chlamydia* infection, or any other major sexually transmitted disease. You don't need to see your health practitioner immediately if you've simply been exposed to herpes, genital warts, or a yeast infection, but since two or more sexually transmitted diseases often occur together, a checkup soon is indicated.

SEE YOUR PRACTITIONER SOON:

- if you have had difficulty starting urination, trouble with a weak or interrupted urinary stream, or dribbling of urine.

CHAPTER 11

HEADACHES

MOST OF US have one or two "weak links"—parts of the body that take the brunt of physical or psychological stress. Some people get colds, some digestive upsets, and a great number are prone to headaches.

Headaches can be a serious health problem. Some people suffer from headaches that are severe or frequent enough to be incapacitating. Certainly, there are times when a headache signals a serious condition. In the great majority of cases, however, the pain of a headache is best seen as a message that your stress level has risen too high. The headache serves as a warning that you need a change—perhaps to rest, deal with an emotional conflict, change your diet, or correct a problem in your personal environment at home or work.

Modern medicine classifies headaches according to the immediate cause of painful stimulation of nerve endings. The types of headaches include muscle-contraction headaches, vascular headaches, and headaches caused by inflammation or structural conditions.

MUSCLE-CONTRACTION HEADACHES

Nearly everyone has had a muscle-contraction headache, more commonly but less precisely referred to as a "tension" headache. Most people assume that the term "tension" refers to emotional stress, and in fact, many times this type of headache is brought on by stress on the job, being stuck in a traffic jam, or other such situations. But the pain of a muscle-contraction headache arises from tightening of the muscles of the upper back, neck, and scalp, which may result from any type of stress, whether physical or emotional. Extremes of heat or cold, hunger, loss of sleep, a tiring drive, and improper posture all are examples of physical stresses that can lead to muscle-contraction headaches.

That the body responds to stress by increasing muscle tone makes sense—it's preparing for a "fight or flight" response. Unfortunately, physical action isn't socially appropriate in many stressful situations, so the muscle tension just builds up. Once it reaches a certain threshold, you get a headache. The pain arises partly because the muscle is simply sore from being overworked, and partly because the tension constricts blood vessels and reduces blood flow to the tiring muscles. It is now thought that in many or most muscle-contraction headaches, the physiological changes that account for vascular headaches also contribute to the pain (see the next section in this chapter).

Typically, the pain of a muscle-contraction headache is a dull, steady ache felt across the forehead, at the temples, or at the base of the head and neck. A sensation of tightness, as if a constricting band were wrapped around the head, may be felt. Often the scalp and neck are tender to touch.

GENERAL HOME CARE

Generally muscle-contraction headaches are easy to treat at home: Simply take a break from the stress that led to the headache, get some rest, and perhaps massage the sore neck muscles. If the headache doesn't respond to these simple measures in a short time, try a homeopathic medicine from the list in this chapter. By helping the body restore order and balance, the correct homeopathic medicine speeds relaxation of the muscles and relief from the pain, without any of the side effects associated with standard painkillers.

There are some steps you can take to prevent recurrent muscle-contraction headaches.

• Learn to recognize and avoid simple physical causes of muscle tension like poor posture, uncomfortable clothing, or unpleasant environmental conditions (an overly chilly room, irritating noise, and so on). Notice whether any of your habits is awkward or causes tension and straining, such as the way you sit at your desk, hold the telephone, or clench your jaw.

- Recognize and deal with emotionally stressful situations in your life. We realize this is easier said than done, but very commonly, headaches are associated with emotional stress.
- Become familiar with the early signs and sensations of tension, both muscular and emotional. If you can sense tension before a bad headache comes on, you can do something to break the cycle before tension increases. Get out of the stressful situation for a few minutes; to help release stored tension, do some physical exercise, meditate, pray, or do anything you find relaxing or joyful (laughter is great for releasing tension).
- Learn to relax the muscles that tense up during a headache, so that you can relax them during periods of stress. We suggest you set aside ten minutes or so, twice a day, for relaxation exercises. Relax your whole body, and your head and neck muscles in particular. Spend the last few moments of each period of relaxation imagining yourself in the situation that causes you the most stress—perhaps it's driving in rush-hour traffic—keeping that relaxed feeling. After a week or so, you'll start to remember the relaxation sessions whenever you're in that tense situation, and before long, you'll find that you can maintain greater tranquillity even then. Biofeedback can help you learn to control various physiological processes that lead to tension headaches, as can meditation.
- Both exercise and massage are great for relieving tension and lifting your mood. The specialty bodywork practices—such as the Alexander technique, chiropractic, Rolfing, or acupressure—also can be helpful in treating or preventing headaches.
- Some people get headaches when they are hungry or when they eat foods that don't agree with them. Pay attention to the pattern of your headaches in relation to diet. We recommend regular meals, with an emphasis on fresh vegetables, whole grains, and, if desired, lean meats. Avoid sweets and caffeine. Specific foods often aggravate vascular headaches, and since many headaches may be of mixed type, it may be useful to avoid these foods.
- If you have any visual difficulties, see an eye specialist. While eyestrain isn't a common cause of headaches, sometimes it is to blame for recurrent headaches.
- Consider a checkup for misalignment or injury of the temporomandibular joints (TMJ). These joints attach the jaw to the rest of the skull on either side, just in front of the ears. One quick test: Try placing a two- to three-inch piece of Popsicle stick or tongue depressor between the teeth to separate the upper and lower jaws. If this relieves

your headache, you may have a TMJ problem. Evaluation is best performed by an ear, nose, and throat specialist or a dentist.

For more information on self-treatment of headaches, we recommend *Headache Help,* by Lawrence Robbins, M.D., and Susan Lang (1995); and *Migraine: What Works,* by Joseph Kandel, M.D., and David Sudderth, M.D. (1996). For more details on learning to deal with stress, see *Full Catastrophe Living: Using the Wisdom of Your Body and Mind to Face Stress, Pain and Illness,* by Jon Kabat-Zinn, Ph.D. (1990); and *PNI: The New Mind/Body Healing Program,* by Elliott Dacher, M.D. (1993).

MIGRAINES AND OTHER VASCULAR HEADACHES

Many people use the word "migraine" to refer to any really bad headache, but migraine headache, as medically understood, denotes that pain resulting from a complex series of specific changes in the blood vessels of the head and brain. During a migraine, the blood vessels first become overly constricted, and then widen abnormally. This sequence of constriction and widening affects the blood vessels on one side of the head more intensely, and often it is especially pronounced in a particular area of the brain.

The symptoms of migraine headaches are directly related to these changes in the blood vessels. During the initial phase of blood vessel narrowing, decreased blood flow to the brain leads to malfunction in the area of greatest constriction. So, before any pain is felt, the typical migraine begins with some sort of warning symptom, called an aura. The most common aura is disturbance of vision, which may take the form of bright or colored zigzag lines, areas of cloudy vision, flashing lights, and so on. Other people have auras with such symptoms as slurred speech, dizziness, weakness or numbness of one side of the body, and other signs of neurological impairment.

The migraine headache pain begins when the previously narrowed blood vessels then open too wide. Normal brain function is restored by the return of blood flow, but stretching of the vessel walls, along with inflammation caused by chemical changes in the blood, stimulate pain-sensitive nerve endings in the vessel walls. At first the pain is localized on one side of the head, but often it spreads to the other side as the headache progresses. The pain is intense and throbbing in character. Accompanying the headache may be symptoms such as nausea, vomiting or diarrhea, intolerance of light, dizziness, and sweating or chilliness.

This description of the migraine applies to the "classic" type, but other forms of migraine are not uncommon. Sometimes the headache begins without a prior aura. On the other hand, "migraine equivalents" may occur; there may be the neurological disturbances (visual changes and so on) or vomiting typical of a migraine, though there is no headache. The tendency to have migraines clearly runs in families and seems to be due, in part, to a genetic predisposition. They first occur before the person reaches the age of thirty, usually in the early teen years. Migraines often start in childhood, particularly around the time of puberty. Even very young children can get migraines. Before the child is old enough to tell you about the headache, the first sign you may see in your two- to four-year-old is recurrent vomiting. The child who gets headaches may well be saying something about a difficulty in her life that she finds hard to express openly. Do your best to identify the stresses your child faces, and work with her to find ways to resolve the conflicts.

A migraine headache is most often triggered by psychological stress, but, curiously, it is characteristic that the attack begins when the stress is relieved. High-pressure businesspeople, for instance, may dread the "relaxing" weekends that bring on their headaches. Other stresses that frequently lead to migraines include going without food, sleeping too long, bright lights, and fluctuations in hormone levels (some women get migraines every month before the menstrual period or when they ovulate). Foods and drinks including nuts, chocolate, coffee, cheese, citrus, and alcohol also may trigger migraines, as do some drugs.

Another type of vascular headache is the "cluster" headache. These are severe, one-sided headaches that occur in spells, most often during sleep. The pain is accompanied by redness and tearing of the eye, and the nostril drops on the painful side.

GENERAL HOME CARE

An untreated migraine lasts at least several hours, often a full day. Many migraine headaches are so severe that simple measures like rest or aspirin offer little or no help. Relaxation measures may bring some relief. Learning to warm the hands by increasing blood flow through biofeedback has been especially effective, probably because the circulatory system in general is affected. Suggesting to yourself that the hands are becoming warm and heavy is the best way for most people to achieve this without a biofeedback device.

Dealing effectively with stress and avoiding the factors that you know lead to your headaches are critical for preventing migraines. Constitutional homeopathic treatment from a professional practitioner is the most helpful preventive approach for those whose headaches don't respond to simple home-care measures or to self-care homeopathy.

Many different conventional medicines are used to treat and prevent migraines; some are strong drugs with many potentially serious side effects. We recommend that you opt for conventional treatment only if your headaches persist after you've tried self-care methods and professional homeopathic treatment.

OTHER HEADACHES

Less common than muscle-contraction and migraine headaches are the various types of headaches caused by infection, inflammation, and structural changes in the face and head. Many of these are serious conditions requiring medical treatment.

For information about acute sinus headaches, see the section on sinus conditions in chapter 4.

CASETAKING QUESTIONS FOR HEADACHES

Onset of symptoms:
- Did anything seem to trigger the headache? For example, exposure to cold or wet weather or to a draft, eating too much or eating something in particular, alcohol or drugs, emotions, overwork, or lack of sleep?

Character of the pain:
- Where in the head is the pain centered, and where does it radiate?
- What is the character of the pain (throbbing, aching, burning, etc.)?

Associated symptoms:
- Has the headache affected the patient's appearance? Is the face pale, or flushed red? Are the pupils dilated?
- How is vision affected?
- Have digestive symptoms such as nausea or vomiting developed?

- Does the headache seem related to the menstrual cycle, occurring prior to, during, or after the periods?

Modalities:
- At what time of day is the headache worse?
- What makes the pain better or worse? How is it affected by hot or cold applications, heat and cold in general, pressure, light, and noise? How do motion and position (lying down, sitting, or standing) affect the pain? Does motion of the eyes affect the pain?

HOMEOPATHIC MEDICINES
FOR HEADACHES OF ALL TYPES

Use homeopathic medicines at home when you or your children have mild to moderate headaches.

It's often difficult to choose the right medicine for a headache. So many headaches are made better or worse by the same factors, and many remedies cover these common modalities. Often the person's general symptoms are your best guide in choosing the medicine. Use only the strongest, most definite headache symptoms in your case analysis, and compare them to the symptoms we list here. If you still have trouble picking the right medicine, we recommend you choose among the first three we cover, *Belladonna, Nux,* and *Bryonia.* One of these three medicines will help the majority who suffer from acute headaches that have few specific symptoms.

Belladonna is indicated for people whose headaches are intense, with violent throbbing pains. The headache causes an extreme sensitivity, and the least bit of light, noise, touch, strong or unusual smell, motion, or jarring brings on a new wave of throbbing and pain. The pain often begins suddenly, and it may go away suddenly as well. It may spread throughout the entire head, or it may be localized anywhere, but it is more typically focused in the forehead; from the forehead it may extend to the back of the head. Often the face is flushed or feels hot, and sometimes the hands and feet are cold. *Belladonna* is thus the most commonly given medicine for headaches associated with high fever. The pupils may be noticeably dilated during a *Belladonna* headache. Firm pressure applied to the head helps (other remedies also have this modality). *Belladonna* is unique in that it suits headaches that are definitely relieved by sitting. *Belladonna* is one of a number of medicines that cover headaches made worse by climbing steps, but it alone fits those also aggravated by traveling down a slope or stairway. Afternoon is more characteristically the time of worse pain. *Bryonia* is best used when the most prominent characteristic of the headache is aggravation with motion. Both *Belladonna* and *Bryonia* cover this marked sensitivity to motion, and many other remedies also fit headaches made worse from motion. For the *Bryonia* patient, however, this is the outstanding characteristic. Even slight motion of the head or eyes worsens the pain. The pain is worse from slight touch, but better from firm pressure. It is generally worse in the morning, and though it may be felt immediately upon waking, it is just as likely to come on only after the person first moves in bed or after she gets out of bed. There is little throbbing with *Bryonia* headaches, unlike those of *Belladonna,* and the pain is described as a steady ache, sometimes with a sense of fullness or heaviness. As with *Belladonna,* the headache is likely to be located in the forehead, extending from there to the back of the head, but it is commonly centered over the left eye, a symptom not shared with *Belladonna.* Nausea, vomiting, and especially constipation may occur in connection with *Bryonia* headaches. The *Bryonia* patient is irritable and irascible and wants to be left alone.

Nux vomica also is a good medicine for irritable people with headaches. The apparent cause of the headache is more often the best indication for *Nux,* since this medicine frequently suits the symptoms of headaches brought on by overeating, the use of alcohol, coffee, or other drugs, or staying up too late and missing sleep. The person with a typical morning hangover headache, who often has indulged in all of these pursuits, frequently is gratefully relieved with a dose or two of *Nux.* Such headaches generally are accompanied by an overall sick feeling and by digestive upsets. The sufferer may have a sour or bitter taste in the mouth in the morning, queasiness, nausea, or vomiting (dry heaves and gas are especially typical *Nux* symptoms). The *Nux* headache also may be brought on by concentrated or prolonged mental work, or by cold air or cold wind. In contrast to *Bryonia* headaches, those of *Nux* are worse in the morning, particularly upon first waking, and tend to get somewhat better after the person is up and about. As with most headaches, motion may aggravate the symptoms, but shaking the head is particularly painful (as in *Belladonna*). Lying on the painful side often makes the pain worse, and the sound of footsteps is particularly irritating to the *Nux* headache patient. Wrapping up the head or being in a warm room may relieve the pain.

Pulsatilla headaches also have been associated with digestive upsets. They often come on after meals and particularly after eating warm, rich, or fatty foods or after eating ice cream. Nausea and vomiting frequently accompany a *Pulsatilla* headache. *Pulsatilla* also is a good medicine for headaches that occur in connection with menstrual periods (before, during, or especially when the period ends), or those that result from a frightening experience. More often the pain is felt in the forehead or on one side of the head, and may change location frequently (as it does with *Sanguinaria*). Throbbing accompanies the headache. Although walking briskly may make the pain worse, generally there is relief from gentle motion, especially walking about slowly in the open air. Pressure relieves the pain, and blowing the nose aggravates it. The *Pulsatilla* individual is emotionally mild and sensitive and may weep from the pains. Though a little irritable, the person is likely to want company and consolation.

Gelsemium headaches generally begin at the back of the head, often extending to the rest of the head or to the forehead. The person may feel as though a band or hood were bound tightly around his head. These symptoms are, of course, characteristic of muscle-contraction headaches. But also *Gelsemium* is one of the fairly few homeopathic medicines that clearly suit headaches preceded by dimness of vision or other visual disturbances, symptoms of migraines. Localized pain on the right side of the head also is covered by this remedy. The *Gelsemium* headache is not much affected by changes of temperature, but other environmental factors (light, noise, motion, jarring) aggravate it. Napping or, curiously, urinating relieves the pain. The person feels dull, tired, heavy, and apathetic. His eyes droop, and he looks exhausted. He is not particularly irritable but wants to be left alone.

The headaches of *Iris* also are preceded or accompanied by dimness of vision or other changes in eyesight. The pain is felt in one side of the forehead, particularly the right side. Nausea and vomiting ensue, and the headache is worse after the vomiting. The pain is made better from walking in the open air. *Iris* has helped many people with periodic migraine headaches such as those that return every weekend. Even if visual disturbance does not accompany the headache, *Iris* may help if its other symptoms fit.

Sanguinaria headaches typically begin at the back of the head but extend to and soon settle over the right eye or on the right side of the head. Right-sided headaches are covered by other medicines (*Iris* and *Gelsemium,* for instance), but *Sanguinaria* is especially noted for this symptom. The pain is sharp, splitting, knifelike, and sometimes throbbing. Once again, nausea and vomiting occur at the height of the pain, but unlike *Iris* headaches, those of *Sanguinaria* are relieved after vomiting. Motion aggravates the pain, whereas sleep and firm pressure relieve it. Like *Iris, Sanguinaria* suits headaches that recur in a consistent pattern, such as every seven days. Homeopathic reference texts do not mention *San-*

guinaria in connection with visual disturbances. However, if you have a classic visual-aura migraine headache that also has the symptoms just mentioned, we certainly recommend that you use this medicine.

The headaches that need *Spigelia* have stitching, burning, and pulsating pains, usually on the frontal part of the head and often on the left side. Lying with the head propped up makes the pains better; stooping, motion, noise, and cold stormy weather make them worse. Washing with cold water can feel good, but usually the pain is worse after you finish. In general, the head pains are worse from warmth and temporarily better from cold (for other pain symptoms of *Spigelia,* the reverse is true). A stiff neck and shoulders accompany the headache and make motion very painful. The person also may experience severe pain in and around the eyes and extending deep into the sockets.

REMEDY SUMMARY FOR HEADACHES

If you find it hard to select a medicine from those listed here, choose among *Belladonna, Nux,* and *Bryonia.*
Give the medicine: Up to every 2 hours; once improvement begins, repeat only when symptoms are worse again or improvement has ceased for an hour or so.
When to try another medicine: If the symptoms are no better after 2 or 3 doses of the first medicine you try.

BELLADONNA ★

Essentials
- Intense headaches with violent, throbbing pains
- Pain aggravated by light, noise, touch, strong or unusual smells, motion, or jarring
- Pain begins and passes suddenly

Confirmatory symptoms
- Pain more typically located in the forehead, from which it may extend to the back of the head
- Face flushed or feels hot, sometimes with cold hands and feet
- Dilated pupils
- Relief from sitting or firm pressure
- Pain worse from climbing steps or descending a slope or stairway, and in the afternoon

BRYONIA ★

Essentials
- Headache aggravated by motion, even very slight motion of the head or eyes
- Steady aching or sense of heaviness with little throbbing

Confirmatory symptoms
- Pain worsened by slight touch, relieved by firm pressure
- Pain worse in the morning, especially after first moving in bed or just after getting out of bed
- Headache centered over left eye
- Headache accompanied by nausea, vomiting, or constipation
- Patient irritable, wants to be left alone

NUX VOMICA ★

Essentials
- Headache begins after overeating; from alcohol, coffee, or other drugs; from loss of sleep; or from excessive mental work
- Headache accompanied by general sick feeling and by digestive upsets including vomiting, gas, or sour or bitter taste

Confirmatory symptoms
- Pain worse on first waking in the morning, improves after getting up
- Pain aggravated by sounds, such as footsteps
- Pain relieved by wrapping up the head or being in a warm room

PULSATILLA

Essentials
- Headache comes on after meals or after warm, rich, or fatty foods or ice cream

  or
- Headaches in connection with menstrual period (before, during, or at end of the period)

Confirmatory symptoms
- Patient wants company and consolation
- Relief with gentle motion, especially walking slowly in open air
- Pain in forehead or on one side; or changes location frequently
- Pain relieved by pressure, worsened by blowing the nose

GELSEMIUM

Essentials
- Pain begins at the back of the head, extending upward or to the forehead

  or
- Headache preceded by dimness of vision or other visual disturbances

Confirmatory symptoms
- Sensation of a band or hood bound tightly around the head
- Pain on the right side of the head
- Pain relieved by napping or urinating
- Headache aggravated by light, noise, motion, or jarring
- Patient feels dull, tired, heavy, and apathetic; wants to be left alone, but not markedly irritable

IRIS

Essentials
- Pain on one side of the forehead, particularly the right
- Migraine headaches that come on at regular intervals

Confirmatory symptoms
- Headache preceded or accompanied by dimness of vision or other visual changes
- Nausea and vomiting follow the headache; headache worse after vomiting
- Pain improved by walking in the open air

SANGUINARIA

Essentials
- Pain begins at the back of the head, extending to right side of the head or right eye
- Headaches recur periodically

Confirmatory symptoms
- Nausea and vomiting; vomiting brings relief
- Pain sharp, splitting, knifelike, or throbbing
- Pain worse from motion, better from sleep and firm pressure

SPIGELIA

Essentials

- Stitching, burning, or pulsating pains, usually on the frontal part of the head, often on the left
- Headache accompanied by stiff neck and shoulders, making motion painful

Confirmatory symptoms

- Pain better from lying with the head propped up; worse from stooping, motion, noise, and cold stormy weather
- Temporary relief from washing with cold water, but pain is worse later
- Pain in and around the eyes or extending into the eye sockets

BEYOND HOME CARE

GET MEDICAL CARE IMMEDIATELY:

- for any very severe headache, particularly if it is unusual for you;
- for headache accompanied by stiff neck or high fever;
- for any headache that occurs after a head injury.

GET MEDICAL CARE TODAY:

- the first time you have a headache preceded or accompanied by visual disturbances, weakness of one side or part of the body, speech disorders, or dizziness. If you have had these symptoms previously, but their pattern has changed significantly, call or see your practitioner;
- for a headache lasting more than 3 or 4 days, even if mild (a call to your doctor may suffice);
- if a headache begins while you're taking medicine, including birth control pills.

SEE YOUR PRACTITIONER SOON:

- for headaches that recur frequently, even if mild;
- for headaches that are consistently worse in the morning or upon waking.

CHAPTER 12

ALLERGIES AND
RELATED CONDITIONS

FOR PEOPLE WITH allergies, symptoms occur when the body's immune system overreacts to substances in the environment. The immune system's ability to identify and remove foreign substances enables it to fight off infecting germs, neutralize poisons, and destroy cancer cells. During an allergic reaction, however, these normally protective defenses are triggered by innocuous substances such as foods, pollens, animal hairs, medicines, and so forth, and uncomfortable, sometimes dangerous symptoms are produced. The most common symptoms of allergic reactions include skin eruptions, stuffy or runny nose, and wheezing or coughing. Generalized allergic reactions, called anaphylaxis, are rare but life-threatening.

While true allergies are reactions to specific substances, the immune system can produce similar symptoms when triggered by nonspecific factors such as temperature or weather changes, overexertion, stress, strong emotions, or infectious illness. Sometimes such symptoms seem to develop by themselves. In this chapter, we cover common conditions of both types: skin problems (contact dermatitis, hives, and eczema) and respiratory disorders (upper respiratory allergies and asthma).

Whether the diagnosis is allergy or a related condition, homeopathy offers a uniquely effective way to treat the person. From the homeopathic perspective, the basic problem is an imbalance in the system as a whole, which leads to the oversensitive state. It is sensible to avoid substances or other influences that trigger symptoms. Often, however, identifying exactly what causes the reaction is nearly impossible. Many times, too, it turns out to be something you just can't avoid completely. Moreover, the underlying weakness remains; the symptoms return as soon as the substance is encountered again.

Professional constitutional homeopathic treatment can help the system correct its imbalance and help free it from its sensitivity. In the home, homeopathic medicines may be used when acute, short-lived allergy symptoms occur in people who are otherwise healthy. Even when constitutional care is needed for recurrent allergies, home treatment during a particularly bad outbreak of symptoms may offer great relief. If you are receiving constitutional care, please consult with your homeopath before using home treatment.

CONTACT DERMATITIS

Any itching skin eruption triggered by exposure to allergenic substances is called contact dermatitis. The most familiar kind is the rash that appears after contact with or exposure to poison oak, ivy, or sumac. Additional common causes of contact dermatitis include other plants, cosmetics, jewelry, and rubber. Some diaper rashes are triggered by contact allergic reactions to laundry detergent or to chemicals in disposable diapers, and others occur as a reaction to contact with irritating urine. Contact rashes may become infected with bacteria or fungi; otherwise the main concern is the itching and unattractive appearance.

Diagnosis of contact dermatitis depends on careful attention to the details of how the rash appeared. Think about what may have touched the skin at the site of the rash, and try to recall any new household chemicals, toiletries, or clothing in use. PABA, found in some sunscreen lotions, and benzocaine, found in many topical pain relievers and antiseptics, are frequent offenders.

Conventional medicine treats contact dermatitis with corticosteroid creams (available over the counter), oral antihistamines for the itching, and in bad cases, short courses of oral steroids. The steroid creams usually don't help much, in our experience. Oral steroids usually work well, and they don't cause major side effects when given for only a week or two (they can cause serious problems when given over the long term, however). But whether topical or oral, steroids suppress the body's natural responses, instead of working with them as homeopathy does.

GENERAL HOME CARE

Once you know what caused the rash, avoid it, and the skin should clear up in a week or two. Meanwhile you can try relaxation and visualization practices to quell the itching and speed healing. Of the many herbal treatments advised for poison-oak rashes, we haven't found one that is consistently successful. Some of the more promising include liberal applications of the juice of the plantain (*Plantago*) or *Grindelia* plants (either fresh or as tinctures available from homeopathic pharmacies), or green clay powder (available in health-food stores). Calamine and similar lotions feel cooling but don't really relieve much itching.

CASETAKING QUESTIONS FOR CONTACT DERMATITIS

Character of the symptoms:
• Is the rash dry, or are there blisters?
• If there are blisters, how large are they? What does the fluid in them look like?
• Where on the body is the rash worse?

Modalities:
• At what time of day or night are the symptoms worse?
• How is the itching affected by heat or cold, hot water, or being in or out of doors?

HOMEOPATHIC MEDICINES

Homeopathic medicines taken internally can work to help the body relieve itching and speed healing of the rash. Some of our severely poison oak–sensitive patients have told us that the homeopathic treatment brought faster and more complete improvement than powerful oral doses of steroid hormones.

Once the rash has begun to subside and itching is less intense, apply one part *Calendula* tincture diluted with three parts water with a cotton swab several times a day. The skin will heal much faster, particularly if it has been open and raw from blistering.

Croton tiglium is indicated when there is a great deal of blistering, inflammation, and itching. If the symptoms are mild, itching may be relieved by gentle scratching or rubbing. However, the rash can become so painful and tender that the patient can't stand to touch it. The *Croton tig.*

rash tends to be worse on the scalp, around the eyes, and on the genitals. *Croton tig.* is the first remedy to try when the symptoms don't point you to a particular medicine.

Homeopathic medicines made from *Rhus toxicodendron* (poison ivy) or *Rhus diversiloba* (poison oak) can be very effective for people who are reacting to these plants, as well as for those with dermatitis caused by other allergens. Typically, the *Rhus* patient has marked burning with the itching, and the discomfort is aggravated by scratching, open air, night, and the warmth of the bed. He often gets relief from the itching by immersing the area in near-scalding water. The skin is intensely inflamed with fluid-filled blisters. The patient is generally restless, irritable, and anxious. One note of caution: Some homeopaths have reported worsening of poison oak or ivy rashes after the patient has taken *Rhus tox.* We haven't observed this, and *Rhus diversiloba* in particular has been extremely helpful for many of our own patients with poison oak. If an aggravation does occur, wait a few hours (it may be a healing response), then move on to another medicine.

Consider *Anacardium* when there are large blisters filled with yellow fluid. The face may be prominently affected by the eruption.

Bryonia can be helpful when the rash is made up mainly of fine, dry bumps, especially on the face. Classically, the *Bryonia* patient's symptoms are made worse by moving around, and the person is irritable and wants to be left alone—but you can give the medicine even if these more general characteristics aren't present.

Sepia is another possibility when the rash is dry (there may be tiny blisters but not large ones). A warm room helps relieve itching, but getting warm in bed makes it worse. The rash may have a brownish or reddish color, and scaling may be evident.

Give *Graphites* when there is much oozing of sticky, honey-colored fluid from the eruptions. Itching is worse at night and in warmth.

Sulphur can help no matter what the rash looks like if the itching is worse in warmth and at night. When some of the general characteristics of *Sulphur* are present—for example, if the person is sensitive to heat and feels warm—then you can be more certain of your choice (see the *materia medica* section).

REMEDY SUMMARY FOR CONTACT DERMATITIS

Give the medicine: Two to 3 times a day for up to 3 days, stopping when there is significant improvement in the itching or the appearance of the rash.

When to try another medicine: If there is no improvement after 24 to 48 hours.

CROTON TIGLIUM ★

Essentials
- Much blistering, inflammation, and itching
- When mild, itching is relieved by gentle scratching or rubbing; when severe, rash is painful and tender, and touch is intolerable

Confirmatory symptoms
- Rash worse on the scalp, around the eyes, and on the genitals

ANACARDIUM

Essentials
- Large blisters filled with yellow fluid

Confirmatory symptoms
- Face prominently affected

RHUS TOXICODENDRON or RHUS DIVERSILOBA

Essentials
- Skin is intensely inflamed, with fluid-filled blisters
- Marked burning with the itching

Confirmatory symptoms
- Itching worse at night and aggravated by scratching, open air, and warmth of the bed
- Itching relieved by very hot water
- Restless, irritable, anxious patient

BRYONIA

Essentials
- Rash mainly of fine, dry bumps, especially on the face

Confirmatory symptoms
- Symptoms worse from moving around
- Irritability, wish to be left alone

SEPIA

Essentials
- Dry rash (possibly with tiny blisters)

Confirmatory symptoms
- Itching better in a warm room but worse after getting warm in bed
- Rash brownish or reddish color, scaly

GRAPHITES

Essentials
- Oozing of sticky, honey-colored fluid from the eruptions
- Itching worse at night and from warmth

SULPHUR

Essentials
- Itching worse from warmth and at night
  and/or
- General characteristics of *Sulphur* are present (for example, the person is generally sensitive to heat and feels warm—see *materia medica* section)

BEYOND HOME CARE

Consult the section on impetigo in chapter 13 if signs of infection (pus, swelling, spreading redness) appear.

HIVES (URTICARIA)

Hives are red, raised swellings, or welts, that appear suddenly with intense itching. The individual welts generally are a half-inch across or larger, and they may run together to form large patches of raised, puffy skin.

Hives may be triggered by food, food additives, medicines, insect venoms, rubbing or scratching the skin, contact with cold objects, or emotional upset. Often the precipitating cause is never found. In most cases, the eruption lasts from several hours to a day or so and disappears as quickly as it came, leaving no trace. Most people get hives only once or twice in a lifetime, but some get them recurrently, and sometimes they become a chronic problem. Recurrent or chronic hives may indicate a serious illness, so you should be checked if this occurs.

Hives themselves are only a nuisance unless the swelling involves the respiratory passages. Occasionally, severe allergic reactions cause hivelike swellings in the throat that impede breathing—this is a true emergency.

GENERAL HOME CARE

Since attacks of hives are generally self-limited, little treatment is really necessary. Applying a cool sponge to the affected area may relieve itching and help bring down the swelling, unless the hives are caused by cold.

HOMEOPATHIC MEDICINES

Recurrent outbreaks are a constitutional problem and should be treated by a homeopath. For an isolated case of hives, choose from among the following remedies, giving two doses an hour apart. If another hour passes without definite improvement, you can try a second medicine.

Apis is the medicine most likely to help the person with hives. The hives are intensely itchy and usually aggravated by warmth. They are worse at night and come on during perspiration, after exercise, or when the body becomes hot; they may begin after any change in weather. *Apis* is particularly indicated when the hives cause swelling around the eyes.

If neither of the medicines listed below is strongly indicated, use *Apis* whether or not its characteristic symptoms are present. Give a dose of the thirtieth potency every three hours, stopping as soon as improvement begins. Often a single dose is enough to bring rapid improvement.

Urtica urens, the stinging nettle, is almost as frequently useful as *Apis.* Unique characteristics of this medicine include hives brought on by bathing, and itching relieved by lying down. As with *Apis,* the hives are worse from warmth or exercise, in this case especially if the exercise is particularly strenuous.

Rhus tox. should help if rubbing or scratching, cold weather, or getting wet seems to bring on the welts. Welts may form also during perspiration.

BEYOND HOME CARE

GET MEDICAL CARE IMMEDIATELY:

• if the hives involve the throat, or if a sense of constriction in the throat is felt, even mildly. Swelling may suddenly increase and interfere with breathing.

SEE YOUR PRACTITIONER SOON:

• for 2 or more outbreaks of hives within 6 months, unless they are clearly a reaction to a particular food or to contact with a specific allergen such as grass or animal fur.

ATOPIC DERMATITIS (ECZEMA)

The term eczema describes any rash that reddens and inflames the skin, causing bumps and tiny blisters, oozing, crusting, or dryness and thickening of the skin. Although many skin conditions cause eczematous eruptions, eczema is more often thought of as synonymous with atopic dermatitis, a chronic skin disorder related to allergies. Because it is a severe, deeply rooted condition, atopic dermatitis should be treated constitutionally by a skilled homeopathic practitioner.

Conventional treatment with corticosteroid-hormone creams should be avoided if at all possible. These medications directly suppress the symptoms, which from the homeopathic view represent the body's effort to cope with an internal imbalance. From a pharmacologic point of view, steroid creams are safe unless applied to large areas of raw skin. In that case, the amount of the drug absorbed into the circulation can be considerable and can profoundly affect the body's hormonal balance.

GENERAL HOME CARE

Don't bathe too often, and use as little soap as possible. Irritating fabrics like wool should be avoided. Launder clothes in mild detergents or plain water. Be sure to keep the skin well lubricated with bland, unmedicated cream or lotion.

UPPER-RESPIRATORY TRACT ALLERGIES

Many people suffer from allergic reactions that involve the nose, throat, eyes, and ears. The symptoms include sneezing, runny or stuffy nose, itchy and watery eyes, as well as itching of the throat, roof of the mouth, ears, or any combination of these. Pollens, dust mites, animal dander, and other inhaled allergens more often are associated with respiratory allergies, though foods and other substances also may be involved. Seasonal reactions to high levels of pollen in the air, which prevails when weeds and trees are in bloom, is called hay fever.

Standard treatment of upper-respiratory allergies includes antihistamines, decongestants, and desensitization shots. Both antihistamines and decongestants directly suppress the body's defenses. Not only do the symptoms come right back as soon as the drugs wear off, but such suppression may force the system to create deeper symptoms to handle the underlying imbalance. Antihistamines cause drowsiness and often dryness of the mouth. When decongestants wear off, there is a rebound effect, and the symptoms become worse than before. Avoid these medicines if possible.

Desensitization therapy (allergy shots) involves frequent injections of known allergens in minute amounts. The dose is gradually increased until the person can tolerate exposure to the allergens in daily life. Though this approach makes more sense to us than symptom suppression, it has its problems. The shots themselves occasionally cause severe allergic reactions requiring emergency treatment. Exposure to allergens by injection does not occur naturally. And if it works, the treatment prevents reactions only to the injected allergens; it doesn't address the underlying tendency toward allergic reactions. We recommend you try homeopathic treatment first.

GENERAL HOME CARE

Avoiding pollens, animal dander, and other things that stimulate your allergies is of course important when possible. Rinsing mucous membranes of the nose and eyes with normal saline solution (it should be sterile if used in the eyes) to remove pollen granules and other allergens may bring substantial relief. You should drink ample amounts of water. Inhaling water vapor from a humidifier can help open swollen air passages.

CASETAKING QUESTIONS FOR
UPPER-RESPIRATORY ALLERGIES

Character of the symptoms:
- Which is the most uncomfortable symptom—runny nose, sneezing, or eye irritation?
- What is the color and consistency of the nasal discharge? Does it irritate the skin?
- Is the nose runny, or stuffy, and is this consistent?
- Are the eyes tearing? Do the tears cause reddened eyes or cheeks?
- Is there itching in the nose or mouth?

Associated symptoms:
- Is the throat affected, and how?
- Is there a cough?

Modalities:
- At what time of day are the symptoms worse?
- How are they affected by heat or cold, being in or out of doors, lying down or being in motion, and eating?
- Are the symptoms seasonal?

HOMEOPATHIC MEDICINES

Constitutional homeopathic treatment is indicated if symptoms of upper-respiratory allergies are recurrent. Still, you can use homeopathic medicines at home to get through the worse parts of an allergy attack. Consult your homeopath first if you are being treated constitutionally.

Read also the descriptions of medicines in the chapter on colds, especially those of *Nux vomica, Arsenicum, Allium cepa,* and *Euphrasia.* If no medicine seems well indicated, start with *Allium cepa.*

Sabadilla covers the typical symptoms of hay-fever allergies, including copious, watery nasal discharge; spasmodic sneezing; itching in the nose; and red, runny eyes. All these symptoms are improved by being outdoors or walking in the open air. There may be a sensation like a lump in the throat, along with a constant urge to swallow.

Wyethia is indicated when upper-respiratory allergies are accompanied by intense, urgent itching of the back part of the roof of the mouth, or itching behind the nose. The nose, nasal passages, and throat feel dry in spite of a continuous, burning, watery flow from the nose.

REMEDY SUMMARY FOR UPPER-RESPIRATORY ALLERGIES

In addition to the medicines listed here, those covered in chapter 4 also can be useful, especially *Nux vomica, Arsenicum, Allium cepa,* and *Euphrasia.* If there is mild wheezing, consider *Arsenicum, Euphrasia, Nux vomica* (described in chapter 4), or *Sabadilla* (covered here). If no medicine seems well indicated, choose *Allium cepa.*

Give the medicine: Up to every hour, but repeat the dose only when symptoms come back. If treatment is needed for more than a day, give the medicine no more than 3 times a day and no more than a week at a time. Be sure not to give any more medicine as long as there is still improvement from the previous dose.

When to try another medicine: If there is no improvement after 4 hours following at least 2 doses of the previous medicine.

SABADILLA

Essentials
• Copious, watery nasal discharge; spasmodic sneezing; itching in the nose; and red, runny eyes

Confirmatory symptoms
• Symptoms improved from being outdoors or walking in the open air
• Sensation like a lump in the throat with a constant urge to swallow

WYETHIA

Essentials
• Nasal allergies accompanied by intense, urgent itching of the back part of the roof of the mouth, or itching behind the nose

Confirmatory symptoms
• Dry sensation in the nose, nasal passages, and throat

ASTHMA

Asthma is a chronic disease in which the basic problem is hyperreactive airways—in response to various stimuli, the small breathing tubes in the lungs constrict when they shouldn't, and inflammatory changes occur in their walls. Although some people get asthma attacks when exposed to allergenic substances, in the majority of sufferers the symptoms are triggered by nonspecific factors such as exercise, cold air, stress, or head colds.

Wheezing, the tight whistling sound so characteristic of an asthma attack, occurs when the breathing passages narrow due to contraction of their muscular walls, swelling of their linings, and accumulation of thick mucus. Air can't flow normally into and, especially, out of the lungs. The chest feels tight, and the person is short of breath, wheezes, and must breathe rapidly with much greater effort. Coughing can be prominent; sometimes, especially in children, it is the only obvious symptom, complicating the diagnosis.

The worse symptoms of an asthma attack may run their course within a day or two, usually clearing without treatment. But you can't be sure this will happen, and an attack of asthma carries with it the danger of suffocation and death.

Conventional medical treatment of asthma includes avoidance of known allergens or other triggering substances, and desensitization shots if specific allergens have been identified (see the previous section on upper–respiratory tract allergies). Drugs are used to widen the constricted airways, reduce inflammation, or prevent asthma attacks from happening in the first place.

Though all conventional drugs carry the risk of side effects, sometimes they are simply necessary. Details of treatment must be worked out with your practitioner, but we recommend that appropriate conventional medications be used if an asthma attack remains severe for more than a brief period or whenever there is doubt that the person is getting enough oxygen.

It should be noted that wheezing can result from conditions other than asthma. An acute allergic response can cause wheezing in people who don't have chronic asthma. Wheezing is common with emphysema and other chronic lung diseases, and frequently occurs when a child inhales a foreign object.

GENERAL HOME CARE

During an attack of wheezing, drinking plenty of liquids is extremely important to replace water lost through rapid breathing and increased perspiration (see the section on dehydration in chapter 8 for more information). The liquids also help loosen sticky mucus in the breathing passages. Relaxation practices often help. Breathing exercises (your practitioner can demonstrate them) are valuable both during acute attacks and when the patient gets asthma recurrently. Because asthma is potentially life-threatening, you should be in close contact with your health-care practitioner during an attack; don't hesitate to seek emergency care.

CASETAKING QUESTIONS FOR ACUTE ASTHMA

Character of the asthma:
- Describe the breathing and wheezing. How does the breathing sound?
- Is there much rattling of mucus in the chest? How easy or difficult is it to expel the mucus?

Modalities:
- At which time of day are the symptoms worse?
- How are the symptoms affected by motion, sleep, exposure to heat or cold, eating or drinking, or position of the body (including lying down)?

Associated symptoms:
- Is there nausea or vomiting? Cough?

HOMEOPATHIC MEDICINES

Asthma is generally a deep-seated, chronic illness, but that doesn't mean the symptoms have to dominate your life. All asthmatics have gone through periods when symptoms were absent or minimal, even though no obvious environmental changes had occurred. Constitutional homeopathic treatment can make these periods of freedom from asthma more frequent and longer lasting. Though you can expect occasional setbacks and you may need standard drugs at times, with treatment overall improvement will come.

Once the diagnosis of asthma is established, and once you are familiar with the pattern of symptoms, you can use homeopathy at home for acute, mild to moderate asthma symptoms. If you are receiving constitutional care, consult your homeopath first.

The strongest indications for the use of *Arsenicum* are fearfulness, restlessness, weakness, and aggravation of the symptoms at or after midnight. It's not at all surprising that the asthmatic grows frightened when he can't get his breath, and *Arsenicum* suits the restless agitation typical of this state. The patient tosses and turns or suddenly springs out of bed to relieve the anxiety and to catch a deep breath. In spite of the urge to move about, a profound weakness often develops, and the person may become too weak to continue his restless behavior and may be unable to move much at all. Most *Arsenicum* patients have a worse time with wheezing and shortness of breath between midnight and 3 A.M. If other symptoms suggest the medicine, however, don't hesitate to try it just because the asthma is worse at some other time of day or night. There may be accompanying cough and cold or hay-fever symptoms. *Arsenicum* patients typically feel quite chilly and are relieved in general by warmth. They tend to be quite thirsty, sometimes for frequent sips of water.

Spongia suits well the classic case of asthma with dry wheezing and little or no phlegm in the chest. Breathing is labored and noisy, sounding like whistling or sawing (typical of asthma but most pronounced when *Spongia* is the remedy). Often the asthma begins after the person has gotten a chill or is coming down with a cold. There may be a sudden onset of wheezing with a feeling of suffocation just as the person begins to fall asleep, or the wheezing may be worse after sleep. Shortness of breath is worse from lying down and from every motion, and it gets better when the person leans the head back. Warm food or drinks also may help relieve the wheezing. A dry barking or croupy cough commonly accompanies the symptoms.

Lobelia is another good medicine for the person experiencing a typical asthma attack with wheezing and a feeling of constriction in the chest. As in *Spongia,* the symptoms may begin after the person gets chilled. However, if breathing cold air definitely makes the wheezing worse, *Lobelia* is a better first choice. The wheezing isn't typically as loudly raspy as in *Spongia.* Some *Lobelia* patients have worse symptoms around noon.

Sambucus can help the person who feels like she is suffocating with the wheezing, especially when the symptoms are worse at or after midnight. Though you would certainly consider *Arsenicum* under these circumstances, the patient probably won't show the extreme fear or marked restlessness of that remedy. However, if those symptoms are present but *Arsenicum* doesn't help, *Sambucus* would be a good medicine to try next.

If the asthmatic is sweet and affectionate or perhaps tearful and clingy, feels oppressed by warm and stuffy rooms, and has little thirst, *Pulsatilla* is the probable remedy, no matter what the respiratory symptoms are. On the other hand, you may give *Pulsatilla* when it is indicated by specific asthma symptoms, including wheezing that begins or is worse in the evening or at night. There is usually an accumulation of phlegm in the chest that must be coughed out (see the description in chapter 4 on colds and coughs). The asthma may be worse after eating, especially fatty or rich foods.

Ipecac. is similarly suited to those whose asthma is accompanied by a great deal of phlegm in the chest. The respiratory distress may be spasmodic and severe, with marked wheezing. You may hear, in addition to the wheezing, much rattling of mucus in the chest as the person breathes. Coughing is common and sounds rattly from mucus deep in the chest. The cough may come in intense spasms that continue until there is vomiting of food or mucus. The asthma may be worse at night. The patient often is nauseated, and vomiting is common even when there is no coughing (see chapter 8 on digestive problems). Exhausted by the illness, the person looks pale and quite sick. Many of these symptoms are similar to those of *Pulsatilla,* but with *Ipecac.,* the buildup of mucus is even greater and the characteristic mental symptoms of *Pulsatilla* are not prominent.

Bryonia may be called for if the symptoms are typical of the remedy in general: aggravation caused by motion is pronounced, and the patient is warm, thirsty, and probably irritable. The wheezing is dry in character, with little phlegm.

Chamomilla should be considered for people with asthma, especially children, when they strongly display the irritability typical of the medicine. *Chamomilla* is a good choice also if the asthma attack began after a period of anger and no other remedy is clearly indicated.

REMEDY SUMMARY FOR ASTHMA

Give the medicine: Up to every hour for 3 doses; after that, repeat whenever the symptoms get worse, up to every 2 hours. Stay in daily contact with your health practitioner.

When to try another medicine: If there is no improvement after the third dose.

SPONGIA ★

Essentials
- Dry wheezing with very labored, noisy breathing—sounds like whistling or sawing

Confirmatory symptoms
- Onset after being chilled or when coming down with a cold
- Symptoms begin suddenly with a feeling of suffocation on falling asleep, or are worse after sleep
- Wheezing worse from lying down or motion; better from warm food or drinks or leaning the head back
- Dry barking or croupy cough

IPECAC. (★ FOR ASTHMA WITH WET COUGH OR RATTLING MUCUS IN CHEST)

Essentials
- Asthma with rattling mucus in the chest
- Deep, rattling cough

Confirmatory symptoms
- Wheezing worse at night
- Cough in continuous spasms resulting in gagging or vomiting of food or mucus
- Wheezing accompanied by nausea or vomiting, even when there is no coughing
- Face pale, person appears ill

ARSENICUM

Essentials
- Fearfulness, restlessness, weakness with the asthma
  and/or
- Aggravation of symptoms between midnight and 3 A.M.

Confirmatory symptoms
- Wheezing accompanied by cough and cold or hay-fever symptoms
- Patient feels chilly in general, relieved by warmth
- Thirst for frequent sips of water

LOBELIA

Essentials
- Dry asthma with shortness of breath and sensation of constriction in the chest

Confirmatory symptoms
- Wheezing worse from cold air or being chilled
- Symptoms worse around noon
- Patient breathes easier while walking rapidly

SAMBUCUS

Essentials
- Asthma in children, with feeling of suffocation

Confirmatory symptoms
- Aggravation of symptoms at or after midnight

CHAMOMILLA

Essentials
- Marked irritability (see *materia medica* section)
  or
- Symptoms begin after anger

Confirmatory symptoms
- Relief from cold air

BRYONIA

Essentials
- Dry wheezing definitely worse from motion
- Patient feels warm, thirsty, and irritable; wants to be left alone

PULSATILLA

Essentials
- General symptoms of *Pulsatilla* are present (mild, tearful disposition, feels worse in warm rooms, little thirst—see *materia medica* section)
  or
- Symptoms begin or are worse in the evening or at night

• Accumulation of phlegm in the chest that must be coughed out

Confirmatory symptoms

• Symptoms worse after eating, especially fatty or rich foods

BEYOND HOME CARE

GET MEDICAL CARE IMMEDIATELY:

• for any severe shortness of breath;
• if shortness of breath is accompanied by severe sore throat with difficulty swallowing, or if you notice that a wheezing child is drooling a great deal.

GET MEDICAL CARE TODAY:

• for a first occurrence of wheezing, or if the pattern of wheezing is different from the established one;
• whenever wheezing occurs in children under 2 years old. For anyone over this age, you should consult with your practitioner ahead of time so that you know how to handle recurrences of asthma that do follow the person's established pattern.

CHAPTER 13

SKIN PROBLEMS
AND RELATED DISORDERS

THE SKIN IS the largest organ of the body. It covers an area of some three thousand square inches on an average adult, and one-third of all the circulating blood is supplied to the skin. Many important physiological functions are performed by the skin: it helps to regulate body temperature and participates in the control of fluid balance; nerve endings sensitive to temperature, pain, touch, and pressure are located in the skin; the outer layer of the skin produces an acidic mantle, or covering, which inhibits the growth of disease-causing bacteria; and the skin eliminates fluids, minerals, and various biochemicals.

Homeopaths believe the skin has other functions as well. According to our understanding, the body uses the skin to express and eliminate internal imbalance through the appearance of skin symptoms. Homeopaths consider the appearance of a skin disorder often as an indication that the body is moving the level of physiological imbalance to the surface. Since the skin is the most external organ of the body, skin troubles are seen as the healthiest symptoms the body can produce as it heals from the inside out. They show that the body is keeping the imbalance as far away from the vital organs as possible.

Therefore, we encourage you not to look at skin symptoms simply as nuisances that should be done away with as soon as possible. There may well be reasons for their appearance, and they may represent a body's healthy response to stress. Certainly you should correct any conditions affecting hygiene, diet, or psychological stress that contribute to your susceptibility, but try to avoid medicines that suppress symptoms. Seek homeopathic treatment that helps rouse the body's defenses to fully restore balance.

Many people with common skin problems can be treated with simple home-care measures and homeopathic medicines. In this chapter we cover boils, styes, impetigo, herpes, shingles, ringworm, yeast infections, and warts (hives and contact dermatitis, such as poison oak, are covered in chapter 12 on allergies and related conditions). We have space enough only for outline descriptions of these conditions. If you're not positive what the problem is, you'll have to rely on other medical self-care books or a visit to your medical professional. People who have chronic skin troubles—such as psoriasis, eczema (also mentioned in chapter 12), or frequently recurring infections—should be treated constitutionally by a professional homeopath.

BEYOND HOME CARE

GET MEDICAL CARE IMMEDIATELY:

- if there is a new rash or skin eruption that looks like blood under the skin, is purple, or does not blanch when pressed. An accompanying fever is an additional danger sign;
- if there is a skin eruption that looks like a burn, or if large blisters appear spontaneously on the skin or mucous membranes.

SEE YOUR PRACTITIONER TODAY:

- if there has been an accompanying fever for more than 24 hours;
- if there is red streaking extending away from the site of an eruption or swollen area;
- if you think the skin eruption may be related to a medication;
- if the urine is red or dark.

BOILS, ABSCESSES, AND OTHER SKIN INFECTIONS

Boils and other skin infections occur when the skin's first levels of defense are breached. The outer layer of the skin serves as a barrier that is usually impenetrable to germs. Once disease-causing bacteria have passed through this outer barrier, they are quickly recognized by the immune defenses and attacked. More blood is brought to the area to increase these immune responses. At the same time, changes in the skin tissue occur that serve to wall off the infected area from nearby healthy skin, preventing the spread of the bacteria.

Boils are one way the interactions of germs and the body's defenses become visibly manifest. As the infection/inflammation process progresses, the skin becomes red, swollen, and warm because of the increased blood brought to the area. Stretching of the swollen skin may cause much pain. The inflammation may resolve without further complication, but when it does not eliminate and absorb the infection quickly, the walling-off process continues, and pus forms in a central cavity of the developing boil. Pus is a mixture of fluid from the blood, dead white blood cells, and bacteria. As the inflammatory process continues to battle aggressive germs, boils can become as large as an inch or two in diameter. A carbuncle is a particularly large boil with multiple centers of pus formation.

In time, the boil comes to a head at the surface of the skin, eventually opening to allow the pus to escape. Once the boil has ruptured and released the pus, pain is relieved immediately and the infection heals rapidly. But sometimes the infected material is permanently enclosed in a protective capsule, from which it may be absorbed by the body. The healthy function of these defenses results in complete healing of the skin or, at worst, a small lump where the infected tissue has been enclosed and reabsorbed.

Any localized collection of pus encapsulated in a cavity is called an abscess. Boils are abscesses in the skin, but abscesses themselves can occur in many other parts of the body. Abscesses you can treat often at home include infections around fingers and toenails (whitlows or felons), and styes on the eyelids (covered later in this chapter).

Boils usually are not serious health problems if the infection remains confined to the area of the swelling. But if the body's defenses cannot contain the bacteria within the boil, germs invade surrounding tissues, where they can spread more quickly and sometimes enter the bloodstream to cause generalized illness.

Cellulitis is the term for an infection spreading within the skin and underlying tissues that is not walled within a specific area. The first hint of cellulitis often is the presence of red streaks extending away from a boil, an abscess, or any other skin infection like impetigo (see the following section). The body continues to fight the infection with inflammation and immunity defenses, but until these defenses prevail, cellulitis develops as a puffy, red swelling that extends from the original infection and that feels warm to the touch. The inflammation of cellulitis is usually too diffuse to cause pus to form anywhere but in the original boil. When bacteria enter the bloodstream in significant numbers, a generalized illness may ensue. The person feels sick with fever, muscle aches, and severe headaches. Shock may occur.

GENERAL HOME CARE

The best home treatment for simple boils is to aid the body's inflammatory defenses with hot compresses or soakings. Applying heat to a well-localized skin infection brings the area even more blood to help kill germs, remove dead cells and debris, and begin the healing process. The heat helps bring the boil to a head and hastens the discharge of pus. Keeping a nutritious diet and getting plenty of rest also are essential.

CASETAKING QUESTIONS FOR SKIN INFECTIONS

Character of the symptoms:
- Has pus formed yet?
- What is the color of the infected area and surrounding skin?
- How painful is the area? What sort of pain is it—throbbing, burning, like splinters?

Modalities:
- How sensitive or tender to touch is the infection?
- Is the pain relieved or made worse by warm or cold applications?

HOMEOPATHIC MEDICINES

Homeopathic medicines help increase the body's natural protective responses to the infection. If the proper medicine is given early enough, the infection will resolve before pus ever forms. Given later, the medicines will help ripen the infection so that the pus is eliminated early and completely.

Use *Belladonna* during the early stages of any localized boil or abscess. There is painful, bright-red, hot swelling, but little or no pus formation yet. Throbbing in the developing boil is characteristic. Given early, *Belladonna* frequently helps the body arrest the development of the boil; healing occurs before pus forms.

If *Belladonna* does not help, or if treatment has begun more than twenty-four hours after the onset of symptoms, choose from one of the following medicines:

Before pus has clearly formed, *Hepar sulph.* often helps the body heal the inflammation by absorbing the boil altogether. If the young boil is very painful and tender to the touch, *Hepar* is especially well indicated. *Hepar* is useful also after pus has formed, again, if the inflamed part is very painful. *Hepar* boils typically are tender to the slightest touch and extremely sensitive to cold air or cold applications. There may be throbbing or, more often, sharp or sticking pains, as if a splinter were stuck in the painful part. *Hepar* also is a good medicine to try when a boil is slow to heal, even after pus has drained (*Silica* is another possibility in this situation).

Once pus has definitely formed and gathered, *Mercurius* is the likely remedy. This medicine helps bring the abscess to a head and speeds the drainage of pus. The boil is painful, but not so sensitive to touch as with *Hepar*. Warmth may aggravate the pain.

Silica is suitable for those boils or abscesses that are slow to heal, even though pus is freely draining. Compared with the *Hepar* boil, that of *Silica* is less sensitive and painful, though there may be relief with warmth. Give *Silica* two or three times a day after a boil or whitlow has been lanced and drained. *Silica* is indicated also when a boil comes on slowly or redness and swelling persist for several days without the development of pus. Firm, red, cystic lumps that persist after a boil has mostly healed often disappear after a dose or two of *Silica* 30c or by taking *Silica* 6x once or twice daily for one to two weeks.

Arsenicum is indicated at any stage of an abscess if there is great burning pain clearly relieved by warm applications. The general symptoms of *Arsenicum* may be present.

Choose *Lachesis* if the abscess and surrounding skin become bluish or purplish. Typically, pus is dark and thin, and the abscess is tender to touch. Be especially careful to discontinue this medicine as soon as improvement begins.

REMEDY SUMMARY FOR SKIN INFECTIONS

Give the medicine: Every 3 to 4 hours while redness, swelling, and pain are most acute, decreasing to 3 times a day until pus is no longer being discharged, swelling has improved, and redness diminishes.

When to try another medicine: After at least 3 doses of the previous medicine have had no effect.

BELLADONNA ★

Essentials
- Early stages of any localized boil or abscess
- Painful, bright-red, hot swelling, but as yet little or no pus formation

Confirmatory symptoms
- Throbbing pain

HEPAR SULPH. ★

Essentials
- After the earliest stage of a skin infection, but before pus has clearly formed
  or
- After pus has formed, if the inflamed part is very tender and painful
  or
- Boils that are slow to heal, even after pus has drained

Confirmatory symptoms
- Boils tender to the slightest touch, painfully sensitive to cold air or cold applications
- Sharp or sticking pains, as if a splinter were stuck in the painful part

MERCURIUS

Essentials
- The leading remedy after pus has formed and gathered into a definite boil

Confirmatory symptoms
- The boil is painful but not so sensitive to touch as with *Hepar*
- Pain aggravated by warmth

SILICA

Essentials
- Boils or abscesses that are slow to heal, even though pus is freely draining

248 Home Care with Homeopathic Medicine

or
- After a boil or whitlow has been lanced and drained
  or
- Boil comes on slowly, with redness and swelling that persist for several days without the development of pus
  or
- Firm, red, cystic lumps that persist after a boil has mostly healed (see text)

Confirmatory symptoms
- Relatively little sensitivity or pain, though there may be relief from warmth

ARSENICUM

Essentials
- Burning pain relieved by warm applications

Confirmatory symptoms
- General symptoms of *Arsenicum* are present (see *materia medica* section)

LACHESIS

Essentials
- Abscess and surrounding skin are bluish or purplish

Confirmatory symptoms
- Dark, thin pus
- Abscess tender to touch

BEYOND HOME CARE

GET MEDICAL CARE IMMEDIATELY:

- for high fever, severe headache, or neck stiffness.

SEE YOUR PRACTITIONER TODAY:

- for infection with fever, malaise, or muscle aches;

- if a boil is located on the head or face;
- if redness or swelling is spreading from the boil area;
- if pain is severe or the boil is extremely swollen with pus;
- if the boil is not improving with home treatment after 48 to 72 hours;
- if the boil has opened but does not appear to be healing after a week.

STYES

A stye is an infected pimple or small boil on the eyelid. The germs, usually *Staphylococci*, grow in the oil or sweat glands of the eyelid. The inflammation surfaces at the margin of the lid as a tender, red swelling. Within a few days, the stye comes to a head and then opens to let pus drain. Pimples similar to styes also may form on the inside of the eyelid and are basically the same type of infection. Occasionally, however, these infections on the inner eyelid may spread and involve the whole lid.

Although they can be quite painful, styes are rarely dangerous and they usually heal by themselves. Occasionally a stye does not heal completely and leaves behind a firm, red, cystic lump in the eyelid. These cysts are not painful themselves, but in some cases they rub against the eye, and new acute styes may develop within them recurrently. Constitutional homeopathic treatment can help strengthen the body's immune system.

GENERAL HOME CARE

Soak a clean washcloth in warm water and apply it to the affected eye for ten to fifteen minutes, three or four times a day. The warmer the water, the better—though you should make sure it isn't hot enough to burn the skin. Expect the stye to improve within forty-eight hours.

CASETAKING QUESTIONS FOR STYES

Character of the symptoms:
- How painful is the stye? What sort of pain is it—throbbing, burning, like splinters?

- Where is the stye located? Note which lid it is on (upper or lower), and whether or not it is near the inner corner of the eye.
- Is there a discharge from the stye, and what does it look like?
- Is the eyelid involved? If so, how—is it just swollen, or are there crusts or scales?

Modalities:
- How sensitive or tender to touch is the stye?
- Is the pain relieved or made worse by warm or cold applications?

HOMEOPATHIC MEDICINES

Pulsatilla is one of the more commonly used medicines for people with styes, and it should be given if no other medicine is clearly indicated. More often, the stye occurs on the upper lid. The stye may not be particularly painful, in spite of the inflammation. It comes to a head and discharges a yellow to green pus.

Staphysagria is indicated when styes come out in crops, one after another, over a period of weeks. The problem may begin after the person suffers nervous exhaustion. It is a good medicine to try also when the symptoms don't suggest a more specific choice.

Hepar sulph. is effective when the stye is hypersensitive to touch, cold air, and cold applications. The pain is throbbing in character, or it may feel as if a splinter were in the eyelid. The pain is relieved by warm applications.

Apis also covers painful styes, especially those that burn and sting and are worse from heat or warm applications. *Apis* should be thought of also if the entire lid becomes red and swollen.

Graphites styes are painful, but not so tender to touch as those of *Hepar.* Thick yellow material may be discharged from the stye. Crusts, scales, and sores on the eyelid are typical of *Graphites.*

Try *Lycopodium* if the stye is near the inner corner of the eye and other remedies listed above haven't helped.

Firm cysts that remain in the eyelid after the acute stage of a stye often heal following a dose or two of the thirtieth potency of *Staphysagria* or *Silica.* Also you can try either of these remedies in a lower strength (3x, 3c, 6x, or 6c) given daily for ten to fourteen days.

Since styes are simply small skin abscesses located in the eyelids, any of the medicines listed in the section on boils and abscesses also may be helpful. If none of the remedies listed here seems to fit the case, read the descriptions in that section for additional options.

REMEDY SUMMARY FOR STYES

Give the medicine: Every 6 to 8 hours for up to 3 days, stopping when improvement occurs. Repeat the dose only if the symptoms worsen again, or if there has been no further improvement for 24 hours.

When to try another medicine: If there is no improvement after 24 to 48 hours.

PULSATILLA ★

Confirmatory symptoms
- Relatively painless styes
- Stye occurs on the upper lid
- Discharges of yellow to green pus

HEPAR SULPH.

Essentials
- Stye is hypersensitive to touch, cold air, and cold applications

Confirmatory symptoms
- Pain is throbbing or feels as if a splinter were in the eyelid
- Pain relieved by warm applications

APIS

Essentials
- Styes with burning or stinging pains

Confirmatory symptoms
- Pain worse from heat or warm applications
- Redness and swelling of entire lid

GRAPHITES

Essentials
- Stye is painful but not so tender to touch as with *Hepar*

Confirmatory symptoms
- Discharge of thick yellow material from the stye
- Crusts, scales, and sores on the eyelids

STAPHYSAGRIA

Essentials
- Styes come out in crops over a period of weeks
  or
- Firm cysts remain in the eyelid after the acute stage of a stye

Confirmatory symptoms
- Styes begin after the patient experiences stress

LYCOPODIUM

Essentials
- Stye near the inner corner of the eye, if other remedies haven't helped

SILICA

Essentials
- Firm cysts remain in the eyelid after the acute stage of a stye

---

BEYOND HOME CARE

GET MEDICAL CARE TODAY:

- if vision is affected in any way;
- if the stye is accompanied by fever, headache, loss of appetite, or lethargy;
- if the swelling is located on or directed toward the inside of the eyelid;
- if the stye persists for more than 48 hours despite the use of warm applications and homeopathic treatment.

Note: Consult the section on conjunctivitis if the white of the eye becomes inflamed.

IMPETIGO

Impetigo is a highly contagious, superficial bacterial infection of the skin caused by *Streptococcus* and *Staphylococcus* bacteria. The eruption consists of small, red, raised bumps that quickly develop into tiny blisters, which then pop and ooze a sticky fluid and leave raw, red sores. Soon the sores are covered with a sticky, golden yellow crust. The infection can spread rapidly, as the bacteria are carried on fingers, clothing, and so on. Crops of crusty sores may develop quickly. Children are more prone to impetigo than are adults, and they can easily pass on the contagious germs to their playmates.

Impetigo is more commonly located on the face. Sores frequently appear on the cheeks, about the lips, and at the nostrils. The sores' appearance is similar to that of cold sores or herpes, but impetigo spreads more rapidly, does not confine itself to one area of the body, and does not affect the inner lips or inside the mouth. Any doubt about which infection is responsible for a given eruption can be cleared up by taking a culture.

Impetigo sores rarely hurt, and eventually most people overcome the infection on their own. But in the meantime the sores may become widespread, and other people may become infected. There also are a number of complications that can develop. These include infection of the deeper layers of skin (see the discussion of cellulitis in the section on boils), and a kidney disease that is caused by the immune system's reaction to *Streptococcus* germs. Only certain strains of the strep bacteria trigger this disease (called glomerulonephritis), so several members of a family, neighborhood, or school group all may come down with it after catching impetigo. Symptoms include malaise, loss of appetite, nausea, headache, reduced urine production, and puffiness and swelling of the face and extremities. This illness almost always clears up without permanent problems.

Conventional practitioners use oral antibiotics, including erythromycin and synthetic penicillin drugs such as dicloxacillin. Antibiotics do not prevent glomerulonephritis, but they do kill the germs and help prevent spread of the infection, and that makes them a valid choice as a public health measure.

GENERAL HOME CARE

Preventing impetigo is difficult, but you should try to keep your children from playing with others who have the infection. If you or a family member has impetigo, avoid touching the sores, and wash your hands immediately if you do. Use warm soakings to remove the crusts, and then wash them and the surrounding skin with gentle soap and water. *Calendula* tincture (diluted 3:1 with sterile water or normal saline) should then be painted on the sores with a sterile cotton swab. Allow the sores to dry, and leave them exposed to the air. Topical antibiotics such as Neosporin rarely help, and creams may delay healing.

CASETAKING QUESTIONS FOR IMPETIGO

Character of the symptoms:
- Describe the sores: Are they primarily crusty, or open sores?
- What color are they, and what color is the fluid?
- Is there burning pain or itching?

Modalities:
- How sensitive or tender to touch is the area?
- How is the pain or the rash itself affected by warmth or bathing?

Other symptoms:
- Are nearby lymph nodes swollen?

HOMEOPATHIC MEDICINES

Antimonium crudum covers the classic symptoms of impetigo. There is an oozing eruption with the formation of thick yellow crusts. The eruption is worse on the face. The individual sores begin to run together into larger patches. They may seem to spread or look more inflamed after bathing. In general the *Antimonium crudum* patient is irritable and may not be able to stand being looked at. The tongue may have a thick white coat.

The person who has impetigo with markedly scabby, oozy eruptions needs *Graphites*. This is especially true if the liquid in the sores is sticky and has the color, though not necessarily the thickness, of honey. The sores are more likely to be worse around the mouth or nose.

Rhus tox. may be indicated when impetigo is maddeningly itchy. The blisters are small but appear in clusters. There may be stinging or tingling in the sores as well. The discomfort is better when the patient is moving around. The discharge from the crusty, oozing sores is sometimes dark but translucent.

Mercurius is indicated if the sores are open and especially deep. The typical yellowish crusts may form, especially around the mouth or on the scalp, but the discharge is of pus rather than of translucent liquid and is likely to smell bad. The discharge also may be streaked with a little blood. Swelling of the lymph nodes of the face and neck is common.

Hepar sulph. can be a good medicine for the person with impetigo if the sores are especially sensitive to touch and to cold. The scabs are often soft and break apart easily. As with *Mercurius,* there may well be pus formation and swelling of the glands. Also similar to *Mercurius,* the sores may be deep and may bleed a little. The typical *Hepar* patient is extremely irritable.

If the sores burn or feel painfully raw, and feel better in warmth or with warm applications, *Arsenicum* probably is indicated. The sores tend to look dark. They exude a thin watery fluid.

REMEDY SUMMARY FOR IMPETIGO

Give the medicine: Every 4 to 6 hours for 2 to 3 days.
When to try another medicine: If there is no change after 24 hours.

ANTIMONIUM CRUDUM ★

Essentials
- Oozing eruption with thick yellow crusts

Confirmatory symptoms
- Sores run together into larger patches
- Sores spread or look more inflamed after bathing
- Irritability; person can't stand to be looked at
- Tongue coated thick white

GRAPHITES

Essentials
- Scabby eruptions oozing a sticky, honey-colored liquid

Confirmatory symptoms
- Sores worse around mouth or nose

RHUS TOX.

Essentials
- Itchy, crusty sores

Confirmatory symptoms
- Small blisters in clusters
- Itching, stinging, or tingling in the sores
- Discharge dark-colored but translucent
- Discomfort is better when the patient is moving around

MERCURIUS

Essentials
- Some sores open, deep
- Discharge of pus rather than of translucent liquid; discharge may be bloody, smells bad

Confirmatory symptoms
- Swelling of the lymph nodes of the face and neck
- General symptoms of *Mercurius* (see *materia medica* section)

HEPAR SULPH.

Essentials
- Sores sensitive to touch and cold

Confirmatory symptoms
- Symptoms similar to *Mercurius*: deep sores, pus formation with some bleeding, swollen glands
- Scabs are often soft and break apart easily
- Irritability

ARSENICUM

Essentials
- Sores burn or feel painfully raw
- Pain is better with warm applications
- Sores tend to look dark

Confirmatory symptoms
- Discharge of thin, watery fluid

BEYOND HOME CARE

GET MEDICAL CARE TODAY:

- if there are more than 3 or 4 sores, or if the sores are large or painful;
- if there is fever, malaise, or muscle aches;
- if redness or swelling extends from the sores;
- if you are infected after exposure to others who have had glomerulonephritis;
- if the sores do not improve within 48 to 72 hours.

HERPES SIMPLEX

Herpes is an infection of the skin and nerves caused by a small virus related to the chicken pox virus. After exposure to the germ, usually in three to six days, the characteristic eruption breaks out, appearing as groups of tiny blisters (vesicles) surrounded by red, angry, inflamed skin. Each individual vesicle is only a millimeter across, while the patches of grouped vesicles are usually about a centimeter (a half-inch) in diameter or less.

At first, each tiny vesicle is filled with a clear liquid, but this may become white or yellow pus. After a day or so, the vesicles pop and merge, leaving a shallow, raw, red sore, which in turn scabs, eventually dries up, and heals.

There are two strains of the herpes simplex virus: Type I usually infects the face and mouth (cold sores or fever blisters), while Type II more often is responsible for eruptions on the genitals and surrounding areas. The virus enters through the skin or mucous membranes. It can live only within the human body, so infection is passed from one person to the next through direct contact with the sores or by being carried briefly on something warm and moist such as fingers or a towel. Recently it has been shown that the virus can survive briefly in bathwater or hot tubs, but it is quickly destroyed when dried. Herpes is more contagious when the vesicles are present or just after they have popped, but it should be considered infectious until the sores are healed completely.

Once you contract herpes, the virus lives permanently in the infected nerve cells. It is estimated that 95 percent of the population harbors the Type I germ. Herpes eruptions are often recurrent; they may break out at regular intervals or in response to a particular stimulus, such as sunlight or sexual activity. The first time the sores appear is usually the worst, as they form in larger, more numerous, and more painful groups of vesicles. About a third of the people with first-time herpes experience fever, muscle aches, headache, and other general symptoms suggestive of a viral illness. These symptoms rarely return with later outbreaks, but generally the sores themselves hurt or itch somewhat.

Herpes is not a serious disease in healthy adults, though it can be painful and annoying. Most people adjust to the virus fairly well, and recurrences generally become less frequent over time. Homeopaths consider most cases of herpes as representing relatively mild illness, the same as the majority of skin diseases. The body's defense mechanism is able to keep the level of physiological imbalance, as manifested in the susceptibility to the herpes infection, at the very periphery of the body, an achievement consistent with good health.

In contrast to the ordinary form of this illness, herpes can be a serious, generalized infection if it occurs in newborn babies or people whose immunity is too weak. Preventing herpes in babies is critical, and mothers prone to recurrent herpes outbreaks should be observed closely by their practitioners. No one with an active herpes sore of either type should be allowed to handle a baby unless the sores are completely covered by clean clothing or a fresh bandage, and then only if the person bathes and washes his hands thoroughly before touching the child. People who suffer from debilitating illnesses or who have seriously decreased resistance also are susceptible to severe herpes infection, and the same precautions apply.

Another serious concern is herpes infection of the eye. The symptoms, including redness and watering, are similar to those of ordinary viral conjunctivitis (see chapter 4), but there is, in addition, marked pain and reduced vision. Herpes sores may or may not be present on the face. This is a serious condition that can cause permanent damage to eyesight if untreated. It represents an emergency and must be treated by a medical professional immediately (see "Beyond Home Care" in the section on conjunctivitis in chapter 4).

In conventional medicine, antiviral drugs such as acyclovir are now being used against herpes. These medicines more effectively treat the rash than previous nonspecific measures. Still, the homeopath's concern is that drug treatment only suppresses the eruption and thereby blocks the body's best strategy of dealing with the underlying imbalance.

GENERAL HOME CARE

Keep the eruption and surrounding skin clean and dry. When practical, cover it with a gauze bandage to protect it from injury and to keep out dirt and bacteria. Check the area from time to time to be sure that a bacterial infection isn't taking hold (indicated by a great deal of pus or redness spreading from around the sores). Take special care to eat well and get ample rest.

CASETAKING QUESTIONS FOR HERPES

Character of the symptoms:
- How painful is the eruption? What is the character of the pain—burning, stinging, or another sensation?
- How large are the blisters and sores?
- Describe any liquid that oozes from the sores.

Modalities:
- How sensitive or tender to touch is the eruption?
- How is the pain or itching affected by warm or cold applications?

Other symptoms:
- Does the person feel generally unwell?
- Are there any general aches and pains?
- Are there cracks in the lips?

HOMEOPATHIC MEDICINES

Rhus tox. is an important remedy for people with herpes. Small inflamed blisters appearing in clusters and filled with a yellowish, watery fluid are typical of herpes and of this medicine, as are intense burning and itching. Outbreaks may be accompanied by a general feeling of sickness and achiness, with aches and pains improved by moving around. *Rhus tox.,* along with *Arsenicum, Natrum mur.,* and *Hepar,* is a primary medicine for people with cold sores around the lips or mouth.

Arsenicum should be thought of if the herpes sores burn intensely but feel better when warmth is applied. The other typical general symptoms of *Arsenicum* also may be present.

Natrum mur. is indicated when herpes blisters containing a clear liquid develop about the lips, appearing like little pearls. The lips may be cracked. Often the cold sores appear during a fever or cold. Though the sores may be painful, pain is not as characteristic as with other medicines like *Hepar* or *Arsenicum*.

Herpes sores that are painfully sensitive to touch or cold suggest *Hepar*. Pus is likely to form rapidly.

Give *Graphites* if the eruptions ooze a translucent, sticky fluid the color of honey. The individual blisters are likely to be large (pea-sized or larger). They usually itch.

Sepia is considered an important medicine for herpes of both the face and the genitals. Unfortunately, however, there are few distinguishing skin symptoms. If the general symptoms of this medicine (as discussed in the *materia medica* section) match those of the person treated, certainly it should be given. Otherwise we suggest you try it if no other medicine seems to fit or if others haven't helped.

Petroleum is especially indicated for people who have herpes sores in the genital area that are moist and that ooze and itch. The itching may be worse in the open air and better in warmth. In men, the eruption may be on the penis, but more characteristically it is on the scrotum or the area between the scrotum and thighs. The medicine is equally appropriate for women with genital herpes.

Apply *Calendula* tincture, diluted 3:1 with water, several times a day after the sores have opened; this helps the skin heal a little more quickly.

REMEDY SUMMARY FOR HERPES

Give the medicine: During an acute outbreak, twice daily for 2 to 3 days, stopping after definite improvement begins.
When to try another medicine: If there is no change after 2 days.

RHUS TOX. ★

Essentials
- Small inflamed blisters appearing in clusters and filled with a yellowish, watery fluid
- Intense burning pain, with or without itching

Confirmatory symptoms
- General feeling of sickness and achiness; aches and pains improved by moving around
- Cold sores around the lips or mouth

ARSENICUM

Essentials
- Herpes sores that burn intensely but feel better when warmth is applied

Confirmatory symptoms
- General symptoms of *Arsenicum* (see *materia medica* section)

NATRUM MUR.

Essentials
- Blisters containing a clear liquid develop about the lips, appearing like little pearls

Confirmatory symptoms
- Cracked lips
- Cold sores appearing during a fever or cold
- Pain, if any, is mild

SEPIA

Essentials
- Use if the general symptoms of *Sepia* are present (see *materia medica* section)
  or
- Use if no other medicine seems to fit or if others haven't helped

PETROLEUM

Essentials
- Herpes sores in the genital area that ooze and itch

Confirmatory symptoms
- Itching worse in the open air and better in warmth
- In men, herpes located on the scrotum or in the area between the scrotum and thighs

HEPAR SULPH.

Essentials
- Sores painfully sensitive to touch or cold

Confirmatory symptoms
• Irritability

GRAPHITES

Essentials
• Sores ooze a translucent, sticky fluid the color of honey

Confirmatory symptoms
• Large individual blisters (pea-sized or larger)
• Itching sores

BEYOND HOME CARE
See "Beyond Home Care" following herpes zoster.

Herpes Zoster (Shingles)

Herpes zoster (shingles) is a skin eruption associated with reactivation of the chicken pox virus. Once a person has had chicken pox, the virus lives on in the nervous system in a dormant state. In some individuals the virus becomes reactivated, travels down a particular nerve, and multiplies at the ends of the nerve on the skin surface. The resulting eruption looks similar to herpes simplex, but typically the individual blisters are bigger and the overall area of skin involved is larger.

Shingles may erupt on nearly any part of the body, but more commonly it breaks out on the trunk or face. The eruptions are always distributed along the course of the infected nerve. In all but rare cases, only a single nerve is involved, and the rash is confined to one side of the body or one part (a leg, an arm, one side of the face or back). The rash itself usually clears up within a few weeks, but many people have severe pain that lasts for weeks or months because of the irritation of the nerve.

Conventional medical treatment for generally healthy people with herpes zoster is limited to symptom relief, using painkillers and antihistamines that must be taken repeatedly. New antiviral drugs are being tested and are used for patients with reduced immunity. Antidepressant and anticonvulsant drugs are recommended by conventional practitioners for the pain that lingers after the rash has cleared.

GENERAL HOME CARE

Pressure on the rash may relieve pain and discomfort, and may be applied with a snug elastic (Ace) bandage. Cool compresses also may help. Protect the sores with a loose, dry gauze bandage when you are active. You should examine the rash to make sure there has been no secondary bacterial infection (the signs would be pus or redness extending from around the rash).

CASETAKING QUESTIONS FOR HERPES ZOSTER (SHINGLES)

Character of the symptoms:
- What is the character of the pain—burning or sharp?
- How bad is the itching?
- Where is the rash located?
- What is the color of the rash?

Modalities:
- How is the pain or itching affected by warmth or cold, motion, breathing, touch, or rubbing?

Other symptoms:
- Does a digestive disturbance accompany the rash?

HOMEOPATHIC MEDICINES

Homeopathic medicines can help the body restore health to the irritated nerves and permanently relieve pain. Untreated, herpes zoster may last three or four weeks; even when homeopathic treatment is successful, the rash may require seven to ten days to heal, although we have seen better results.

Rhus tox. is indicated by intense itching as well as pain. Pea-sized blisters filled with a yellowish but watery fluid appear. Gently rubbing the inflamed areas may give some relief, and moving around lightly also helps.

Ranunculus bulbosus often proves helpful during an attack of shingles, particularly when it involves the chest or back. The pain is severe, especially between the ribs, and is made worse by touch or motion. Breathing deeply or lying on the rash also may aggravate the pain.

Arsenicum is an especially important medicine for people with herpes zoster. The eruption burns intensely, there is relief from warmth, and aggravation from cold air or cold applications. The general characteristics of the *Arsenicum* patient may be in evidence.

Lachesis should be considered if the rash is very dark red or especially if it looks bluish or purplish. The eruption is very painful and extremely sensitive to touch. Typically, *Lachesis* eruptions are worse on the left side of the body.

Mezereum should be considered when there are burning pains or sharp lightninglike pains, especially when the pains remain after the eruption is gone. The pains are worse while the patient is eating or in bed, and from touch. People who need *Mezereum* are chilly and sensitive to cold air.

Iris versicolor may be appropriate if the rash involves the right side of the abdomen or chest. An unusual feature sometimes seen is the appearance of small blisters with dark points. Digestive upsets may accompany the rash.

Apis, Mercurius, Hepar sulph., and *Sulphur* all are sometimes indicated for the person with zoster. Consult the *materia medica* section and the references to these medicines elsewhere in this chapter if none of the above descriptions seems to fit.

REMEDY SUMMARY FOR HERPES ZOSTER

Give the medicine: Every 8 to 12 hours for 2 days; if symptoms return, repeat the medicine no more than twice a day.
When to try another medicine: If there is no change after 2 days.

RHUS TOX. ★

Essentials
• Eruptions are painful and itch intensely

Confirmatory symptoms
• Relief from gentle rubbing of the inflamed areas
• Relief from steady, gentle motion

RANUNCULUS BULBOSUS ★

Essentials
• Zoster on the chest or back with marked pain worse from touch, motion, or breathing deeply

Confirmatory symptoms
• Severe pain between ribs

LACHESIS

Essentials
- Zoster that appears very dark red, bluish, or purplish
- Much pain, extremely sensitive to touch

Confirmatory symptoms
- Eruptions on left side of the body

MEZEREUM

Essentials
- Burning or sharp lightninglike pains; pain remains after eruption heals

Confirmatory symptoms
- Pains worse while eating, in bed, and from touch
- Patient feels chilly and dislikes cold air

IRIS VERSICOLOR

Essentials
- Zoster on the right side of the abdomen or chest

Confirmatory symptoms
- Small blisters with dark points
- Skin symptoms accompanied by digestive upset

ARSENICUM

Essentials
- Eruption burns intensely

Confirmatory symptoms
- Relief from warmth; aggravation from cold air or cold applications
- General symptoms of *Arsenicum* (see *materia medica* section)

BEYOND HOME CARE

These indications are for herpes simplex and herpes zoster.

GET MEDICAL CARE TODAY:

• if an apparent herpes eruption is located on the face, especially if near the eye;
• if you have any sores on the genitals or develop an eruption after sexual contact, unless you're sure it is a recurrence of herpes you've had before;
• if the rash has lasted longer than a week without improvement;
• if there are signs of secondary bacterial infection: much pus, spreading redness, or swelling.

SEE YOUR PRACTITIONER SOON:

• the first time you get any eruption you think may be herpes;
• if you are pregnant and have a rash that may be herpes.

CALL YOUR PRACTITIONER TODAY:

• if you are in the last trimester of a pregnancy and this is the first outbreak.

Note: Some pus in the herpes sores is expected, even when there is no significant bacterial problem (see "Beyond Home Care" in the sections on boils and impetigo).

WARTS

Warts are overgrowths of skin cells triggered by a viral infection. As the body reacts to the virus, regulatory control of cell division is disrupted and the infected skin cells begin to grow and divide abnormally, building upon themselves till they form the familiar cauliflower shape of a wart.

Warts are caused by a closely related group of viruses. There are several types of warts, including common warts, which most often appear on the hands, feet, and face; venereal warts, which grow on the genitals, anus, and surrounding areas; plantar warts, which form on the soles of the feet; flat warts—smooth, barely elevated, oval spots on the face; and molluscum contagiosum—smooth, rounded bumps with a central pit, or plug.

Wart viruses are contagious, but some people are extremely susceptible to infection, others very resistant. Children get warts more easily than adults, and venereal warts are more contagious than other types. The ordinary wart virus is so common that there is no way to prevent your exposure to it. You should not be overly concerned about contact with others who have warts.

People who already have them do notice that the warts readily spread to nearby areas, especially if the skin is cut or scraped. Shaving cuts are notorious for "seeding" warts, and a whole crop may grow on the throat of a susceptible man. Children with finger warts may spread the infection by pulling on hangnails or biting their nails.

Warts cause no pain or other symptoms unless they are subjected to pressure or friction. Plantar warts usually cause pain during walking, and warts on the writing fingers of schoolchildren may hurt.

Conventional treatment of warts involves applying topical agents that chemically dissolve the warts, destroying them with electricity, or freezing them with liquid nitrogen. Warts should not be removed surgically, since the virus can easily spread to cut skin. We recommend that you avoid these suppressive measures at least until you've already tried homeopathic medicines or suggested treatments.

GENERAL HOME CARE

Warts will disappear sooner or later, and it is fine to leave them alone if they are not causing pain. The best treatment for warts is one that makes the body "take notice" of the virus. Once the body starts to fight the virus, warts shrivel up quickly, often in just a day or two, no matter how long they have been there. The power of suggestion is particularly effective in rousing the body's defenses against the wart virus. You might try visualizing the warts disappearing, saying a spell over them, or any other safe "ritual" treatment that appeals to you.

HOMEOPATHIC MEDICINES

Homeopathic medicines have been very successful in helping people rid themselves of wart infections. The placebo effect is of course at work here, too, but in our admittedly biased observations we have seen many rapid and dramatic successes with homeopathic medicines, more than we've seen with other treatments. You should use homeopathic treatments for yourself or a family member if the warts are numerous, painful, or if their appearance really bothers you. The person may receive home treatment if he has no significant concurrent health problems.

The best homeopathic medicine for someone with warts is the constitutional prescription. It's preferable to have professional care if it is available. If not, try a medicine from the following list. Give it in the 6x or 6c potency twice a day for a week, or give a single dose of the thirtieth potency. Allow at least two weeks before trying another medicine.

Thuja warts may be anywhere on the body and of any type, but those that especially indicate this medicine are on the chin, genitals, or anus. These are often soft warts and may be painful or bleeding. (You can also try painting any wart with *Thuja* tincture twice a day.)

Causticum symptoms include fleshy warts anywhere, but especially near the fingernails or on the face (often near the lips), and warts with extra growth on stalks above the main part.

Dulcamara may help with warts on the backs of hands or fingers or on the face. They tend to be large, smooth, and flat.

Antimonium crudum warts are horny and hardened, or they can have a smooth surface. In our experience this medicine has been consistently helpful to otherwise healthy people with plantar warts.

Another remedy that is effective in treating a wide variety of plantar warts is *Ruta,* though it tends to be more useful to people whose plantar warts are sore or have a smooth surface.

Nitric acid is another important medicine when warts appear on the genitals or anus. There may be warts on the lips. Soft warts; irregular shapes or irregularities on stalks; great pain, especially sharp, sticking pains; and bleeding warts, especially of the genitals, all are symptoms that may indicate this medicine's use.

RINGWORM, ATHLETE'S FOOT, AND RELATED FUNGAL INFECTIONS

"Ringworm" is the common name for a fungal skin infection that results in rough, dry, slightly raised eruptions that occur usually in circular patches. The infected area is slightly reddened. As the eruption gradually enlarges, the central portion begins to heal and clear, while the advancing border remains slightly raised and reddened, thus creating the ringlike appearance that gives the infection its name. This is the typical pattern, but ringworm infections sometimes occur without having the clearing in the center or without being circular in outline. Pus does not form, and if the eruption is left alone, it does not become raw or scabby.

Ringworm is known medically as *tinea corporis.* Other related fungi also cause skin infections. *Tinea capitis* is ringworm of the scalp; athlete's foot, jock itch, and fungus infections under the nails all are called *tinea cruris*. A similar skin fungus causes *tinea versicolor,* an infection of the face, trunk, and extremities, consisting of light or fawn-colored, oval, slightly scaly patches that do not tan. Children seem particularly prone to ringworm of the body and scalp, but athlete's foot, jock itch, and *tinea versicolor* occur in individuals of all ages.

Severe itching is the worst potential symptom of these infections, but often there is no itching at all. There are no serious complications, and all of these fungal infections are only moderately contagious. Even people who have direct contact with the eruptions may not develop the infection themselves. On the other hand, contact with the lesions, or with clothing, personal articles, or locker-room floors used by infected individuals does spread the fungi. Those with *tinea* infections should be careful to avoid spreading the germs. If you have athlete's foot, avoid stepping barefoot on locker-room floors.

Conventional medical treatment involves antifungal creams, ointments, powders, or sprays. These topical medications have few side effects, but still we recommend you first allow the body to do its own housecleaning before you resort to conventional treatments.

GENERAL HOME CARE

Ringworm and related fungal infections do eventually clear up if untreated, but usually you can hasten their departure. Simple home measures include keeping the infected area dry and, if possible, exposed to light (this is especially important for jock itch and athlete's foot). Wear clean clothing and socks. Painting the area with vinegar diluted with equal parts of water once or twice a day may help the skin to clear more quickly.

CASETAKING QUESTIONS FOR RINGWORM

Character of the symptoms:
- What is the color of the rash?
- Are there scales or crusts? Does fluid ooze from the rash, and if so, how does it appear?
- Is there pain or itching?

Modalities:
- How is the pain or itching affected by warmth or warm applications?

HOMEOPATHIC MEDICINES

People who have ringworm but few other symptoms are difficult to treat with homeopathy, since the skin problem itself usually causes so few symptoms. If there are other problems in addition to the fungus infection, you should receive professional constitutional care. Otherwise, choose a medicine from those listed in this section.

Sepia is probably the most commonly useful medicine for those with simple ringworm infections. The circular, scaly patches are dry and brownish or brownish-red. There may be itching, which changes to burning after scratching.

Tellurium is indicated when the ringworm is more red than brown. The rings are therefore well marked and prominent. Tiny blisters that itch and release a thin liquid may appear on the rings.

Graphites helps some people with ringworm; use it as your first choice if the scales are quite thick or if there is significant oozing. *Graphites* is strongly indicated if the fluid is sticky and honey-colored.

Sulphur may be indicated if the eruption itches a great deal, more so if warmth causes itching. General symptoms of *Sulphur* may be present.

Arsenicum is indicated for those who have very dry ringworm with rough scales. Burning and itching are characteristic. There may be a discharge of clear liquid after scratching.

All of the above medicines may be helpful when the ringworm is on the scalp. Two medicines also particularly indicated for ringworm of the scalp are *Calcarea* and *Dulcamara*. Both cover thick crusts on the scalp that may be accompanied by swelling of the lymph nodes in the neck and head.

REMEDY SUMMARY FOR RINGWORM

Give the medicine: Once a day for 3 days, stopping before then if the symptoms change.

When to try another medicine: After a week if the eruption hasn't changed.

SEPIA ★

Essentials
• Circular, dry, scaly patches, brownish or brownish-red in color (itching may be present)

Confirmatory symptoms
• Itching changes to burning after scratching

TELLURIUM

Essentials
• Ringworm more red than brown; the rings are therefore prominent and well marked

Confirmatory symptoms
• Rash has tiny itching blisters that release a thin liquid

GRAPHITES

Essentials
• Ringworm with thick scales or oozing

Confirmatory symptoms
• Sticky, honey-colored fluid

SULPHUR

Essentials
• Very marked itching

Confirmatory symptoms
• Warmth causes or worsens itching
• General symptoms of *Sulphur* (see *materia medica* section)

ARSENICUM

Essentials
• Dry ringworm with rough scales
• Burning and itching

Confirmatory symptoms
• Discomfort relieved by warmth
• Discharge of clear liquid after scratching

BEYOND HOME CARE

SEE YOUR PRACTITIONER SOON:

• if an apparent ringworm eruption lasts longer than a couple of weeks, or if you need help in diagnosis.

CANDIDA (YEAST INFECTIONS)

The eruption that results from a *Candida* fungus (known commonly as yeast) infection is quite different from those triggered by the ringworm, or *tinea,* fungi. It may start as small, red, raised dots that grow together or spread out from a single infected area. Before long the rash turns into a raised patch or patches of angry red. Between and surrounding the larger patches, small new spots erupt, and the patches spread outward and toward one another. The eruption is initially dry, without blisters or pus formation, but the inflamed skin looks raw, and shallow open places may develop and begin to weep. Bacteria can invade, leading to pimplelike bumps or pus in the open areas.

Candida eruptions tend to spread faster than ringworm infections, at least when they involve areas of the body conducive to growth of the fungus. When the infected person is otherwise healthy, the *Candida* fungus thrives only in warm, dark, moist places on the skin. Common sites are the groin, under the arms, under the breasts, and in skin folds of overweight individuals. Considering these environmental preferences, one can easily see why the *Candida* fungus is so often involved in diaper rashes. The diaper keeps the skin warm and moist, providing the perfect conditions for growth of the organism. In addition, the prolonged contact with the moisture and irritating chemicals of urine weakens and inflames the skin, allowing the fungus to enter. Even when a diaper rash is caused initially by simple irritation from contact with urine, the *Candida* fungus usually becomes involved within a few days.

The same *Candida* fungus also is involved in vaginal infections (see chapter 9) and in the thrush infections of the mouth so common among babies. Thrush is characterized by off-white, elevated patches that may occur anywhere in the mouth. If you scrape off a patch, the underlying lining of the mouth bleeds. Breast-feeding mothers often get *Candida* of the nipples from their children's mouths.

The resistance of the individual is of course a major factor that determines whether or not a person gets a *Candida* infection. Some babies, for instance, never have a problem with diaper rashes, while others get them all the time, in spite of parents' best efforts to keep them clean and dry. Most of the time, even really bad or recurrent *Candida* infections result from a specific susceptibility to the particular fungus, and the person is not sickly in any other way. At times, however, frequent or severe *Candida* infections are the first warning of a serious general illness, like diabetes or an immune disorder. Your health practitioner should check for such illnesses if you or a family member is prone to severe or recurrent *Candida* infections or when adults or older children get thrush.

Over the past fifteen years or so, there has been popular concern about the possibility of subtle *Candida* infections of the whole system in people with normal immune defenses. Some practitioners have claimed that these undetected systemic *Candida* infections are responsible for a wide range of symptoms and illnesses. Whether this actually is true or not is not the primary issue. An underlying imbalance or susceptibility must exist to allow any infection to become established, and treating the infecting germs does nothing to restore balance. Constitutional care should be sought for individuals susceptible to infection and for those with recurrent symptoms, regardless of the supposed cause.

GENERAL HOME CARE

Exposing the affected area to dry air and light usually enables the body to heal the infection quickly. Babies' diapers should be changed frequently and whenever they become wet. Clean and dry the diaper area carefully before rediapering the child, and allow her to stay out of the diapers as much as possible. Vinegar retards the growth of this fungus and neutralizes the alkalinity of the urine. If you use cloth diapers, try adding a cup of vinegar to the last rinse. It may also help to paint the affected area with vinegar diluted to quarter-strength (make sure it doesn't sting the raw skin). Apply sparingly either *Calendula* ointment or *Calendula* tincture diluted 3:1 with water to any raw areas a few times a day.

Adults and older children sometimes find that strictly avoiding sweets helps prevent and quickly heal *Candida* infections. Homeopathic treatment usually is not necessary unless there is a constitutional susceptibility to frequent infections. Conventional medicine treats *Candida* infections with various antifungal drugs applied directly to the skin or given orally.

CASETAKING QUESTIONS FOR CANDIDAL INFECTIONS OF THE SKIN

Character of the symptoms:
- How does the skin appear—is it simply red and swollen, are there raw areas, or are there pimplelike eruptions?
- Is there oozing from the affected area, and if so, does the fluid appear to irritate the skin?
- How painful is the rash, and what type of pain is it?
- How much does the rash itch?

Modalities:
- How sensitive or tender to touch is the rash?
- How is the pain or itching affected by bathing or warm applications?

HOMEOPATHIC MEDICINES

Belladonna is indicated if the skin is bright red and swollen with inflammation but is not raw or oozing.

Chamomilla is probably the correct medicine if a baby with diaper rash also has the marked irritability and other emotional symptoms typical of this medicine.

If the rash burns and itches greatly, *Arsenicum* may help, especially if it is relieved by warmth or if the general symptoms of the medicine are present. The skin may be cracked or raw, and the watery fluid that oozes out is acrid and inflames the skin.

As with other skin conditions, *Graphites* is indicated if the rash oozes a sticky, often honey-colored fluid. Raw areas become crusted, or the skin may appear simply dry, rough, and cracked.

Hepar should be considered if there is a secondary bacterial infection, and if pimples develop or pus forms in the raw areas. Discharges smell bad. Extreme tenderness of the inflamed parts and relief brought on by warm bathing also indicate *Hepar.*

Severe itching made worse by heat or bathing suggests *Sulphur.* The skin may be rough and dry, or there may be pimples and pus (as with *Hepar* rashes).

Candida albicans is a homeopathic medicine made from the *Candida* organism itself. Some homeopaths have found this effective when other seemingly well-indicated medicines haven't acted.

For thrush infections of the mouth:
Borax is probably the best remedy to begin with if symptoms don't clearly indicate another. The child cries when pulled away from the breast or bottle, because of the pain. There may be raw sores on the mucous membrane (as with *Mercurius*), especially on the tongue. Although there may be increased saliva, dryness of the mouth is more typical. Compared to *Mercurius, Borax* has less swelling and bleeding. *Borax* children sometimes have a strong dread of downward motion or falling.

Choose *Mercurius* if the sore, inflamed mouth smells offensive. There is a great deal of drooling and salivation, the gums are spongy and bleed easily, and there may be white lines on them. The tongue is puffy and flabby and is imprinted by the teeth. It is heavily coated with a black, white, or dirty-yellow color.

Sulphur is indicated by burning and soreness especially during eating. Symptoms are similar to *Mercurius,* but the gums and tongue are not so spongy and weak. The general symptoms of *Sulphur* may be present.

Hydrastis should be tried when there is a great deal of thick mucus in the mouth and collected on the tongue. The tongue feels as though it had been burned.

Chamomilla is appropriate if the emotional symptoms of this medicine, described in the *materia medica* section, are prominent.

REMEDY SUMMARY FOR CANDIDA INFECTIONS

Give the medicine: Twice daily for 2 or 3 days, stopping as soon as you see improvement.

When to try another medicine: If there has been no improvement within 3 days.

BELLADONNA ★

Essentials
• Skin bright red and swollen but not raw or oozing

CHAMOMILLA

Essentials
• Diaper rash with marked irritability and other emotional symptoms typical of this medicine (see *materia medica* section)

GRAPHITES

Essentials
- Rash oozes a sticky, often honey-colored fluid
- Raw areas become crusted, or skin appears dry, rough, and cracked

ARSENICUM

Essentials
- Much burning and itching

Confirmatory symptoms
- Skin cracked or raw
- Fluid oozing from the rash irritates the skin
- Symptoms relieved by warmth
- General symptoms of *Arsenicum* are present (see *materia medica* section)

HEPAR SULPH.

Essentials
- Secondary bacterial infection—pimples develop or pus forms in the affected areas

Confirmatory symptoms
- Inflamed areas very tender
- Pain relieved by warm bathing
- Discharge from the rash smells bad

SULPHUR

Essentials
- Severe itching made worse by heat or bathing
- Skin may be rough and dry, or there may be pimples and pus

Confirmatory symptoms
- General symptoms of *Sulphur* are present (see *materia medica* section)

CANDIDA ALBICANS

Essentials
- May be tried when well-indicated medicines have not helped

REMEDY SUMMARY FOR THRUSH OF THE MOUTH

BORAX ★
Essentials
- Child cries in pain when pulled away from the breast or bottle
- Raw sores in the mouth, especially on the tongue

Confirmatory symptoms
- Strong dread of downward motion or falling
- Dryness of the mouth typical, but salivation may be increased

MERCURIUS
Essentials
- Sore, inflamed mouth that smells offensive

Confirmatory symptoms
- Much salivation and drooling
- Gums are swollen, "spongy," and bleed easily
- Tongue is puffy and flabby and is imprinted by the teeth; coated with a black, white, or dirty-yellow color

SULPHUR
Essentials
- Burning and soreness, especially during eating

Confirmatory symptoms
- Symptoms similar to those of *Mercurius,* but the gums and tongue are not so spongy and weak
- General symptoms of *Sulphur* are present (see *materia medica* section)

HYDRASTIS
Essentials
- Thick mucus in the mouth and on the tongue

Confirmatory symptoms
- Tongue feels as though it had been burned

CHAMOMILLA

Essentials
- Irritability and related emotional symptoms characteristic of this medicine (see *materia medica* section)

BEYOND HOME CARE

SEE YOUR PRACTITIONER SOON:

- if you get frequent or severe *Candida* infections;
- if you are not sure of the diagnosis;
- if pus forms (see sections on boils and impetigo);
- if home treatment fails and the infection is severe;
- if an adult or older child develops thrush (*Candida* infection of the mouth).

ACNE

Acne is always a manifestation of an internal imbalance. The bacteria involved are present on everyone's skin, so they alone don't explain the eruption of pimples. Topical and oral antibiotics are effective in killing these bacteria and often reduce the number of eruptions, but of course such treatments do nothing to change the underlying disorder. Other drugs, both topically and internally taken, work by suppressing the physiological mechanisms that produce the acne; from a homeopathic standpoint, they are even worse.

We encourage those with mild acne to follow simple measures of cleanliness and good diet—and leave it at that. Those who have more severe cases should seek constitutional homeopathic care before resorting to conventional drugs.

CHAPTER 14

ACCIDENTS AND INJURIES

ACCIDENTS CAUSE FAR more deaths and serious injuries to children and young adults than all diseases put together. We strongly recommend you give accident prevention high priority in your family's plan for good health.

If someone in your family does suffer from an injury, your first priorities are to apply the proper first-aid measures and to get medical help if necessary. The Red Cross offers first-aid classes in most localities. Every household should have a current, basic first-aid manual such as the Red Cross *First Aid Textbook*. You should also maintain a home first-aid kit (see the Red Cross book for details) as well as a kit of homeopathic first-aid medicines.

The correct homeopathic medicine can complement the standard first-aid measures taken, as it reduces pain and speeds healing remarkably. Even if an injury requires medical care, you can use homeopathy once the injured person's condition is stable.

Homeopathic treatment of injuries is easy compared with that of the various acute diseases with their highly individualized symptoms, as injuries do not require such detailed casetaking. Homeopaths have found that only a small number of medicines need be considered for each type of injury.

CUTS AND SCRAPES

Cuts (lacerations) and scrapes (abrasions) are among the more common of life's mishaps.

GENERAL HOME CARE

One of the first priorities is to stop any significant bleeding by applying firm, direct pressure on the wound or the appropriate pressure point for that part of the body (see a good first-aid manual for details).

If the wound is minor enough to be cared for at home, cleanse it with soap and water once bleeding has stopped. Be gentle but thorough, and don't leave any dirt in the wound. Cleaning the wound gently with a Water Pik dental appliance is particularly effective for removing tiny bits of debris.

After the wound has been thoroughly cleansed, apply *Calendula* or *Hypericum* externally as indicated later in this section. If the cut is wide, you may need to bring its edges together with a steristrips or a butterfly closure before covering it with a gauze bandage. The bandage is needed to protect the cut while it heals. Try to leave the bandage on for at least three days. Take the bandage off by pulling it in the same direction that the cut runs.

Shallow scrapes generally should be allowed to heal without bandages; it may help if you apply one thin layer of *Calendula* ointment just after your initial cleansing of the wound. Do not repeat the application, however. Remember that the scab forming is the body's way of protecting the wound as it heals. Just let it fall off naturally.

HOMEOPATHIC MEDICINES

Calendula, applied topically, promotes granulation of tissues to heal wounds and burns, helps stop bleeding, and inhibits infection. It is used for shallow injuries, such as scrapes and sores. *Calendula* is available in several different preparations.

Calendula tincture is a mixture of the *Calendula* plant juice and alcohol. The tincture is used in the treatment of any wound that breaks the skin. Since the tincture is prepared with alcohol, to prevent stinging it should be diluted with water or, preferably, sterile normal saline (available in drugstores). Mix one part tincture with three to four parts water or saline. After cleansing, use a medicine dropper to apply the diluted tincture to the wound. Cover with a bandage and repeat the application three or four times a day.

Calendula also is available in a nonalcoholic solution of the plant juice, glycerin, and water. Like the tincture, the solution is used for wounds that break the skin, but dilution is not necessary. Likewise, *Calendula* in gel or spray form can be applied directly to the injury.

Calendula ointment, or cerate, is an extract of the plant juice with a petrolatum base and is good for scrapes and for roughened or chapped skin. It is not appropriate for deeper cuts. The ointment should be applied thinly to scraped knees, chapped lips, diaper rashes, and the like. *Calendula* oil, prepared from the plant extract in mineral oil, is an alternative to the ointment for rough or chapped skin.

Hypericum tincture may be substituted for or mixed with *Calendula* tincture for cuts that seem to be infected. Dilute it the same way as you would the *Calendula* tincture. You may apply it three or four times daily, or you may soak a cotton pad in dilute *Hypericum* tincture and place it over the wound to use as a compress under the bandage. It's okay to combine topical preparations of *Calendula* and *Hypericum* preparations. (For the treatment of infected wounds with internal homeopathic medicines, consult the section "Boils, Abscesses, and Other Skin Infections" in chapter 13.)

In conjunction with the appropriate external application, *Hypericum* may be taken orally for deeper cuts, or if there is much pain or tenderness to touch. Besides lessening pain, *Hypericum* speeds the healing process. *Hypericum* also should be given orally if the injuries involve parts of the body that are richly supplied with nerves, such as the fingers, toes, and spine, or if shooting pains accompany the injury.

Give *Arnica* internally for deep or ragged cuts, or when cuts occur in conjunction with bruises or other injuries (see the section on bruises on page 282).

BEYOND HOME CARE

GET MEDICAL CARE IMMEDIATELY:

- if profuse bleeding occurs, or if there is numbness, tingling, or weakness in or near the wounded part (there is a good chance that important internal structures have been injured);

- for cuts on the chest, back, abdomen, and face, unless they are very shallow. Vital organs and nerves are fairly close to the surface in these areas;
- if the edges of the wound cannot be held together with tape or adhesive bandages (stitches may be required). Stitches should be avoided if possible, since they can cause further injury. Deep, long, or jagged cuts, or those over the joints are most likely to need stitching. Facial cuts, except very superficial ones, usually should be stitched to prevent scarring that would affect appearance. Wounds must be stitched soon after the injury occurs, usually within the first 8 to 12 hours;
- for cuts on the hand or fingers, unless they are very superficial. Such cuts are particularly likely to become infected, and these infections can be severe and spread rapidly;
- if you cannot remove deeply embedded dirt.

GET MEDICAL CARE TODAY:

- if you notice much redness, swelling, or pus buildup in or around the wound, if there are red streaks extending from around the wound, or if fever has occurred;
- if the person is not up to date with tetanus shots. Grown-ups need them only every ten years, though severe or dirty wounds may require repetition earlier. Children need a series of shots to maintain immunity.

CALL YOUR PRACTITIONER:

- if you are not sure whether you need a booster immunization.

BRUISES

A bruise is a superficial injury caused by a blow that does not break the skin. The blow breaks blood vessels and causes black and blue discoloration under the skin.

GENERAL HOME CARE

Apply ice packs to the injured parts for twenty to thirty minutes if the injury is more than mild. This will help reduce swelling and speed the healing process. See your health-care practitioner soon if you bruise very easily or without apparent injury.

HOMEOPATHIC MEDICINES

Arnica is the main medicine for bruises. It helps reduce pain and speeds the absorption of blood under the skin. The more severe the bruise, the more frequently you should take *Arnica*. If the bruise needs treatment but is minor, take *Arnica* two or three times a day. To treat severe bruising, it should be taken every hour or every other hour the first day, and then less frequently the next couple of days. In any case, stop after five days.

Use *Ledum* instead of *Arnica* as your first choice for black eyes or for severe bruises that feel cold and numb, especially if cold applications help. Take the same dosage recommended for *Arnica*.

Ruta is indicated for bruises of the periosteum, the membrane that covers the bones. *Ruta* often relieves the pain that follows bruising of the shin, kneecap, or elbow.

PUNCTURE WOUNDS

A puncture wound is a wound that is deeper than it is wide. Puncture wounds are particularly dangerous for four reasons: (1) they may penetrate deeply into the body; (2) they may push foreign bodies deep into the tissue, where the material can be difficult to find and remove; (3) they are difficult to clean and thus more susceptible to infection; and (4) they provide a perfect environment for the tetanus germ to thrive and multiply, since this bacteria can grow only in the absence of oxygen.

GENERAL HOME CARE

Clean the wound as thoroughly as you can, using soap and water. Unlike cuts, a puncture wound should be allowed to bleed as long as it can so that foreign bodies, dirt, and germs can be carried out of the wound. You should not stop the bleeding unless it is severe or it seems as though some pressure is forcing the blood to squirt from the wound. If, in such cases, there is any chance at all that a foreign body has remained in the wound, carefully apply pressure not directly to the wound, but to the pressure point over the artery of the wounded area (see a good first-aid manual for instructions). Use the pressure point so you don't push a foreign object in deeper, further cutting internal structures.

Soaking the wounded part is advisable, as it keeps the wound open to facilitate the exit of germs and other material and brings blood to the area to speed healing. Use warm water and soak the part for fifteen to twenty minutes, four times a day, while there is still pain. If there is any opening in the skin, cover the wound with a sterile gauze bandage and inspect it twice a day for signs of infection.

HOMEOPATHIC MEDICINES

Treat people with deep or painful puncture wounds with both an external remedy and an internal medicine. *Hypericum* tincture, the external remedy, should be diluted with water and applied directly to the wound every half hour or so, and *Ledum, Apis,* or *Hypericum* should be given internally every four to six hours.

Ledum is the most commonly used homeopathic medicine in the treatment of puncture wounds, and you should use it if there are no strong indications for the other medicines. *Ledum* is particularly valuable when there is redness, swelling, and throbbing pain, and when the wound feels cold to touch but is relieved by cold applications. However, *Ledum* is likely to help puncture wounds even when these specific symptoms are not present.

Give *Apis* when the puncture wound feels warm or hot, with stinging pains that are made better by cold applications. There is much swelling at the site of the wound.

Hypericum is valuable in the treatment of puncture wounds if there are sharp, shooting pains.

Staphysagria is the leading remedy for stabs from a knife, especially to the abdomen (of course, medical care should be sought immediately). *Arnica* also is usually necessary for the mental and physical shock of such injuries.

BEYOND HOME CARE

GET MEDICAL CARE IMMEDIATELY:

- for puncture wounds in the abdomen, chest, back, neck, genital region, or head (anywhere except the extremities);
- for particularly deep puncture wounds;

- for puncture wounds in the joints, especially in the knee, since this may cause infection of the joint. Signs of joint infection are redness, swelling and pain in the joint, and inability to move the joint normally.

GET MEDICAL CARE TODAY:

- for puncture wounds in the hands (not the fingers);
- for puncture wounds that remain tender for more than 2 days, that become red or swollen, or that discharge pus;
- if the person is not up to date with his tetanus shots.

STRAINS, SPRAINS, AND OTHER INJURIES TO LIGAMENTS AND TENDONS

Joints are surrounded and held together by fibrous tissues: ligaments, which connect the bones of one joint to another; and tendons, which attach muscles to the bones near joints. A strain occurs when a ligament is overstretched; a sprain when a ligament is partially torn loose. More severe stress can completely separate the ligament from the bone, resulting in a torn ligament. Similar injuries can occur in tendons.

GENERAL HOME CARE

Strains, sprains, and torn ligaments or tendons require rest, ice application, elevation, and firm (but not excessive) pressure on the injured part. These measures apply even if the bone is broken. Immediately after the injury, elevate the injured part to help reduce swelling. Apply an ice pack or cold pack: Cover the ice with a cloth and place it over the injured area, wrapping it firmly with an elastic bandage. If you've wrapped the bandage too tightly, the part may become blue and numb, and the person may complain; if so, rewrap a little less tightly. After a half-hour, unwrap the bandage to allow blood to circulate freely for fifteen minutes. Repeat this sequence for three hours or so, after which you can apply the ice pack without the pressure wrap for twenty minutes at a time to help ease the pain.

After twenty-four to forty-eight hours, you can switch to warm applications or soaking the injured part in warm water if this brings pain relief, but continue using ice if the injured person prefers it. Gentle, careful massage is sometimes soothing to a mildly injured joint. We do not recommend the use of liniments containing camphor or other similar medications (Vicks, Heet, Tiger Balm, and other strong-smelling liniments), since camphor tends to neutralize homeopathic medicines.

Rest is extremely important in protecting the injured joint and facilitating healing. It is crucial to avoid any activity that hurts. Crutches, slings, and splints can help keep the joint relatively motionless while still allowing the person to get around. Elastic (Ace) bandages do not really limit motion, so you should not do anything with one on that you wouldn't do without it. The mild pressure and support they provide feel good, though, and they can remind you not to use the weak joint and thereby help prevent further injury.

As the injured tissues heal, begin using the joint slowly and carefully. Ligaments and tendons take longer to heal than tissues like skin and muscle, which are softer and better supplied with blood. Four to six weeks or more may be required. Protecting the joint from sudden motion or stress is required throughout that time.

HOMEOPATHIC MEDICINES

Even if medical care is needed for a joint injury, homeopathic medicines can be very effective in speeding the healing process. Give the remedy every three hours or so during the first two days after the injury, and twice a day for several days after that. Stop as soon as there is significant improvement.

Arnica oil, ointment, or gel can be applied externally, in addition to the appropriate internal medicine. Rub it into the painful area twice a day.

Arnica taken internally is indicated when there is considerable swelling, bruising, and inflammation of the soft tissue around the joint. It is a valuable first medicine for many people, even those with torn ligaments, when the swelling is more prominent. Once the swelling and bruising have improved, you should switch to *Rhus tox.* or one of the other medicines described below to help heal the remaining injury of the fibrous tissue itself.

Rhus tox. is the most common medicine used for strains, sprains, torn ligaments, and tendonitis. It is called the "rusty gate" remedy, since the pains and stiffness are particularly worse during initial motion and become better as the person continues to move and limber up. *Rhus tox.* is especially valuable to people who incur injuries after lifting something or overexerting themselves.

Consider *Bryonia* if the pain is greatly worsened by the slightest motion, and continued motion only makes it hurt more. There is swelling of the injured joint, but not so prominently as with *Arnica* injuries.

Ruta is a valuable medicine for tendons or ligaments that have been torn or wrenched. It is generally best used after the most severe initial swelling and pain have begun to decrease. Select *Ruta* if *Rhus tox.* has not helped, or if the injured part is neither definitely worse during initial motion nor relieved by continued motion. *Ruta* often is effective for people with tennis elbow.

Ledum is valuable for ankle sprains, particularly when the injured part feels cold or numb and is made better with cold applications.

BEYOND HOME CARE

GET MEDICAL CARE IMMEDIATELY:

- if there is any obvious distortion, deformity, or instability (wobbling or looseness) of the joint;
- if there is severe pain or massive swelling;
- if it is impossible to straighten the joint;
- if the injured part, or the limb beyond the injury, is cold, blue, or numb, or if the limb beyond the injury can't be used.

GET MEDICAL CARE TODAY:

- if the limb cannot be used or cannot bear any weight within the first 12 hours after the injury;
- if use of the joint or its bearing weight is significantly difficult after 72 hours;
- if a child suffers injury to the wrist after falling on an outstretched hand. Such wrist injuries are common, and fractures of the bones of the wrist are not unusual. They are difficult to detect even with X rays, and your practitioner may want to see the child again or get a follow-up X ray just to be sure no bone is broken.

CONTACT YOUR PRACTITIONER SOON:

- if symptoms do not steadily improve.

LOW BACK INJURIES AND PAIN

Back pain is one of the more common and debilitating health problems people endure. In addition to direct trauma to the back, responsible factors include poor posture, inadequate exercise, overuse and misuse of the back, and emotional stress. The basic design of the human body also plays a role—walking on two legs rather than four puts lots of pressure on the lower back.

Physiologically, most low back pain results from injury to the soft tissues in the back—muscles, ligaments, and tendons—or to the gelatinous discs that separate the spinal bones. In soft tissue injuries, the primary symptoms include stiffness and pain in the lower back itself. When damage to the disc occurs, the back discomfort often is overshadowed by sciatica, pain or sensations of numbness or tingling radiating into the buttock or down the leg. These symptoms are caused by irritation of or pressure on the nerves of the leg as they branch off from the spinal cord. A "bulging" disc can press on the nerve enough to cause significant sciatica, while a full-scale disc "rupture" often produces excruciating pain in the hip or leg, often accompanied by true numbness and even paralysis.

Once common, back surgery now is reserved mostly for cases involving paralysis and other marked neurological impairments. Research has shown that in the absence of paralysis, sciatic pain eventually improves on its own; results with surgery are no better. At best, surgery for most soft tissue problems is useless.

Low back pain occasionally can signal a more serious problem such as infection or cancer. Pain higher in the back—at or above the level of the belly button—often stems from soft tissue or disc injuries, but it is more likely than low back pain to stem from other, potentially serious, medical problems (see "Beyond Home Care").

GENERAL HOME CARE

Avoiding strain on the back is critical to prevent back problems in the first place and to keep them from recurring. Learn how to lift properly, with your legs, not your back, by bending at the knees rather than the waist. Simple back exercises also can help; these strengthen the abdominal muscles and thereby take some of the load off the back.

When you do injure your back, you may find it necessary to stay in bed for as much as a day during the most acute pain. In general, though, remaining active is the surest and quickest path to recovery. Obviously, you shouldn't overdo it. However, research has shown that people who resume activity at a cautious pace heal faster than those who just rest. Be careful to move slowly and gently to prevent further injury, letting the pain tell you how active to be. Applying heat or cold can mitigate the pain. Sleeping on a firm mattress or the floor may help, too.

HOMEOPATHIC MEDICINES

Give the medicine you choose from those described below every six to twelve hours for several days, less often as the symptoms improve. If the patient isn't better after two to three days, try another medicine.

Immediately after an injury to the back, try *Arnica*. Consider *Hypericum* instead when there are shooting pains, or after a blow to the coccyx.

Nux vomica helps when back pain is aggravated by movement, especially turning over in bed. *Bryonia* is another good choice for back pain with marked aggravation from any motion, though in this case turning over in bed usually doesn't cause worse pain.

By contrast, give *Rhus tox.* when the patient finds relief from continued motion. The low back feels stiff and painful at rest, and the pain may be especially bad when the person first gets up. After a few minutes of limbering up, though, the back feels better. Damp, cold weather may make the symptoms worse, while heat may relieve them. Sciatica may be present.

Among medicines especially helpful during sciatica, try *Tellurium* first when there is marked aggravation from coughing, sneezing, or during a bowel movement. The pain is more often on the right side.

Use *Gnaphalium* instead if the pain is accompanied by a great deal of numbness, or if the pain and numbness alternate. Muscle cramps may occur in the affected leg. The pain is aggravated by movement and is better from rest or sitting down.

If sciatica improves when the patient lies on the painful side or bends at the hip, *Colocynthis* may help. The pain is more often on the right and is typically aggravated by touch and the warmth of the bed.

BEYOND HOME CARE

GET MEDICAL CARE IMMEDIATELY:

- if patient is unable to urinate or defecate;
- if pain in the mid-back comes on suddenly, especially if accompanied by faintness, coldness, or decreased pulses in the legs or feet;
- for back pain following a fall or a blow to the back.

GET MEDICAL CARE TODAY:

- if the pain is accompanied by fever, abdominal pain, or urinary symptoms (urinary pain or frequency, or blood in the urine);
- for any severe back pain.

GET MEDICAL CARE WITHIN A FEW DAYS:

- if the pain is accompanied by weakness or paralysis;
- if the pain began spontaneously, with no obvious strain;
- for persistent pain in the mid- or upper back.

SEE YOUR HEALTH PRACTITIONER SOON:

- for low back pain that doesn't start to improve within a week or that lasts longer than two weeks.

DISLOCATED JOINTS

The bones of a joint may sometimes slip out of position following a fall or blow or after an extremity has been pulled. A rare occurrence, dislocation can cause partial or total loss of function and significant deformity. A common dislocation injury in young children is the partial dislocation of the elbow, which can occur if the child is pulled by the arm. Symptoms of dislocation include swelling, deformity, discoloration, or tenderness of the affected area, along with pain during motion or inability to use the part.

GENERAL HOME CARE

Generally, dislocations should not be treated at home and should receive immediate medical attention. While waiting for help, you should carry out the other home treatments mentioned in the section "Strains, Sprains, and Other Injuries to Ligaments and Tendons."

HOMEOPATHIC MEDICINES

Arnica is a medicine par excellence for dislocated joints. It does *not* take the place of having the dislocated parts put back in place. However, it does allay much of the pain and begins the healing process.

If the person still is experiencing some pain after the first two days, consider giving one of the appropriate medicines listed in the section "Strains, Sprains, and Other Injuries to Ligaments and Tendons."

FRACTURES

You can't always tell whether a bone is broken by looking at the injured part. Whenever an injury involves a great deal of pain and tenderness, swelling and bruising, or difficulty moving the injured part, there's a good possibility it's a fracture. Usually an X ray is necessary to make this determination. Resetting of a broken bone often is required, for without it the bone may heal in a deformed way.

GENERAL HOME CARE

Initial treatment of any injury in which fracture may have occurred involves rest and ice packs. Apply ice as directed in the section on strains and sprains using gentle pressure. Since movement of the broken ends of the bone can cut nearby blood vessels or nerves, use a makeshift splint to prevent the injured bone from moving. Splinting is particularly important if the person must be moved. See the Red Cross or AMA first-aid books for instructions. Initial home treatment of a potential fracture is safe if the guidelines listed in "Beyond Home Care" are followed carefully.

HOMEOPATHIC MEDICINES

Immediately after a possible fracture injury, homeopathic treatment can help minimize pain, swelling, and shock. Give the first medicine—either *Arnica* or *Eupatorium perfoliatum*—every three hours during the first two to three days, cutting back to one dose daily thereafter until discomfort is minimal. Once the fractured bones are reset, time and rest will allow healing to take place, and the correct homeopathic medicine will speed the healing process along.

As with any severe injury, *Arnica* generally should be the first medicine given, since it is so effective in treating the initial reactions to the trauma, both local and general. Bruising, swelling, and tenderness of the injured area, along with a dazed, "shocked" mental state, are the characteristic symptoms of this medicine.

If the main symptom of a fracture is pain and there is not so much bruising, you may give *Eupatorium perfoliatum* instead of or following *Arnica* during the period immediately after the injury.

Once the initial pain and swelling have diminished, give *Symphytum*. *Symphytum*, or comfrey, is the herb that has been known for centuries in Europe as "knitbone" because of its ability to aid the healing of fractures. Give *Symphytum* 6x twice a day for two to three weeks, or *Symphytum* 30x or 30c once a day for seven to ten days.

Bryonia often is helpful for the pain of fractured ribs. Give it as directed for *Arnica* above, but give a dose or two of *Arnica* before starting the *Bryonia*.

Silica is an excellent medicine if small chips have been broken from the bone. Give the 6x potency twice daily for two weeks.

BEYOND HOME CARE

GET MEDICAL CARE IMMEDIATELY:

- if there is obviously a serious injury, a possible neck or back fracture, or if the person is unconscious. Do not move her. Stay with her while someone else goes for medical help. Treat her for shock according to the Red Cross or AMA guidelines while you wait for help to arrive;
- if the possibly fractured part or the limb beyond the injury is bluish, numb, or cold, or cannot be used;
- if the person feels faint or abnormally thirsty or is sweaty or pale;
- if the injured area is obviously distorted or deformed;
- if the possible fracture involves the thigh or pelvis.

GET MEDICAL CARE TODAY:

- if there is marked bruising or bleeding under the skin in the area of the injury, or if the injury was caused by severe force;

- if the limb cannot be used or cannot bear any weight within the first 12 hours after the injury;
- if there is still significant pain 48 hours after the injury, or if use of the joint or its ability to bear weight is significantly difficult after 72 hours;
- if a child injures the wrist after falling on an outstretched hand. Such injuries are common, as are fractures of the wrist bones. They are difficult to detect even with X rays, and your practitioner may want to get a follow-up X ray just to be sure no bone is broken.

SEE YOUR PRACTITIONER SOON:

- if symptoms do not steadily improve.

HEAD INJURIES

Dr. Spock has said that the child who has never bumped his or her head is being watched too closely. Most of these head injuries are minor. Even if a "goose egg" develops, the injury usually is only a slight bruise to the skull and scalp—the severity of the injury does not depend on how big the bump is. Occasionally, however, bleeding underneath the skull or within the brain, or damage to brain tissue can occur.

GENERAL HOME CARE

Many of the symptoms indicating serious problems do not begin for hours or sometimes a couple of days. During this period, unless the injury is just a minor bump on the head, you should check the injured person regularly for the symptoms listed in "Beyond Home Care." Whenever a bad fall or blow to the head has occurred, remember also to check for injuries elsewhere on the body.

If none of the danger symptoms is present, apply an ice pack to the injured area to minimize swelling.

HOMEOPATHIC MEDICINES

Arnica is the first medicine to consider for treating those with head injuries. Give a dose every three hours for the first couple of days, but give the medicine less often or stop altogether if there is notable improvement.

People who have any chronic or recurrent symptoms that began after a head injury may try a single dose of *Natrum sulph.* 200c or IM. We recommend this treatment only if: (1) you have significant symptoms related only to the head injury; and (2) you do not have access to professional homeopathic care.

BEYOND HOME CARE

GET MEDICAL CARE IMMEDIATELY:

- for any obviously severe injury, or if there is a definite soft or deformed area in the bones of the head or face;
- if there is any loss of consciousness, even momentary, resulting from the blow, or if the person cannot remember the events surrounding the accident;
- if there is diminished mental alertness. Increased lethargy or unresponsiveness, slurred or difficult speech, abnormally deep sleep, and your own difficulty rousing the person from sleep are danger signs. A person who has sustained a blow to the head should be awakened from sleep every 30 minutes during the first 6 to 8 hours;
- if there has been a seizure or convulsion. During a seizure, the person should be placed on his side so that he cannot fall or choke on saliva or vomit. Stay with him while someone else gets medical help;
- if there is severe or persistent vomiting. Vomiting once or twice after a head injury is to be expected and does not necessarily indicate severe problems. If there is repeated vomiting, especially after the first few hours, there may be a more serious injury;
- if there is severe or persistent headache;
- if there is blurred or double vision, other visual disturbance, or difficulty moving the eyes normally;
- if the pupils are of unequal size, unless the person's pupils are normally so;
- if there is difficulty moving all the extremities equally well;
- if there is clear or bloody fluid coming from an ear or nostril;
- if the pulse or breathing is slow, irregular, or weak.

BURNS

Burns can be caused by excessive heat, acid or alkaline substances, electricity, or radiation. When the only apparent damage results in pain and redness of the skin, the injury is a first-degree burn. Burns caused by the sun or brief contact with a hot pan are typical examples of first-degree burns. A second-degree burn causes blistering of the skin as well as redness and pain. When all the layers of skin are burned through and the skin appears deathly white or charred black, a third-degree, or "full thickness," burn has occurred.

GENERAL HOME CARE

Since burns are the second leading cause of accidental death among children under age four, and the third leading cause among older children, prevention of burns is essential. Keep matches and cigarette lighters out of children's reach. Don't have gasoline or other flammables in the house, and if you do, keep them locked up. Install child-proof plugs in electrical sockets. Be sure you never smoke in bed, and have a good smoke alarm system installed in the house. And finally, keep a working fire extinguisher.

Treatment of first-degree and not so extensive second-degree burns ordinarily may be carried out at home. Treatment of these burns includes immediately applying cold water to the affected part for at least five minutes or until the pain stops. Immersing the burn in a sink or bucket of ice water is best.

A bandage is not necessary unless the burned part is liable to be bumped or rubbed. Blisters will protect the burn and prevent infection, and thus, if possible, should not be broken. If a blister is large, it should be broken only antiseptically. Although we recommend you leave the skin of the collapsed blister in place to protect the raw area below, some authorities think it should be removed to prevent infection. Either way, you should treat the wound with topical homeopathic remedies, changing the dressing twice a day until healing is clearly under way.

Chemical burns also require immediate treatment. Remove any clothes affected immediately. Most chemical containers have information on them about treating burns. Follow their instructions. If the instructions aren't available, wash off the chemical with large amounts of water and get medical attention.

The use of local anesthetic creams or sprays is not recommended for treating burns, since these tend to slow the healing process.

HOMEOPATHIC MEDICINES

Burn injuries can benefit from both external applications and internal medicines. First-degree burns, including sunburns, should be treated with topical applications (tincture, gel, or spray) of *Calendula, Urtica urens,* or both. *Urtica urens* also may be used internally every few hours for pain if needed. Stop whenever improvement continues.

For second-degree burns, use topical *Hypericum* spray or dilute tincture (one part tincture to three parts water) before the blisters have broken. If you don't have the spray, apply the dilute tincture gently by holding a medicine dropper just over the burn, letting the liquid run over the injury. *Cantharis* or, if it isn't available, *Urtica urens* may be given internally, according to the directions for *Urtica urens* above. After the blisters have been popped, apply *Calendula* via the spray, gel, or dilute tincture two or three times a day, keeping the area covered by a cotton gauze bandage.

For third-degree burns, *Cantharis* should be given internally. Do not use any external applications. With the permission of your health practitioner, you may try *Calendula* (as recommended above) during the latter part of the healing process to speed the regrowth of the outer skin and to reduce the chance of scarring.

Phosphorus, given two or three times daily for several days, is the medicine of choice after an electrical burn.

BEYOND HOME CARE

GET MEDICAL CARE IMMEDIATELY:

- for any third-degree burn. Do not try to remove charred clothing from the burned tissue. Treat for shock while awaiting medical care;
- for second-degree burns that cover an area larger than the hand or that occur on the face, hands, or genitals;
- for an electrical burn. Do not use your bare hands to pull the person away from the source of the electrical burn—use a nonconductive material (a board, mop, wooden chair). Apply mouth-to-mouth resuscitation or CPR if necessary;

- for any radiation burn;
- for any chemical burn, unless obviously minor.

GET MEDICAL CARE TODAY:

- if there is evidence of infection, such as pus or increasing swelling and redness around the burn (see the section on skin infections in chapter 13).

SHOCK

Technically, shock is the disorder that occurs when blood flow is reduced to below the levels needed to maintain vital functions. Obviously, shock can occur during serious injuries or illnesses that involve loss of blood or other body fluids, but it can occur also during infection, allergic reaction (anaphylaxis), or malfunction of the nervous system. In a sense, every significant injury is accompanied by some degree of shock because the nervous system's acute reaction to the stress of the injury alters blood flow.

You should keep in mind the possibility of shock when caring for any injured person. If there is much bleeding, major burns, or a head injury, treatment for shock should be an especially high priority. Symptoms of shock include general weakness; cold, pale skin; rapid, weak heart rate; reduced alertness; confusion or unconsciousness; and shallow, irregular breathing.

GENERAL HOME CARE

Have the patient lie down with his legs elevated somewhat above the head. Don't bend the legs. Loosen clothing at the neck, chest, and waist. Protect the patient from extremes of warmth and cold. If there is any chance a serious injury has occurred, do not move him. Get emergency help immediately. Let him take sips of fluids only if he is fully conscious and alert; do not give him solid foods.

HOMEOPATHIC MEDICINES

Arnica is the first medicine to give for the general effects of an injury, including shock. Once urgent first-aid measures have been taken, give a dose every one-half to two hours the first day if the symptoms are marked. The tiny #10 granules are preferable; just let them stick to the tongue. Or, dissolve a larger pellet or tablet in a teaspoon of water and limit the dose to a single drop.

Arnica is sometimes helpful also for the aftereffects of an injury. If symptoms of any kind can be dated back to a serious injury, and if you don't have access to a professional homeopath, you may try a single dose of *Arnica* 30, 200, or a higher potency.

BEYOND HOME CARE

GET MEDICAL CARE IMMEDIATELY:

• if shock is suspected.

HEAT EXHAUSTION (HEAT PROSTRATION)

Heat exhaustion, also called heat prostration, can develop gradually after the body is exposed to hot weather if it loses water and salt through profuse sweating or intake of alcohol. The result is mild shock. Common symptoms of heat exhaustion include tiredness, cold and clammy skin, pallid complexion, headache, nausea and vomiting, dizziness, and muscle cramps. Body temperature may be normal or slightly elevated, and you may notice more rapid pulse and breathing. Blood pressure falls.

GENERAL HOME CARE

Get the person to lie down in a cool, darkened area. Raise the feet and rub his legs to aid circulation. Apply wet cloths to his head and body, and fan him. Add a half-teaspoon of salt to a glass of water and get him to drink it, repeating this every fifteen to thirty minutes for the first three hours. If fainting or unconsciousness occurs, treat for shock immediately and be sure that an extremely high temperature has not developed (if it has, see the section on heatstroke). After the patient recovers, be sure he avoids further exposure to heat, for he'll be abnormally sensitive.

HOMEOPATHIC MEDICINES

Veratrum album is the most common medicine prescribed for heat exhaustion. The symptoms are profuse, clammy sweat; great weakness, perhaps even collapse, faintness, or actual fainting; extreme coldness of the body, especially of the feet, hands, and face; pallor; nausea; rapid pulse; and general stiffness of the body.

Cuprum metallicum has many symptoms similar to *Veratrum album*'s, but with *Cuprum*, cramping is especially pronounced. Stupor with jerking of the muscles and convulsions may occur.

BEYOND HOME CARE

GET MEDICAL CARE IMMEDIATELY:

- if there is significant dullness or loss of consciousness;
- if the symptoms do not get better within an hour, or if they get worse.

HEATSTROKE (SUNSTROKE)

Heatstroke can come on suddenly when the weather is very hot. Its most frequent victims are older individuals and people who exercise in the heat. This is a life-threatening emergency. A failure of the heat-regulating mechanisms of the body results in high fever (104°F or higher) and sometimes an inability to perspire. The skin is red, rather than pale, and is hot. Perspiration may be absent, but other times it is profuse. The pulse is fast and forceful. Confusion, stupor, and unconsciousness are common. If conscious, the person may complain of headache, nausea, or visual disturbances, and sometimes experiences convulsions.

GENERAL HOME CARE

The body must be cooled immediately. Remove the person's clothing and put her in a cool, shady place. As soon as possible, immerse her in a tub of cold water and stir the water frequently. If you haven't a tub, apply ice packs to the body. If neither a tub nor ice is available, sponge the skin with water or alcohol, or spray the person with water. Continuously fan her to further the cooling. Rub the arms and legs vigorously to get the blood flowing again. Make sure breathing is not obstructed.

As soon as the patient's temperature drops to 102°F (be sure not to over-chill her), dry her off and take her immediately to the nearest emergency room. If you have help, you may be able to transport her while you or others continue the efforts to cool her. If you are alone with the victim, your first priority is to get the temperature down.

After the person recovers from heatstroke, exposure to hot temperatures must be avoided for some time.

HOMEOPATHIC MEDICINES

When treating people suffering an acute case of heatstroke, give the medicine as frequently as every fifteen to thirty minutes the first couple of hours, then diminish it to every hour or every other hour as the person recovers, and stop altogether after twelve to twenty-four hours. Later, constitutional homeopathic treatment from a professional can help reduce abnormal sensitivity to heat.

Belladonna and *Glonoine* are the two more common medicines for individuals suffering the effects of heatstroke. Both cover such heat exposure symptoms as fever, throbbing headache, reddened face, and stupor. Though both medicines tend to be good for individuals with throbbing headaches, *Belladonna* patients tend to have greater burning of the skin than *Glonoine* patients. *Belladonna*'s symptoms are made better by bending the head backward, sitting silently, and keeping the head uncovered, while *Glonoine*'s symptoms are made worse by bending the head backward and applying cold water (which sometimes causes spasms), and better by uncovering and being in the open air.

BEYOND HOME CARE

- Heatstroke is a medical emergency that requires immediate professional treatment.

INSECT AND SPIDER BITES AND STINGS

Human beings usually have the advantage when they encounter other creatures. But painful, sometimes dangerous bites and stings serve to remind us that our dominance isn't absolute. Biting, stinging insects and other arthropods (insects, spiders, ticks, and mites) are found everywhere.

After a bite or sting, local reactions to the venom or the insect's saliva are usually the main problem. Ordinarily, the temporary pain, itching, and discomfort of a local reaction do not seriously endanger health.

In fact, the inflammation serves to localize the venom or saliva to keep it from affecting other parts of the body. Of course, truly poisonous bugs such as black widow spiders and scorpions do exist. And, though rare, systemic allergic reactions to bites and stings also occur, producing hives or rashes, wheezing or other breathing problems, and fainting or loss of consciousness. Obviously, emergency medical attention is required under these circumstances. Arthropods also can carry infectious diseases, such as Rocky Mountain spotted fever, Lyme disease, and malaria. Treatment of such illnesses is beyond the scope of this book, but we can advise you to be aware of those that occur in areas where you live or plan to travel.

GENERAL HOME CARE

Avoiding bites in the first place is the best approach. In areas where bugs are common, wear long sleeves and pants. Light-colored clothing deters ticks. When appropriate, use a good repellent—citronella oil works as well for some people as synthetic chemicals.

If the insect's stinger has penetrated and remains in the skin, it should be removed immediately by flicking it out with a fingernail. Pulling it straight out sometimes causes additional venom to be injected into the skin. Place a cold application on the stung or bitten part to slow circulation and keep the problem localized.

HOMEOPATHIC MEDICINES

Choose a homeopathic medicine from the following list, and give it every one to three hours. Stop as soon as any substantial improvement is noted, and repeat only if improvement ceases.

Ledum is the medicine most commonly used to treat bites and stings from insects and their kin, and is especially good for bee stings. It helps relieve the redness, swelling, stinging, and pricking pains that accompany a bite or sting. Give *Ledum* routinely unless some other medicine is distinctly indicated. Characteristically, the affected part feels cold yet is relieved by cold applications, but still you may use *Ledum* whether or not this symptom is present. *Ledum* often brings relief even when the swelling involves the whole hand, foot, or limb.

Apis is indicated if the bite causes marked redness and swelling, especially if the affected part is very hot and the pain is worse from heat. Use *Apis* if the sensation of hotness is marked or if *Ledum* has not reduced the pain and swelling after four hours. Also, *Apis* is the medicine to use if hives develop after a bite or sting (*Urtica urens* is an alternative medicine for people with hives after a bite or sting).

Staphysagria is an excellent medicine for children who get mosquito bites that become large and irritating.

BEYOND HOME CARE

GET MEDICAL CARE IMMEDIATELY:

- if you suspect a bite is from a poisonous spider;
- if there is any difficulty breathing;
- for fainting, confusion, or loss of consciousness;
- if there is swelling in the mouth or throat;
- if there is severe or rapidly spreading swelling;
- if any of the above symptoms have previously occurred after a bite or sting by the same insect.

SNAKE BITES

The venom of a poisonous snake contains a highly toxic mixture of enzymes and other proteins that can cause capillary destruction, internal bleeding, paralysis of the nervous system, shock, and death. Obviously, a bite from a poisonous snake requires an immediate trip to the emergency room.

GENERAL HOME CARE

When treating a person who has been bitten by a poisonous snake, keep him at rest—exertion and muscle contraction will pump the venom through the body more quickly. **Get medical care immediately whenever poisonous snake bite is suspected.** Even if the bite occurs while the patient is some distance from medical care, it's usually best to have him wait for help. Excitement and strong emotion also can stimulate blood flow, so help the person relax, reassuring him with a soft, gentle voice.

If possible, position the person in such a way that the bitten part is below the level of the heart. Remove every piece of jewelry and any clothing that is the slightest bit constricting to the bitten area. The bitten part should not be moved except when absolutely necessary. Be sure not to give any medication, including aspirin or alcohol. Drugs can cause complications when antivenom medicine is given later in the emergency room. Contrary to what most people have heard, tourniquets and immersion in ice do little or nothing to slow the effects of the venom. In fact, their use increases the chance that an amputation will be necessary. The "cut-and-suck" method for extracting venom should not be used.

ANIMAL AND HUMAN BITES AND SCRATCHES

Bites from dogs, other animals, and people are kinds of lacerated or puncture wounds; you should refer to the sections on cuts and punctures for general principles of treatment. These bites can be infected more easily than other wounds. Human bites in particular require early medical attention, since people's mouths are so laden with bacteria. Any laceration of the hand caused by a bite must be cared for professionally. A dog or wild animal that bites must be caught so health officials can be sure it is free of rabies. Squirrels, skunks, and foxes are the more common carriers of rabies. If the animal cannot be apprehended, your health practitioner will consider a variety of factors to decide whether rabies shots should be given.

HOMEOPATHIC MEDICINES

Consult the earlier sections on cuts, bruises, and puncture wounds, and pick the medicine based on the type of bite you're dealing with. For bites and cat scratches that penetrate the skin, creating puncture wounds, *Ledum* generally is the best option. If the skin is cut or torn, choose *Hypericum* or *Arnica*.

BEYOND HOME CARE

GET MEDICAL CARE IMMEDIATELY:

- for any animal bite on the hand;
- for any human bite.

GET MEDICAL CARE TODAY:

- if bitten by a wild animal;

• if bitten by a domestic animal not known to be fully immunized against rabies, or one that cannot be caught.

Note: See also the criteria listed in the sections on cuts and puncture wounds.

DENTAL PROBLEMS AND PROCEDURES

Homeopathic medicines can be helpful both before and after a trip to the dentist, soothing and healing the injuries caused by tooth decay and by the dentist. The list below offers quick tips on medicines to try. Give the medicine every two to three hours for a few days, less often as the symptoms improve.

For toothache:

PLANTAGO: Tooth painfully sensitive to cold air and slightest pressure; may be better from eating.

KREOSOTE: Pain due to tooth decay without other clear symptoms.

STAPHYSAGRIA: Bad toothache worse from cold air or food or slight pressure (very similar to *Plantago*).

COFFEA: Severe toothache driving the patient to distraction; pain aggravated by heat or hot food, relieved by cold or ice.

CHAMOMILLA: Extreme pain—the person can't stand it and may be crying out or screaming. Classically, the symptoms are better in cold air and worse from warm food or warm drinks.

MERCURIUS: Pain due to inflammation or abscess in the root.

For problems related to dental procedures:

RUTA: The first medicine for pain after most dental procedures.

ARNICA: Pain within the first few days after having a tooth filled or pulled.

HYPERICUM: Persistent or shooting pain after a dental procedure.

PHOSPHORUS: Continued bleeding, especially of bright-red blood, following a tooth extraction.

A dose or two of a homeopathic medicine can sometimes calm the person who is afraid of going to the dentist in the first place. Try *Aconite* for intense fear or abject panic, especially if it begins suddenly. Those who are "just" anxious, perhaps a little weak in the knees, may benefit from *Gelsemium*.

CHAPTER 15

EMOTIONAL DISTRESS AND
SLEEP PROBLEMS

EMOTIONAL UPSETS

Emotional upsets are part and parcel of human life. Even the most well-adjusted people need time to recover from grief, disappointment, sudden fright, or extreme anger. While distress in the wake of such events is completely normal, homeopathic home care often can help restore normal emotional balance.

Sometimes an acute emotional shock leads to chronic depression, anxiety, or other such symptoms. In addition, many people experience recurrent or ongoing psychological difficulties that are not so clearly related to specific traumas. Professional homeopathic care is required in such cases.

Your health-care practitioner (or an experienced mental-health professional) should evaluate symptoms that don't gradually improve after an acutely stressful event, or that come on for no clear reason. Of course, medical attention also is warranted any time severe mental or emotional symptoms occur. The professional can help decide whether the symptoms deserve further monitoring or treatment, and also can rule out the uncommon cases in which medical problems lead to psychiatric symptoms.

HOMEOPATHIC REMEDIES

Give the thirtieth potency of the appropriate medicine every two hours during intense emotional experiences, and every four hours during mild ones. The correct remedy usually will not require more than four doses. If relief is not observed after twenty-four hours, consider another remedy. Seek professional homeopathic or psychological care if symptoms are particularly intense or if they persist.

Ignatia often brings marvelous relief when grief or a broken heart causes anguished emotional pain. The person's feelings are sensitive and easily hurt. She sighs or yawns frequently, perhaps as a sign of her efforts to suppress her feelings. Despite these efforts, she may cry uncontrollably. The typical person who needs *Ignatia* doesn't want to be consoled, and in fact, attempts to reassure may make her feel worse.

Give *Aconite* for acute states of anxiety and panic that follow some terrible shock, such as being the victim of—or narrowly escaping—a car accident, crime, or natural disaster. The patient can't calm down and remains terrified and restless. He may be in terror specifically of death, and may even predict his own death. In such circumstances, give *Aconite* in as high a potency as you have available.

Opium also should be considered when a sudden fright deeply affects the patient. In this case, though, the person is unnaturally calm, peaceful, and "dreamy," as if in shock or denial. Dullness, confusion, and sleepiness are common. Each of these symptoms sometimes alternates with an overexcited state of mind. The symptoms also may appear after very exciting or joyous experiences. *Opium* can be helpful as well for neurological symptoms such as tremor or even apparent seizures that develop after a frightening experience. (At present, *Opium* is not available in the U.S., even in homeopathic doses. We have chosen to include information on it in this book because we feel that it is a useful and safe remedy and because we hope that the illogical prohibition against it will be lifted in the near future.)

Nux vomica often is the remedy for acute emotional states arising from working too hard under too much pressure, or from frustrated ambition. Irritability is the hallmark of this remedy. The *Nux vomica* individual may be simply impatient and irascible, or may become violent, breaking things when she is crossed. She is greatly bothered by noises, light, or other sensations. Temperamentally, the typical *Nux* patient is driven and competitive.

Physical or emotional complaints that come on after getting angry often improve with a few doses of *Chamomilla*. After the acute anger has abated a bit, the patient remains hostile, complaining vehemently. He doesn't want to be touched. He may feel that he wants something, yet nothing satisfies him. Sometimes he throws things, often things he has just demanded. It's common for headaches or other pains to come on after anger, and *Chamomilla* is a good remedy when this happens. Marked hypersensitivity to pain also is very characteristic.

When surprise, joy, or any emotional stress leads to an overexcited state of mind, try *Coffea,* a homeopathic medicine made from coffee beans. The patient's thoughts race, and she can't relax, but she's not especially anxious. Like the *Chamomilla* or *Nux* patient, she is uncomfortably sensitive to noise, touch, taste, and other sensations; any little pain drives her to distraction (headaches are common). On the other hand, while she may be slightly irritable at times, she is basically mild-mannered and there is none of the open anger you'd expect with *Chamomilla* or *Nux.*

BEYOND HOME CARE

GET MEDICAL ATTENTION IMMEDIATELY:

- for any serious thoughts of suicide or of hurting yourself or other people.

SEE YOUR PRACTITIONER SOON:

- if you feel depressed or anxious much of the time for more than a week or so;
- if you experience recurrent guilty thoughts or feelings of hopelessness;
- if you take little or no pleasure in life for more than a week or so;
- if your sleep is disturbed (either too little or too much sleep) for more than a week or so;
- for "attacks" of panicky feelings or severe anxiety.

INSOMNIA

Everyone has trouble with insomnia once in a while. For some people, however, getting to sleep or staying asleep is a recurring battle. Insomnia is a frustrating experience—you're tired when you go to bed, but you toss and turn and just can't get to sleep. A few simple self-care measures along with a dose or two of the correct homeopathic medicine can help you get the sleep you need. The inability to sleep soundly more often is caused by acute or chronic psychological stress. Obviously a noisy room, an uncomfortable bed, or pain from physical illness also can prevent or disturb your sleep. Drugs of all sorts are known to interfere with restful sleep as well. Sleeplessness itself causes no permanent harm to your health. Occasionally, insomnia accompanies or is caused by other, more serious conditions. Sleeplessness can be a symptom of thyroid, liver, kidney, heart, and lung conditions. It can occur also with depression and other ongoing psychological problems. Rarely, insomnia signals another sleep disorder such as sleep-related myoclonus (jerking in sleep) or sleep apnea. If you frequently have trouble getting restful sleep, you should see your health-care practitioner for a checkup.

GENERAL HOME CARE

Don't assume you have a sleep problem just because you can't stay asleep for eight hours a night. As long as you feel refreshed when you awaken and can put in a full day of work or play without feeling deeply fatigued, you're getting enough sleep. Many people find that they need less sleep as they get older; on the other hand, the age-related decline in hours of sleep does lead to discomfort and daytime fatigue for some older people.

Alcohol, caffeine, and other drugs—both prescription and otherwise—can cause sleep difficulties, and you should avoid them whenever possible. Stimulants, of course, often are to blame; remember that some soft drinks, over-the-counter cold medicines, and pain relievers contain caffeine. Decongestants and asthma medications also are common offenders. Alcohol may make you feel drowsy and even help you fall asleep, but it can disrupt your sleep cycle, causing early or frequent waking during the night.

When sleeplessness strikes, don't fight it—*trying* to get to sleep only makes the problem worse. After about twenty or thirty minutes, you should get out of bed and read, listen to music, iron, or do other repetitive chores. Go back to bed only when you start to feel sleepy. You may need to repeat this process several times the first night, but before long, it should break the cycle.

If insomnia is a recurrent problem, your best bet is to establish a regular sleep routine. Make a ritual of locking the doors, putting on your pajamas or nightgown, and brushing your teeth, and follow this pattern every night. Also, be sure your bedroom is comfortable, and avoid using it for anything other than restful activities.

Here are some additional suggestions for preventing and alleviating insomnia.

• Avoid large meals just before bedtime.
• Do your jogging, speed walking, or other workout several hours before you go to bed, since vigorous exercise has a stimulating effect (gentle stretches just before bedtime should be fine).
• Take a hot bath to relax shortly before bedtime.
• Avoid daytime naps (if you're tired during the day, exercise instead).
• Use your bed only for sleep and intimacy—avoid watching TV or doing "brain work" in bed.
• Learn a relaxation technique and practice it both during the day and at night.
• If you can't stop thinking about worrisome concerns, write them down as a promise to yourself to deal with them tomorrow.
• Jobs that require shift changes can cause major disruptions in your sleep cycle. Ideally, you should stay on the same shift for several weeks before changing to another. When you do move to another shift, it's better to go to one that starts later rather than earlier in the day.

A last resort—short of sedative drugs or a trip to a sleep clinic—is a sleep restriction program. Set a time several hours after your normal bedtime and force yourself not to go to bed until then. You'll probably find that you worry more about how to stay awake that long than about your inability to fall asleep. What's more, you'll be tired the next day, which should help you fall asleep more easily the following night. Each night, move your bedtime ten or fifteen minutes earlier. By the time you're back to your original bedtime, you'll probably have forgotten about your insomnia.

CASETAKING QUESTIONS FOR INSOMNIA

Character of the symptoms:
• What seemed to cause the sleeping problem—an emotional upset, being overworked, physical pain, or something else?
• Is the person irritable or anxious while trying to get to sleep?
• Is the mind overactive?

• Is the person restless? Does the bed or pillow feel uncomfortable?
• If the person is able to fall asleep initially but wakes up during the night, at what time does he awaken?

Associated symptoms:
• Is there frequent sighing or yawning?
• Does the person sob or weep during sleep?

HOMEOPATHIC MEDICINES

You should seek professional homeopathic care if you suffer from recurrent or chronic insomnia (though the medicines listed here may help, relief may be temporary). When sleeplessness is the result of physical discomfort, review the chapter related to that condition for appropriate homeopathic treatment and get medical care for the condition as necessary.

We all know that coffee is a stimulant, and yet, in homeopathic doses, it can help relax an overactive mind. When sleep won't come because of racing thoughts, *Coffea* often brings relief. This state of mind often follows good or bad news or other sudden emotions, and *Coffea* is renowned for restoring natural sleep under such circumstances. Also, *Coffea* sometimes can help you get to sleep if you drank too much coffee, tea, or other caffeinated beverages earlier in the day.

Nux vomica is effective when insomnia results from abuse of coffee, alcohol, or drugs of any type. *Nux* also helps insomnia after mental strain or excessive study. *Nux* is clearly the choice when the patient is quite irritable and is hypersensitive, unable to fall asleep due to even slight noises, lights, or other distractions. In the typical case, the patient is sleepy in the evening but awakens at 3 or 4 A.M. He can't fall back asleep until daybreak, and when he eventually awakens, he feels unrefreshed.

If attacks of anxiety and fear drive you out of bed, *Arsenicum* is the medicine to try. Patients who need *Arsenicum* may feel that they are anxious even when asleep, and they often have anxious dreams. Restlessness in bed (both before and during sleep) is very characteristic of this medicine. *Arsenicum* is indicated also when the patient is "too tired" to fall asleep or is worn out by mental exertion.

Pulsatilla should be considered if the patient can't sleep because of a "fixed idea," one specific melody, thought, or experience that won't leave the mind. This medicine is probably best given if the typical *Pulsatilla* personality characteristics are present (a gentle, mild disposition; a wish to be comforted and consoled). The patient may weep over being unable to go to sleep. Sometimes the person sleeps with her hands over the head.

Passiflora may be the closest to a generic homeopathic medicine for insomnia in children and older people. It is indicated for those who have a hyperactive mind, and is best taken in the 1x or 3x potencies.

When the bed or pillow feels too hard, *Arnica* may help. The patient moves about restlessly, seeking a more comfortable position. The problem may be the result of being overextended physically or mentally.

Chamomilla is good for anyone who can't sleep because of extreme irritability or physical pains. It also can help those who have become dependent on sedatives. The patient may weep during sleep.

If the insomnia is caused by grief, *Ignatia* often is the remedy. One obvious indication for *Ignatia* is frequent sighing or yawning. Sometimes the patient sobs or whimpers during sleep.

REMEDY SUMMARY FOR INSOMNIA

Give the medicine: Up to every 30 minutes for up to 3 doses.

When to try another medicine: If still sleepless after 2 or 3 doses. Don't use more than 2 medicines in any one night.

COFFEA ★

Essentials
- Overactivity of the mind prevents sleep (patient is not markedly irritable or anxious)

  or
- Insomnia after hearing good or bad news or from other sudden emotions

  or
- Insomnia after drinking coffee or other caffeinated beverages

ARSENICUM

Essentials
- Sleepless because of anxiety and fears; driven out of bed by anxiety, or feels anxious while sleeping

  or

- "Too tired" to sleep (for example, after physical or mental overexertion)

Confirmatory symptoms
- Restless before and during sleep
- Insomnia after midnight; waking between midnight and 1 A.M.

NUX VOMICA

Essentials
- Insomnia after abuse of coffee, alcohol, or other drugs, or following mental strain or excessive study
- Irritability
- Hypersensitivity to even slight noise or distraction

Confirmatory symptoms
- Waking at 3 or 4 A.M. with ideas crowding the mind; can't return to sleep
- Finally falls asleep at daybreak; awakens later feeling unrefreshed

PULSATILLA

Essentials
- Kept awake by one specific repeated thought

Confirmatory symptoms
- Weeping because of the inability to go to sleep
- Hands held over the head during sleep

IGNATIA

Essentials
- Insomnia from grief

Confirmatory symptoms
- Sobbing or whimpering during sleep
- Frequent sighing or yawning (while awake)

CHAMOMILLA

Essentials
- Insomnia due to irritability
  or

- Insomnia from physical pains
or
- Insomnia in people dependent on sedatives

Confirmatory symptoms
- Weeping in sleep

PASSIFLORA

Essentials
- Insomnia with few specific symptoms in children and older people
- Overactive mind

ARNICA

Essentials
- Bed or pillow feels too hard
- Restless in bed, can't find a comfortable position

BEYOND HOME CARE

SEE YOUR PRACTITIONER SOON:

- if you have significant difficulty falling asleep or staying asleep for more than 10 days;
- if you are unable to sleep as the result of a painful or uncomfortable condition.

PART 3

HOMEOPATHIC

MATERIA MEDICA

THE MEDICINES LISTED HERE include those more commonly employed in acute care. The psychological and physical general symptoms of each medicine are described, sometimes along with prominent physical symptoms that may accompany any illness for which the medicine is used. When other medicines share the given symptoms, these other medicines are listed in parentheses. For more detail on specific physical symptoms, turn to the appropriate chapters in part 2 of this book.

Although many more homeopathic medicines are used by experienced homeopaths, only the remedies included in the clinical chapters of this book are covered here. There also are a number of medicines included in the clinical chapters that are not included here, either because the medicine is not known to have significant psychological or physical general symptoms, or because the essential information is covered sufficiently in the clinical section.

The symptoms in these *materia medica* descriptions are condensations intended for use in acute care situations only. Many symptoms that pertain to constitutional treatment are omitted. For more information on medicines listed here, see one or more of the books suggested in part 4.

Aconite
Monkshood

The symptoms of *Aconite* come on quickly, violently, and intensely. *Aconite* is particularly useful at the beginning of a high fever, during the initial stages of inflammatory conditions, and immediately after the shock of injury or surgery. The symptoms generally begin a short while after exposure to cold or after experiences of sudden fright, anger, or shock. Because it is normally used at the very onset of an illness, *Aconite* is more often prescribed by laypeople at home than by professional homeopaths. By the time the patient gets to the homeopath, the condition has progressed beyond the *Aconite* stage.

The emotional state of those who need *Aconite* is characterized by acute, panicky fear and anguished restlessness. They may fear death, darkness, crowds, or some unknown, impending evil. In extreme cases they are sure that they will die and may even predict the hour of death. They are very restless, both physically and mentally, and toss about without relief. Their senses are overly acute. Pain drives them to despair, and they are sensitive to light touch, light, and noise. Their sleep is restless; they toss and turn and wake up full of fear, thinking they will die.

Aconite can help restore emotional balance quickly when acute fear and panic follow any sudden, severe stress, such as a car accident or natural disaster. *Aconite* is just as useful when such symptoms occur after a close call with catastrophe, even though nothing terrible actually has happened.

Aconite patients may have stomach pain that is made worse by cold drinks (*Arsenicum, Rhus tox.*). During fever, the head may feel hot and full, while the body feels cold.

Although we do not specifically mention *Aconite* in some of the chapters on acute illnesses, this medicine certainly should be considered if the early stages of an earache, sore throat, urinary tract infection, or any other illness are marked by the violent onset and general symptoms typical of *Aconite*.

Though both *Aconite* and *Belladonna* cover sudden onset of intense symptoms, people who need *Aconite* are fearful, even panicky, and mentally hyperalert, whereas those who need *Belladonna* are delirious, confused, and less aware of their surroundings. The *Belladonna* patient may fear imaginary things and internal hallucinations, but the fear is not the overriding characteristic as in the *Aconite* case. The *Belladonna* patient is much more likely to be violent and destructive when delirious. Physically, the *Aconite* patient has a flushed, red face, but often this alternates with paleness, or one cheek may be flushed while the other is pale. The

Belladonna patient's face is consistently flushed. Dilation of the pupils is a symptom more consistent with *Belladonna*. *Aconite* patients are more likely to experience extreme thirst and usually want plenty of cold water. It is not uncommon for *Belladonna* to be indicated after *Aconite* if the latter remedy was given too late or is only partly effective.

Arsenicum is another medicine similar to *Aconite,* and both cover fear and restlessness. But *Aconite* is primarily helpful in the earlier stages of generalized illnesses, those involving the whole system, whereas *Arsenicum* conditions arise later and usually involve a localized infection (sore throat, digestive illness, and so on). *Aconite* patients generally are not afraid to be alone, but, instead, are afraid of people or crowds. *Aconite* patients have less general sensitivity to cold or drafts than do *Arsenicum* patients, though the symptoms may have begun after exposure to cold. Both medicines cover extreme thirst, but *Arsenicum* patients may specifically desire frequent sips of water.

What Makes Aconite Symptoms

Worse: cold dry wind, rising, night, noise, light, jarring, lying on the painful side

Better: perspiring

Apis Mellifica
The Honey Bee or Bee Venom

The familiar stinging, burning pain of a bee sting and the hivelike welt it produces are the key symptoms of *Apis* in acute-care situations. Any acute inflammation may call for *Apis* if there is much stinging and burning, marked redness and swelling, and sensitivity of the inflamed part to any form of heat. People with sore throats, hives, conjunctivitis, styes, or insect bites often need this medicine.

Any application of heat makes the pain more intense, and the *Apis* patient gets relief from cold baths or anything cool applied to the inflamed part. The sore throat is relieved by cold drinks and made worse by warm liquids.

The inflammatory swellings most typical of this medicine have a puffy, water-filled appearance. An inflamed eyelid with a stye looks like a red bag of water, just as if it had been stung by a bee. The inner linings of the eyelids or the surface layers of the eye itself may swell greatly during an eye infection. The throat and palate of the *Apis* patient with a sore throat are red and puffed, and the uvula hangs as though swollen with water.

Those who need *Apis* usually have little thirst, although sometimes they crave milk. The skin is likely to be hot and dry, and it can be sensitive to touch, even when it has no eruptions. Sometimes symptoms appear initially on the right side of the body and then move to the left as they progress.

Sadness and depression can accompany the physical symptoms. The person may weep constantly and without cause. He may be extremely irritable as well, and he may be suspicious and jealous for no apparent reason. He may claim that he is well and doesn't need medical attention even when he is quite ill.

Apis should be considered when illness follows jealousy, fright, rage, or disappointment.

What Makes *Apis* Symptoms

Worse: all forms of heat, hot applications, warm drinks, closed or heated room, the right side, touch, pressure, 3 to 5 P.M., after sleep

Better: cool or cold applications, cold baths, open air, uncovering

Arsenicum Album
Arsenious Acid; White Arsenic

The distinctive symptoms of *Arsenicum* include great restlessness and fear, severe weakness and exhaustion, intense chilliness, burning pains, and aggravation of the symptoms at night. Whenever this distinctive group of symptoms appears, *Arsenicum* is the curative medicine, whatever the local symptoms may be.

The *Arsenicum* patient experiences marked weakness and exhaustion, which is often out of proportion compared with the rest of the illness. She becomes exhausted from the slightest exertion. But often this great weakness is accompanied by anxious restlessness. The patient keeps in constant motion until she becomes completely worn out; her agitation makes her toss about in bed or drives her from bed to pace the floor.

Arsenicum patients often feel intense anxiety and fear. A penetrating anxiety about health is common. The patient may be terrified of dying from her illness or from some other catastrophe. Whatever her ailment, she may think it is much more serious than it really is. Her fears are worse at night, when she also may be tormented by fear of the dark. She is afraid to be alone and must have company for reassurance, else her fears will escalate intolerably. Yet she may not be able to bear being looked at.

She may become possessive about people and things because of her insecurity. She also can be extremely fastidious, and she may be unable to rest if the environment is not meticulously clean. Cleaning and tidying help allay her constant anxiety.

Burning pains are a key symptom of *Arsenicum*. Any part of the body may burn, but especially the throat, eyes, and stomach. Discharges, like a runny nose or diarrhea, burn and irritate the skin. Characteristically, all these burning pains are made better by heat. A warm room may help, or the person may want to use a heating pad on a painful infection. Warm drinks relieve burning in the throat and stomach.

In general the *Arsenicum* patient is extremely cold, despite her burning pains. Coldness of any form aggravates her general condition and all her individual symptoms (except the headache, which is made better with cold applications). She craves warmth, which eventually makes her feel much better. Icy coldness of individual parts of the body—forehead, face, chest, knees, hands, or feet—is common.

Most of the symptoms are worse at night, especially between midnight and 2 A.M. The sick person may have trouble falling asleep because of anxiety and restlessness or because of the physical symptoms, such as cough or vomiting, which are worse at night. She sleeps restlessly and has frightening dreams.

Arsenicum patients have a burning thirst, though they may want only sips of water at frequent intervals. They may have a craving for either warm or cold drinks, including milk, though sometimes milk makes them worse.

What Makes *Arsenicum* Symptoms

Worse: coldness of any kind, open air and drafts, night, midnight to 2 A.M., cold food or drink, physical exertion, sea air, right side of the body, fruit

Better: warmth, warm applications, warm food or drinks, the company of others

Belladonna
Deadly Nightshade

Often you can tell when someone needs *Belladonna* just by looking at him. His face is flushed and the skin is bright red and dry. His eyes are glassy and glaring, and the pupils are dilated. He looks feverish and dull or even stuporous.

Generally *Belladonna* is a medicine for the acute early stages of inflammatory illnesses characterized by high fever and severe pain. *Belladonna* conditions begin suddenly and violently, worsen rapidly, and then
leave as abruptly as they started. Fevers, earaches, sore throats, painful
menstrual cramps, urinary tract inflammation, and skin infections are
some of the more common conditions for which *Belladonna* has been
used successfully. *Belladonna* is given commonly to infants and children
for many of the inflammatory conditions they experience, and parents
often are extremely amazed by the rapid beneficial results this remedy
creates when used accurately.

Intense heat, redness, throbbing, and swelling are the key symptoms
of *Belladonna*. Fever makes the skin so hot it seems to radiate heat. It is
said that *Belladonna* is indicated when your fingers remain hot after you
have touched the patient's skin. The skin is bright red, maybe even shiny
at first, though a dusky flushed complexion may develop with time. Inflamed parts (throat, skin, eardrums) are bright red and swollen but with
no pus formation. Swelling develops rapidly during the sudden onset of
inflammation, and it causes severe pain. With all the blood brought to the
inflamed area, the part burns and throbs intensely.

The *Belladonna* patient experiences heat, throbbing, and a sensation
of fullness of the head along with his fever, even while his extremities
may be ice-cold. In general, though, he is usually less sensitive to the
temperature around him than are those who need medicines such as *Arsenicum, Pulsatilla,* or *Nux vomica.* The skin and mucous membranes are
ordinarily dry, but if the sick person is perspiring heavily and other
symptoms suggest *Belladonna,* you still can give this medicine. What little
mucus, pus, or other discharge there may be is clear and thin. Though
they have dry mouths, *Belladonna* patients are generally not that thirsty.

Usually *Belladonna* patients are dull and tired only during the fever.
Characteristically, their senses are overly acute, and they may be startled
or bothered by noise, touch, light, or jarring motion. In general, however, the patient's attention is inwardly focused, and he is much less responsive to things that happen around him.

Fever often makes the *Belladonna* patient somewhat delirious. In
home-care situations, this usually does not progress beyond that dull,
dazed mentality, or perhaps it leads to some moaning or speaking non-
sensically. If the fever is high enough or lasts long enough, however, more
severely excited delirium may develop. Scary imaginings and hallucinations may haunt the patient, especially when he closes his eyes. Wild,
frightful dreams trouble his sleep. He moans incessantly or his speech

wanders or becomes completely unintelligible. He may be startled or may jerk in his sleep or cry out as if he had been shocked. He may become even violent and destructive, breaking things around him, striking at people or imaginary things, or even biting or kicking. This sort of behavior suggests serious illness, not a home-care situation, but a dose of *Belladonna* given en route to your health practitioner's office may arrest the crisis.

Belladonna pains are severe, most often of a throbbing or burning type, but the medicine suits any type of pain. The pains are made much worse by sudden jarring motion; even his own walking or someone else touching his bed may jar him intolerably. Sudden touch or pressure increases the pain, but gradually applied pressure may relieve it. Sensations of constriction are common, such as feeling as though a band or strap were wrapped around the head or chest. The person may experience a sensation similar to having a ball inside various parts of the body, especially the throat, bladder, or abdomen. The head, extremities, eyes, or uterus (during menstruation) may feel heavy.

Twitchings of the extremities or other parts of the body may accompany fever. The symptoms may be worse on the right side of the body.

What Makes *Belladonna* Symptoms

Worse: touch, jarring, motion, bright lights, noise, lying on the painful side, rising, letting the affected part hang limply, uncovering the head

Better: lying down, lying on the abdomen

Bryonia
Wild Hops

The most distinctive characteristic of *Bryonia* is aggravation from motion. Any type of motion makes the symptoms worse. Walking is intolerable. Simply moving the eyes is unbearable to the *Bryonia* patient with a headache. Deep breathing brings on a coughing spell along with sharp chest pain, and talking also can cause coughing. Swallowing irritates the throat. Even slightly changing the position of some remote part of the body may cause muscular or neuralgic pain. Passive motion, being jarred or carried for instance, also brings on increased pain. When *Bryonia* patients are acutely ill, they want to lie completely still.

Bryonia individuals also are irritable, easily angered, and morose. They don't like to be disturbed and resent being questioned. Adults who need *Bryonia* prefer to be left alone. Sick children are, of course, less likely to want to be completely by themselves, but *Bryonia* children don't want much contact or affection.

Bryonia patients are likely to be somewhat confused or dull. They may be disinclined to think. Sometimes they feel homesick and say that they want to go home, even when they are already there. They may have business or school affairs on their mind. Even though they are too sick to work, they may talk at length about business or school.

People who need *Bryonia* commonly have headaches, respiratory problems, digestive disorders, or musculoskeletal pains. Motion of any kind may aggravate all of these conditions. On the other hand, firm pressure on painful spots feels good, and lying on the painful part also brings relief.

Many of the *Bryonia* patient's symptoms can get worse after eating. For example, eating aggravates the headache, cough, and abdominal pains. The classical *Bryonia* patient wants plenty of liquids to drink for long intervals. In any case, she is likely to be markedly thirsty. The abdomen becomes painfully distended after eating. The patient may crave milk, sweets, or sour foods. She may be worse after eating fruit, bread, beans, or milk. Although she usually prefers cold drinks, her stomach complaints may be relieved by warm liquids.

Various symptoms of the muscles and joints are likely to appear in the person who needs *Bryonia*. A generalized muscular soreness, which is made worse during motion, commonly accompanies *Bryonia* colds and flus. Joint paints made worse from motion may indicate *Bryonia*, whether they occur during a fever or after an injury.

Dryness is another symptom characteristic of *Bryonia*. The individual often has dry lips, mouth, tongue, and throat. The stools are typically large, hard, and dry, and are difficult to expel. The cough is usually dry. The tongue is dry and may have a white, furry appearance.

In general, *Bryonia* patients tend to be worse in heat, in warm rooms, in the sun, and in the summertime, and are usually better in cool or open air and also after cold applications. The headache, cough, and muscle and joint pains are worsened by warmth. The *Bryonia* patient may get dizzy in warm rooms and may have trouble falling asleep if the room is stuffy. Cool environments and open air may help relieve anxiety and confusion. Some complaints begin after exposure to cold, however.

The symptoms of people who need *Bryonia* develop somewhat slowly, as compared with the rapid onset of symptoms occurring when *Aconite* and *Belladonna* is indicated. Many of the pains are worse on the right side of the body.

What Makes *Bryonia* Symptoms

Worse: motion, exertion, jarring, rising, becoming heated, warm rooms, the sun, eating, evening or night, cold (sometimes)

Better: rest, lying still, firm pressure, lying on the painful side, lying down, cold drinks (except when these are stomach complaints), cool rooms, open air

Calcarea Carbonica
Carbonate of Lime or Calcium Carbonate

Calcarea carb. sometimes is used during acute conditions, though it is given more commonly as a constitutional medicine. We give instructions for its use in the sections on vaginitis in chapter 9 and skin infections in chapter 13.

People who need *Calcarea carbonica* are physically and mentally weak. Commonly, *Calcarea carbonica* is given to people who are plump and fair skinned, have flabby muscle tone, and are prone to swollen lymph nodes. These individuals have strong chills and difficulty keeping warm. They are averse to cold, open air, which seems to go right through them. Exposure to damp, cold weather is aggravating, and an acute illness may develop after being out in the rain.

Calcarea carbonica patients are frequently tired and tend to sweat easily. Perspiration of isolated parts of the body is common. The head often perspires during sleep, usually shortly after falling asleep. They may sweat also on the abdomen, upper torso, genitalia, feet, or palms. Perspiration, discharges, and stools often smell sour.

A strong craving for eggs is a classic symptom of those who need *Calcerea carbonica,* but they may crave also raw potatoes, milk, sweets, salt, and indigestible items such as dirt or chalk. On the other hand, they may be averse to milk or meat. They are thirsty, usually for cold or iced drinks.

Calcarea carbonica patients often are passive and complacent people, but they may become surprisingly stubborn if asked to do something they don't want to. They are slow, methodical, plodding individuals who don't like to be rushed. Though their energy may be low, they persevere and usually complete their projects. They prefer sticking to routine and are stressed by change. They may be afraid of the dark, being alone, becoming ill, or going crazy.

See also chapter 9 on women's health and chapter 13 on skin problems.

What Makes *Calcarea Carbonica* Symptoms

Worse: cold, damp weather, exertion, fright

Better: warmth, lying down

Chamomilla
Chamomile

Chamomilla patients are cross and irascible, probably the most irritable among the homeopathic remedy types. Infants particularly are given to the open displays of irritability and discontent so typical of *Chamomilla,* so they may require this medicine more often than adults. Nothing pleases the *Chamomilla* patient, and everything seems to bother him. He demands to have something, but when he gets it, he rejects what he so urgently desired and becomes even more upset. He is stubbornly disagreeable and refuses to do anything asked of him. His irritability increases until a screaming tantrum ensues, and a *Chamomilla* child may strike out at anyone within range during one of these fits. He hates to be touched, spoken to, or even looked at, and he bursts into renewed screaming if these attentions are offered. He is extremely sensitive to pain, and screams as he suffers it.

Chamomilla people are inconsolable. Soothing words and affectionate touch don't calm them and are likely to make them even more upset. The only thing that may help a *Chamomilla* child feel better is being carried about or rocked. He may fall asleep in your arms and then start fussing again as soon as you stop the motion.

The head, face, and feet are especially hot. Often one cheek is hot and red while the other is cold and pale. In spite of the internal warmth, becoming cold is eventually aggravating. These people are generally very thirsty, especially for cold water. Sometimes a sense of numbness accompanies the pains.

What Makes *Chamomilla* Symptoms

Worse: warmth of the bed, anger, night, touch, lying down, lying on the painless side, eating, milk, warm food, open air, wind, cold

Better: being carried, passive motion (such as being rocked), fasting, perspiring, cold applications

Ferrum Phosphoricum
Phosphate of Iron

Ferrum phos. is indicated in the first stages of various inflammatory conditions. People who need *Ferrum phos.* have symptoms similar to those of *Aconite* and *Belladonna*; however, the onset of the symptoms of *Ferrum phos.* may not be as rapid or violent. *Ferrum phos.* is more commonly prescribed for people with fever, colds and other viral illnesses, and earaches. It should be chosen when the person doesn't have clear, distinguishing symptoms that would indicate another medicine.

The *Ferrum phos.* patient is flushed and hot with the fever. Classically, there is well-defined, circular redness on the cheeks (usually the entire *Belladonna* face is flushed). She may be sensitive to cold and cold air. She is tired and easily exhausted by physical exertion, and sometimes her illnesses begin after overexertion. She may have a tendency to bleed easily. There may be bright-red blood coming from the nose or gums at the onset of a feverish illness, or a dry cough may bring up a little blood-streaked mucus.

Ferrum phos. patients are more alert than those who need *Belladonna*, less anguished and fearful than *Aconite* patients. They pay attention to what is going on about them, and even during a high fever follow everything happening in the room with their eyes. Sometimes there is a tendency toward loquacity and mirth. They'll joke and chat as though they aren't ill. The fever can make it difficult for them to concentrate, and sometimes they become forgetful, dull, and indifferent as they tire. These symptoms are like those of *Phosphorus,* but *Phosphorus* is more useful later in the course of an illness and has many other individual symptoms.

What Makes *Ferrum Phos.* Symptoms

Worse: cold, night, exertion, standing

Better: gentle motion

Gelsemium
Yellow Jessamine

Drowsiness and mental and physical weakness are the prominent symptoms of the *Gelsemium* patient. The patient dreads movement, not because it's painful, but because it's just too much effort. The body feels heavy and tired. The limbs in particular feel heavy, and the legs tire easily from walking or other exertion. Sometimes there is weakness of individual parts of the body. The eyelids may feel heavy and droop notice-ably, and the face looks sleepy and weary. The limbs are weak and heavy, and the legs tire easily from walking or other exertion.

The mental weakness of the person with a *Gelsemium* illness corre-sponds to this physical condition. The mind is sluggish, and the person becomes dull, forgetful, and indifferent. She doesn't want to be spoken to, and just wants to be left alone in a quiet room. She is really too tired to be irritable.

The *Gelsemium* person with a flu or fever often feels achy all over. There may be stiffness of the neck and upper back. Headache may ac-company the symptoms, classically beginning in the neck and back of the head and extending to the forehead or the entire head. She may experi-ence temporary relief of her symptoms after urinating.

Gelsemium patients often feel chills running up and down the back. They want heat in general, though exposure to the sun may bring on headache. They usually experience little or no thirst. The face may be flushed a dusky red color.

Anticipation, nervousness, and similar emotions may bring on the symptoms. A *Gelsemium* condition may begin, for instance, because of anticipation of an examination or public performance, or after receiving bad news.

What Makes *Gelsemium* Symptoms

Worse: anticipatory anxiety, bad news

Better: perspiration, urination

Hepar Sulphuricum
Hahnemann's Calcium Sulphide*

Physical hypersensitivity and mental irritability characterize those who need *Hepar sulph.* These people are exquisitely sensitive to touch, cold, and pain. Any infected part (such as a boil, stye, or swollen gland) is extremely tender to touch, and the slightest pressure causes sharp pain—as though a splinter or bit of glass were pushing into the affected part. There is a sensation similar to having a splinter or fishbone caught in the throat, and the pain increases upon swallowing.

Hepar patients are so cold that the slightest exposure causes chills.

*Hahnemann developed this medicine by burning a mixture made from the inner layer of oyster shells (a source of calcium carbonate) and flowers of sulphur.

Even a hand or foot sticking out of the blankets may bring on symptoms. Cold air or applications to an infected area make the pain of the inflammation much worse. Dry, cold air may be the least tolerable. The *Hepar* patient is overly sensitive to pain in general, and pain may make him faint. *Hepar* patients are irritable, impatient, and discontented. Everything bothers them, nothing pleases. They are cross and easily angered, and may pick fights for no apparent reason. They may have sudden violent impulses, and at times their anger can get out of control. *Hepar* children, however, are somewhat less apt to hit or scream than children who need *Chamomilla*.

The *Hepar* patient commonly has an offensive or sour smell. His sweat, stool, and discharges also smell sour or offensive. Discharges from the nose, pus from boils, and phlegm that is coughed up are profuse and of a thick yellow or cheesy character.

The *Hepar* patient loves vinegar, pickles, and other sour foods, as well as spices and strong-tasting foods. He may dislike fats. He may be more thirsty than usual.

What Makes *Hepar* Symptoms

Worse: cold, a single part becoming cold, uncovering, lying on the painful side, pressure, night, dry weather, motion, exertion, tight clothing

Better: warmth, hot applications, wet weather, lying on the painless side

Ignatia
St. Ignatius Bean

Although we have recommended *Ignatia* in only two of the chapters dealing with acute care, we include it in this *materia medica* section because of its unique applicability to conditions brought on by acute emotional stress. Whether the symptoms represent disordered nervous system function or the body's response to an infectious illness, *Ignatia* may be the curative medicine if the condition was precipitated by grief, fear, anger, embarrassment, or a scolding. *Ignatia* is an especially good remedy for people who become ill after a romantic disappointment. It may be indicated also after physical or sexual abuse, and for the various emotional and physical symptoms that tend to ensue.

The *Ignatia* patient usually tries to avoid really breaking down in front of others, but she is given to frequent, loud sighs that betray her inner anguish. Though some *Ignatia* patients never cry, more often, when they are alone, they break into involuntary, racking sobs, perhaps punctuated with spasmodic laughter. The patient feels worse when consoled. She is likely to be inordinately sensitive to reprimand, yet she will often inflict severe self-criticism if she doesn't do something right.

Because of her emotional upset, the *Ignatia* patient is often unable to sleep well. Feeling a lump in the throat is common among emotionally distraught people, and this is characteristic of *Ignatia* as well.

Seemingly contradictory symptoms are distinctive of *Ignatia*. Nausea may be made better by eating, while eating may make hunger more intense. Simple fruits cause indigestion, and heavier foods may be more easily tolerated. Ordinary foods may be repugnant to the *Ignatia* patient, and she may crave indigestible things instead. She may want to be uncovered and to drink when she is cold, just as she may be thirstless during the height of a fever. A roaring noise in the ears may get better when she hears music.

The *Ignatia* patient often craves fruit, although it may cause indigestion. She may jerk and twitch out of nervousness. The senses may be overly acute. Sometimes only one cheek is flushed (also a sometime symptom of *Chamomilla, Nux vomica,* and *Pulsatilla*).

If you decide that *Ignatia* should be given during an acute emotional crisis, give a single dose of the 30x or 30c potency and observe the results for six to eight hours. If the symptoms are unchanged, you may repeat the dose one more time, but if there is still no result, try to find another medicine that fits the symptoms. If *Ignatia* seems to help, repeat it only when the symptoms have grown decidedly worse, and do so no more than twice a day for three days.

What Makes *Ignatia* Symptoms

Worse: suppressing grief or other emotions, consolation, tobacco smoke, pressure on the painless side

Better: eating, lying on the painful side

Kali Bichromium
Bichromate of Potash

Thick, stringy discharge from mucous membranes is the most distinctive symptom of those who need *Kali bichromium*. Although many other homeopathic medicines also cover the thick yellow or green discharges that are typical of *Kali bi.*, a marked sticky, gluey quality is more characteristic of this medicine than of any other. A discharge from the nose, for instance, tends to adhere to the nasal passages and throat and may be so gelatinous that it can be pulled away in stringy lengths (described in the older homeopathic literature as "ropy"). Sometimes the material is discharged in nearly solid globs. *Kali bi.* should be considered whenever discharges of this character are found, whether they come from eyes, ears, nose, or throat.

Other characteristics of *Kali bi.* are symptoms that come and go suddenly and pains that are limited to small parts of the body or that wander from place to place. Commonly, joint paints alternate with digestive problems, diarrhea, or respiratory difficulties.

Kali bi. patients generally get cold easily, but they feel worse in hot weather. These temperature reactions are not as marked as those associated with other medicines we've discussed. The patient in general, and especially his cough, often is worse between 2 A.M. and 3 A.M.

Psychologically, those who need *Kali bi.* tend to be low-spirited, ill-humored, irritable, and indifferent. Often they are listless, with a great disinclination for mental or physical labor.

Since the strong symptoms are localized "particulars" and since the general symptoms of *Kali bi.* are not well marked, look first for medicines that match any strong general symptoms of the illness before you give *Kali bi.* When a thick, stringy discharge is a prominent symptom, *Pulsatilla* may be indicated if the person is weepy, thirstless, and uncomfortable in warm rooms. *Mercurius* may better suit the patient who is more irritable, thirsty, sweaty, and bothered by both heat and cold. Use *Kali bi.* if your first choice hasn't helped or if the only striking aspect of the illness is the thickness and stringiness of the discharge.

What Makes *Kali Bi.* Symptoms

Worse: cold, hot weather, 2 to 3 A.M., undressing

Better: heat, motion, pressure

Lachesis
Venom from the Bushmaster or Surucucu Snake

Symptoms that are worse upon waking, during sleep, on the left side of the body—along with a unique "volcanic" mental state—are the primary indications for *Lachesis.* Acute home-care situations in which *Lachesis* is more commonly useful include sore throats, boils and abscesses, and menstrual pain.

Whenever the symptoms of any of these conditions are more intense upon first waking or during sleep, *Lachesis* may be the correct medicine. In fact, people who need *Lachesis* may dread going to sleep, because they anticipate the increased suffering they must endure when they awake. Pain or inflammation that is much worse on the left side of the body, or that begins on the left and moves to the right, is equally characteristic.

The psychological state of the *Lachesis* person has been described as volcanic and intense. The individual is loquacious, jealous, high-strung, and suspicious. Excitability and a vivid imagination are typical, and the patient talks nonstop, jumping from one idea to another, sometimes even before finishing his sentence. Unwarranted suspicions and jealousies may arise, and he may believe that others are conspiring against him or that his lover has been unfaithful. Sadness that comes with the morning, especially upon waking, also is a common *Lachesis* symptom.

People who need *Lachesis* are sensitive to any type of restriction, psychological or physical. They are driven to express themselves and can't stand being told what to do. Physically, they hate restrictive clothing and are especially intolerant of even the slightest pressure on the neck or waist. Even the slightest contact with clothing can be extremely distressing; sometimes the pressure of the blankets aggravates the bedridden *Lachesis* patient.

Lachesis patients usually crave open air, so they may open windows even in cold weather. They prefer cool temperatures and want few clothes or covers. Extremes of either heat or cold may cause weakness.

Inflamed areas, whether in the throat, on the skin, or elsewhere, have a dark bluish or purplish appearance. Similarly, the face may look somewhat purplish during the fever or other acute illness.

One interesting characteristic occasionally seen in people who need *Lachesis* is a tendency of the person's tongue to tremble when it is stuck out, just like when a snake sticks out its tongue.

What Makes *Lachesis* Symptoms

Worse: sleep, waking, touch, pressure, clothing, heat, warmth of the sun, warm rooms, lying down

Better: warm applications, open air, after a discharge, hard pressure, cold drinks, loosening clothing

Lycopodium*
Club Moss

Lycopodium is a frequently used medicine in a wide variety of both acute and chronic illnesses. Though you should not attempt to treat chronic conditions at home, *Lycopodium* may be the indicated medicine during home-care situations involving earaches, sore throats, digestive conditions, and urinary tract problems.

Several key general symptoms of *Lycopodium* indicate its use no matter what the specific problem is. Conditions that are definitely worse on the right side, or that begin on the right and then move to the left, strongly suggest *Lycopodium*. The symptoms often are worse between the hours of 4 and 8 P.M. Craving sweets is also characteristic, as is desiring warm drinks, which relieve symptoms such as cough, sore throat, or stomach discomfort.

Lycopodium patients are particularly prone to disorders of the digestive system, more often suffering intestinal gas and bloating, along with whatever other symptoms they may have. The distension and gas are worse after eating, and the abdomen is sensitive to the pressure of clothing. The appetite is confused. The *Lycopodium* patient may feel hungry sitting down to a meal, but then a bite or two makes him full. Or he may have a ravenous appetite soon after a big meal (a symptom shared with *Phosphorus*). Sometimes intense hunger wakes the *Lycopodium* patient from sleep, and he may get a headache if he doesn't eat. *Lycopodium* patients tend to be averse to meat as well as generally aggravated after eating oysters, onions, cabbage, or milk.

Lycopodium patients may be warm or chilly, though they usually desire open air and dislike warm rooms. Occasionally one foot is hot while the other is cold. Though they prefer warm drinks, they often have little thirst.

The *Lycopodium* psychology is characterized by insecurity and cowardice. The person becomes anxious and doubts his ability to perform new or challenging tasks. He is especially nervous in social situations and worries about what people think of him. He fears rejection and may think that he is being observed critically. He often tries to hide his insecurity by bluff and bravado, and he may resort to domineering behavior, especially over those younger, weaker, or less intelligent than he. He may not like the company of others, but also he can be afraid to be alone; clas-

---

*Lycopodium should not be given immediately after *Sulphur*.

sically, the *Lycopodium* patient wants to know that someone is nearby but not in the same room.

People who need *Lycopodium* don't like to show weakness. Even though they may be quite ill, they deny that there is any problem. They usually try to seem much stronger and smarter than they are feeling. They are beset by performance anxieties. They worry whether people like them, and they worry about their work and whether they will succeed. They worry most when they are alone, and like to have someone else around, even if there is little interaction.

The *Lycopodium* patient can be afraid also of the dark, of crowds, and of death. Often his anxieties are felt in his stomach. He may be cross and peevish, especially when he first wakes in the morning. Fright, anger, or embarrassment may bring on his illness.

What Makes *Lycopodium* Symptoms

Worse: 4 to 8 P.M., waking, warm rooms, eating, pressure of clothing, onions, oysters, cabbage, fruit, milk, cold food or drink

Better: warm food or drink, midnight and later hours, cool or open air, uncovering the head

Mercurius Vivus and *Mercurius Solubilis*
Mercury or Quicksilver

Mercurius vivus, the simple elemental form of mercury, and *Mercurius solubilis,* a soluble preparation of mercury created by Hahnemann, are considered essentially identical medicines by homeopathic authorities. They are used on the basis of the same indications, though the chemical compositions of the two remedies differ.

Mercurius is more likely to be required during acute conditions characterized by marked inflammation of the skin and mucous membranes, along with pus formation and perhaps raw, open areas. Examples of these conditions include eye infections with discharges of thick pus; bacterial ear infections with pus buildup behind the eardrum; sore throats with much pain, pus formation, and even open sore spots; urinary infections; and skin infections such as boils and herpes.

In these conditions and others, the person's whole illness follows the distinct pattern of *Mercurius's* general symptoms. Although there are times the decision to give *Mercurius* may be based on the particular symptoms alone, you can be sure of your choice if the key general symptoms of the medicine are present. These include: heavy perspiration that often makes the patient feel worse; foul-odored perspiration, breath, and entire body; much salivation, so much that when the patient drools he gets his pillow wet; and aggravation of the symptoms at night, often beginning after sunset.

Mercurius patients, in fact, are aggravated by almost every environmental influence and are comfortable only over a narrow range of conditions. Like a mercury thermometer, they are very sensitive to temperature, and they are bothered whenever it gets even slightly too hot or too cold. They are bothered by open air and drafts, but warm air or a warm bed also makes them feel worse.

Trembling is another general *Mercurius* symptom. The hands, tongue, all the limbs, or any other part of the body may tremble or jerk visibly, especially when an effort is made to use them. The *Mercurius* patient generally is weak and tires easily with exertion. The vital responses of the body are weak and slow, and infected tissues are slow to heal and look unhealthy.

On the mental and emotional level, there may be an undirected agitation, restlessness, and hurriedness, along with rapid talking and rushing to get things done. There is an inability to concentrate, which results in impulsiveness as ideas come to mind. At times these impulses can be violent; past *Mercurius* patients have been seized with impulses to commit suicide or murder. The mind is generally dull and sluggish, so the patient may take a long time to answer questions.

Whatever the specific condition afflicting him, the *Mercurius* patient is likely to have prominently swollen lymph nodes as a result of the inflammation. In addition to the salivation and drooling, inflammation and soreness of the mouth is typical, and there is often a metallic taste there as well. The gums are swollen and spongy, and blood oozes from them when they are touched or during eating. The tongue is puffed up and flabby and shows imprints of the teeth.

Often *Mercurius* patients are averse to sweets, meat, fats, or butter, though sometimes they crave buttered bread. They can be thirsty, and they may well have a craving for cold drinks.

What Makes *Mercurius* Symptoms

Worse: heat, cold, dampness, warm air or warmth of the bed, open air, sunset to sunrise, sweating, sweets, motion, lying on the right side

Better: moderate temperature

Natrum Muriaticum
Sodium Chloride (Table Salt)

During an acute illness, *Natrum muriaticum* may be indicated by the specific physical symptoms, even if its general symptoms are not evident. If the psychological or physical general symptoms are present, your choice of this medicine is all the more certain.

Natrum muriaticum patients often become ill after experiencing some type of emotional trauma. They have particular difficulty dealing with loss or rejection—the breakup of a relationship or the death of a loved one—which may weaken their system and precipitate an illness. They also tend to get symptoms after being reprimanded. Although these people are emotionally sensitive and their feelings are easily hurt, they have difficulty expressing their emotions. They hold in grief, anger, disappointment, or frustration and rarely weep in front of others. When alone, however, they may break down and weep loudly. The *Natrum muriaticum* patient may avoid intimacy to prevent being hurt. He wants to be alone when ill, and he feels uncomfortable and irritable when others try to console him.

Sudden noises, like the ringing of a telephone or the slamming of a door, may unduly startle the *Natrum muriaticum* patient, and he may even feel weak and ill afterward. He may be deeply affected by music.

The person tends to be physically warm and is bothered by heat. He is often sensitive to the sun, which may cause exhaustion or a headache. He feels better in the open air or perhaps after a cold bath.

The classic *Natrum muriaticum* patient craves salt, salty foods, and possibly bread. Sometimes, however, he is averse to bread or salt, and more often will dislike fats or slimy foods.

Dryness of the skin and mucous membranes is common, but the face and the hairy parts of the body may be oily. Stools also are often dry and become hard and difficult to expel.

What Makes *Natrum Muriaticum* Symptoms

Worse: grief, heat, sun, 10 A.M., noise, music

Better: open air, cold bathing, fasting

Nux Vomica
Seeds of the Poison Nut Tree

Nux patients are irritable, quick-tempered individuals who get sick after overeating, indulging in alcohol or drugs, or doing too much mental work. Although you may decide to use *Nux* during an acute illness on the basis of the particular symptoms alone, if these key general attributes of the *Nux* patient are present, your choice is confirmed.

Impatient irritability marks the *Nux* patient's psychology. He is prone to argue and may start quarrels over any imagined offense. He feels hurried and driven to accomplish things. He can't stand to wait for others. He is likely to be critical and quick to reproach anyone who doesn't live up to his demanding standards. He can snap sharply when irritated. Or instead, he may try to keep his annoyance to himself, but his displeasure shows in his blunt, undiplomatic language and the frown on his face. He prefers to be left alone and hates having to depend on others less capable than he. He hates to be questioned. Often very competitive, he plays to win.

The *Nux* patient is fastidious and fussy over little things, and he may have a compulsion to arrange his environment according to his own precise sense of order. His nervous system is overly sensitive. Slight noises, such as the sound of people talking or even the sound of footsteps, drive him to distraction, and he can't stand bright lights or unpleasant odors.

Nux patients are particularly chilly and are made worse by cold weather, especially dry, cold weather (a symptom shared with *Hepar*). When they are feverish, they get severe chills and cannot warm themselves even when sitting by a heater. During the fever they cannot stand to uncover or undress, and any slight movement of the covers sets off a new wave of chills.

Sleep is difficult for the *Nux* patient. He may have trouble getting to sleep because of an overactive mind or because he notices every little noise. Or he may wake early in the morning and be unable to get back to sleep. He is especially irritable when awakened.

The digestive system is often a weak area for the *Nux* patient. Even if the main problem is respiratory illness or involves some other system, it is usually accompanied by some of the typical *Nux* digestive disorders. The digestive system is generally weak, and the *Nux* patient is intolerant of many foods. Indigestion, heartburn, nausea, fullness and bloating of the abdomen, gas, and constipation or diarrhea may beset the *Nux* patient in any combination.

A craving for stimulants, alcohol, and other drugs is common to *Nux* patients. Very often overindulgence in drugs brings on the symptoms. Because it so closely covers the common symptoms of an alcoholic hangover, including the typical headache and digestive distress, *Nux* is a more effective medicine for people with that condition. We recommend that if you take it under those circumstances, you do so only very occasionally.

Nux patients are known also to crave fats, spicy foods, and milk. They can be quite thirsty, though drinking may cause bloating of the abdomen.

Other characteristic *Nux* symptoms include a tendency toward twitchings or spasms of various muscles (including muscles of the eyelids, limbs, back, and abdominal wall); headaches; and lower back pain that is particularly aggravated by turning over in bed.

What Makes *Nux Vomica* Symptoms

Worse: anger, mental exertion, morning, cold, eating or overeating, spices, rich food, stimulants, narcotics, alcohol

Better: resting, evening

Phosphorus
Phosphorus

Phosphorus is a deep-acting medicine that is rarely used during the beginning of an illness. In acute care it is more commonly given for coughs and digestive problems. The physical symptoms typical of *Phosphorus* patients include a restless, overexcited state that leads to weakness and exhaustion, chilliness combined with a thirst for cold drinks, and burning pains.

Equally characteristic are the mental symptoms. People who need *Phosphorus* are cheerful, friendly, open, and impressionable. They are bright, and their perceptions are quick. Even during acute illnesses, *Phosphorus* patients are likely to be much more alert and interested in their surroundings than you might expect. They have active imaginations. They are expressive and animated. They are overdramatic when demonstrating their emotions. Their senses are acute; they are bothered by light and noise and are easily startled. They may be intuitive and even psychic. Nervousness and fear are quick to develop in their active, impressionable minds. They may fear the dark, thunder, imaginary things, illness, or death. Fearing the worst, they tend to exaggerate their symptoms. They dread that something bad might happen, and because they tend to believe in the power of intuition, they assume that what they fear will indeed come true.

Phosphorus patients are sociable and crave company. They are often fearful when they are alone. They seek sympathy and attention and feel better when they get it, but compared to *Pulsatilla* patients, they more often want to actively return affection. They can get frightened or upset easily, but reassuring words or distractions help them forget their troubles quickly.

On the other hand, they pick up on the fears of others around them. In general, they tend to have trouble maintaining a definite, individual identity. Their personality changes, sometimes dramatically, depending on who they're with. They often feel another's pain as though it were their own, and they are trusting to the point of being gullible. They tend to believe both sides of an argument because they sympathize with both parties.

Although they are enthusiastic, *Phosphorus* patients lack stamina and easily become tired both mentally and physically. At first, the patient may hardly seem ill, with energy and vitality unusual for a sick person. He may be overexcited and physically restless, and he may begin many projects. But excitement gives way to exhaustion, depression, or irritability, and the projects are left unfinished.

Phosphorus patients usually feel cold, and their symptoms are made worse by cold and better by heat, though sometimes the opposite is true. They are sensitive to sudden changes of weather. Open air may either aggravate or relieve the condition.

Phosphorus patients crave salt, spicy foods, and ice cream (which relieves stomach pain). They are generally thirsty for plenty of cold or iced drinks, though these may cause vomiting as soon as they become warm in the stomach.

Burning pains may occur anywhere in the body, but particularly in the head, stomach, abdomen, chest, and along the spine. There is a tendency to bleed easily, and small wounds may bleed bright-red blood freely. Nosebleeds are common and often accompany a cold or cough.

What Makes *Phosphorus* Symptoms

Worse: cold or heat (either or both), lying on left or painful side, thunderstorms

Better: massaging or rubbing, cold food and drinks

Pulsatilla
Windflower

Pulsatilla is one of the more commonly used medicines for people with acute illnesses of all kinds. Often it is selected primarily because of the patient's emotional nature: those who need *Pulsatilla* tend to have gentle, mild, yielding dispositions along with a desire for attention. Characteristic physical symptoms include lack of thirst, pains that wander from one part of the body to another, and constantly changing symptoms in general. The symptoms are aggravated by heat and improved with slow movement. *Pulsatilla* is commonly indicated for people with colds, coughs, digestive troubles, eye and ear infections, as well as many other conditions.

Vulnerability, weepy sensitivity, and a desire for affection and consolation characterize the *Pulsatilla* personality. The *Pulsatilla* child, for example, becomes clingy, whiny, teary, and fussy. Though she might be fussy and irritable, she is almost never given to full-blown temper tantrums (as inconsolable *Chamomilla* or *Hepar* children are). The *Pulsatilla* patient wants people around her and craves comforting attention. She seeks sympathy and feels better when she gets it. She may be fearful of being alone or in the dark.

Changeable emotions are typical of people who need *Pulsatilla.* They tend to be moody—happy and laughing one moment, sad and crying the next. They cry easily, even at the thought of pain, and when sick they may break into tears for no apparent reason. They are easily hurt emotionally; receiving slight criticism, being ignored, or hearing loved ones argue may deeply affect them.

In general, *Pulsatilla* patients are sweet and likable, and they like people to like them. They are sensitive to what others think about them, and they do what they can to please others. They tend to be generous, and they may tell you what you want to hear to get your approval.

The sweet and loving disposition of the *Pulsatilla* patient makes it easy for people to offer comfort and support. In turn, the *Pulsatilla* patient thrives on the attention. There is a tendency to be self-pitying, and the person who is sick may whine, "Why does this always have to happen to me?" or, "Why don't people understand me more?" Offer a little sympathy, however, and she quickly forgets these worries.

These people are often indecisive. They may ask for something, but once they get it, they want something else. They are easily led and easily swayed and don't tend to be stubborn.

The physical symptoms of *Pulsatilla* patients are as changeable as the psychological ones. Symptoms shift from one part of the body to another or change character frequently. The pains may appear suddenly and disappear gradually. Sometimes the stools have a different consistency or color with every bowel movement.

Physically, *Pulsatilla* patients are "warm-blooded"—that is, they don't need much clothing and even prefer cold weather. They are sensitive to heat and to warm rooms, and they become less energetic and develop physical symptoms when exposed to heat. They have difficulty sleeping if the room is warm. They thrive in cool, open air, as it relieves many of their symptoms. However, they may get sick from being chilled during warm weather, and they sometimes develop symptoms after eating ice cream.

Slow, gentle motion, especially in the open air, is beneficial to the *Pulsatilla* patient. Walking about slowly often relieves the headache, digestive symptoms, or aches and pains, and it makes the person feel better in general.

Even if they are feverish, *Pulsatilla* patients are rarely thirsty. In fact, during acute illnesses they are usually less thirsty than normal and must be reminded to drink enough liquids.

Puslatilla is known for body discharges that are thick in character and yellow to green in color. Mucus from a runny nose, phlegm brought up with a cough, and discharges from the eyes, ears, or vagina all have these characteristics. These secretions are produced in large quantity but do not irritate the skin.

The *Pulsatilla* patient often has digestive problems. Her abdomen becomes bloated and sensitive to touch, especially after she's eaten. Digestive symptoms may start shortly after eating rich or fatty foods, pork, ice cream, fruit, or cold things. She wants something to eat, but can't decide what she wants. She may crave foods she can't digest or that make her feel bad. Usually the patient is averse to fat, pork, meat, milk, or bread.

What Makes *Pulsatilla* Symptoms

Worse: warm or closed rooms, foods rich in fat, hot food or drinks, eating, evening, lying on painless side

Better: cool and open air, cold applications, cold food or drinks (though the patient is not thirsty), lying on painful side

Rhus Toxicodendron
Poison Ivy

Relief of symptoms by motion is the fundamental characteristic of *Rhus tox.* This applies as much to the various individual symptoms as to those of the person as a whole. In particular, painful joints and muscles hurt when at rest and when first moved, and then get much better as they grow limber during continued motion. In general, the *Rhus tox.* patient is restless and anxious and cannot be comfortable unless she is moving about. She restlessly tosses and turns in bed, and she feels mentally restless and anxious as well.

The restlessness and anxiety make sleep difficult for the *Rhus tox.* patient. Generally symptoms are worse in the evening, as well as during the night, when the patient also may feel more irritable and fearful. In addition, she may be very depressed and tend to weep easily.

Generally *Rhus tox.* patients are chilly and are aggravated by cold and damp weather. Symptoms worsen if even a single part of the body is uncovered or otherwise becomes cold.

Rhus tox. markedly affects fibrous tissues: joints, tendons, ligaments, and connective tissues. The characteristic pains, worse on first motion and better by continued motion, may be felt during acute illnesses, like the flu, or may be caused by an injury. In fact, even though the pains are better during motion, sustained or vigorous exertion can be difficult for *Rhus tox.* patients. Symptoms often begin after overexertion—for example, after lifting heavy boxes or working out too strenuously.

The pains in the muscles and joints are achy, sore, or needlelike in character. The joints are stiff and perhaps swollen as well as painful. The pain is usually made worse by cold of any form (cold air, cold baths, or cold applications) and by damp, cold weather. Warmth relieves the symptoms. Firm pressure also can make the painful parts feel better, and *Rhus tox.* backaches feel better when the person is lying on something hard.

As anyone who has had poison ivy knows, *Rhus tox.* strongly affects the skin. Eruptions are red and inflamed and itch terribly, especially after scratching, at night, and from the warmth of the bed. Usually there are inflamed blisters with a *Rhus tox.* eruption, ranging in size from tiny pinpoint vesicles on up. The blisters may be filled with clear fluid or with pus, and the eruptions usually ooze. These *Rhus tox.* symptoms often are experienced when people have chicken pox, herpes, and, of course, poison ivy or poison oak.

The *Rhus tox.* patient is usually thirsty, often for cold drinks or milk. Cold drinks, however, may aggravate the symptoms. A peculiar *Rhus tox.* symptom is the presence of a triangular red area at the tip of the tongue.

What Makes *Rhus Tox.* Symptoms

Worse: initial motion, prolonged rest, overexertion, cold, cold and damp weather, uncovering, getting wet, night

Better: continued motion, change of position, perspiration, warm applications, warm covering, pressure, rubbing

Sepia
Inky Juice of the Cuttlefish

A lack of vitality, even a sense of lifelessness, is characteristic of *Sepia.* The person feels sluggish and lacks energy. Yet, when she does muster her strength to exercise, she feels much better. Dancing, walking rapidly, or other vigorous exercise improves the person's general condition and many of her specific physical symptoms. The lack of vitality of the *Sepia* person is evident also in her intolerance of cold temperature.

The lifelessness typical of the *Sepia* physical condition may be apparent also in the psychological state. The person becomes withdrawn, emotionally cold, easily angered, and depressed. She may feel an emptiness inside, a sense of indifference or apathy. This may become so strong that she feels indifference or even aversion to her own spouse, children, or siblings. She becomes uninterested in affection and sex, and she may actively dislike lovemaking.

Sepia patients can be moody, feeling sad, gentle, and yielding at one moment, disagreeable, excitable, and stubborn at the next. They are easily offended and can be mean to those around them. They are often averse to company yet may dread being alone. Their defenses are brittle and they weep easily. They are aggravated by efforts to comfort them.

Sepia patients may be so averse to food that they cannot stand its smell, and the smell of food may cause intense nausea. They may have a gnawing hunger or a sensation of emptiness in the stomach or abdomen that food does not satisfy. On the other hand, sometimes nausea improves after they've eaten, and they may feel generally better after a meal. *Sepia* patients are often constipated. They tend to crave sour, bitter, pungent, and spicy foods; they may strongly dislike bread, fats, milk, meat, or salt. Eating bread, fats, fruit, milk, pork, or sour foods may make them feel worse.

Sepia patients sometimes experience a sensation of a ball inside the body. They may have this feeling in the throat, abdomen, rectum, or uterus. *Sepia* women may experience a feeling of pressure and bearing down, as if things were protruding from the vagina. When this happens, they have a strong need to keep the legs crossed.

What Makes *Sepia* Symptoms

Worse: cold, 4 to 6 P.M., morning, menstruation, smelling food, beginning to move, milk, pork, fats, bread, fruit, sour foods, thunderstorms

Better: dancing, walking rapidly, vigorous exercise, hard pressure, eating

Silica
Flint

"Weakly" might be the best one-word description of people who need *Silica*. During an acute illness, a lack of mental and physical stamina prevails, whether the person is normally vigorous or feeble. When he is ill, the *Silica* patient's physiological defenses lack vigor. His symptoms develop slowly and without violence, though eventually he may become very sick.

Often *Silica* patients are intelligent and perceptive, but their minds tire easily and become dull, sluggish, and confused. Though they may have trouble thinking and concentrating, they have a tendency to become preoccupied with insignificant details. They doubt their abilities, though if they push themselves, they usually meet a challenge successfully. The *Silica* patient is timid, fainthearted, and yielding. He is not likely to assert his own opinions and generally won't push himself on others. He is happy to be seen and not heard.

Despite this passivity, however, he can be stubborn and irritable. He resents interference and withdraws into himself if asked to do something he doesn't want to. He is irritated by attempts to console him. Although nervous and perhaps fidgety, the person who needs *Silica* is not really anxious and is rarely troubled by intense fears.

Silica patients lack physical stamina. They are easily tired and easily chilled. Their hands and feet get cold and can't be warmed. Open air and drafts aggravate this, and like *Hepar* and *Rhus* patients, they may develop symptoms if a single part of the body is uncovered or gets cold. Inflamed parts, however, are not so sensitive to cold as those of *Hepar* patients.

This lack of vitality also is evident in other symptoms. Little wounds tend to become infected, and skin infections are slow to heal, leaving reddened cysts rather than clearing completely. Constipation is common. The body lacks the strength to completely expel the stool, and the stool recedes into the rectum.

Some specific symptoms include frequently swollen lymph nodes; profuse, offensive perspiration, especially on the feet, hands, head, and lower back; in *Silica* children, sour-smelling perspiration on the back of the head and the neck, and vomiting after drinking milk, even breast milk; and sometimes a sensation as though a splinter or stick were caught in the throat or other inflamed areas. Again, the similarity to *Hepar* is evident, but *Silica* infections, though painful, are not tender to touch as are those of *Hepar.*

Silica patients may dislike meat, milk, and warm foods. Children may refuse even mother's milk. Thirst may be increased, especially at night, though cold food or drinks may make symptoms worse.

What Makes *Silica* Symptoms

Worse: cold, open air, winter, damp weather, uncovering, coldness or uncovering of a single part of the body, getting the feet wet, cold food or drinks, lying on the painful side, suppressed perspiration, eating

Better: warmth

*Sulphur**
Sulfur

Sulphur is one of the more commonly prescribed homeopathic medicines for chronically ill people. It is prescribed for acute illness only occasionally, but it should be considered during fevers, skin conditions, and a variety of other conditions whenever the overall *Sulphur* picture is present.

Usually *Sulphur* patients are invigorated by cold weather and by being in the open air. They feel worse when it is warm, in warm rooms, and in warm beds. Along with this internal heat, burning pains and discharges that cause burning discomfort often are experienced. The eyes, ears, nose, throat, stomach, anus, or the top of the head may burn. More characteristically, the soles of the feet burn. The *Sulphur* patient may need to stick the feet or hands out of the covers. The lips and other mucous membranes are red and dry. The skin in general, and particularly the face, is reddened.

Discharges, whether from the nose, skin, eyes, ears, or elsewhere, are likely to have an offensive odor. The breath, stool, and sweat also smell bad. The patient is often unaware of his odor, though at the same time he may be overly sensitive to other odors around him. Some *Sulphur* patients find their own odor extremely offensive, even after they bathe. Often the patient doesn't like to wash, and bathing may aggravate some of his symptoms, especially those on the skin.

Suphur patients are often robust and emotionally thick-skinned; they are less emotionally sensitive than patients who need medicines such as *Pulsatilla* or *Nux vomica*. When they are acutely ill, they may be impatient, hurried, and quick-tempered, yet they tend to be lazy and averse to business or any systematic work. They become sloppy and disorganized and allow home and work environments to become messy. The disorder doesn't bother them, however, since they claim to know where every-

---

* Sulphur should not be given immediately after *Calcarea*.

thing is when they need it. People who need *Sulphur* are "pack rats," keeping old possessions because of the special meaning each has. The *Sulphur* patient's appearance also is messy. His clothes are disheveled and dirty, and his hair is unkempt.

While he ignores his external environment, the *Sulphur* patient may become obsessed with abstract concepts, religious or philosophical issues, or other subjects that do not have definitive answers. He may become preoccupied with obscure facts and details or with grand pipe dreams, though often he is unproductive.

Sulphur children are self-centered and demanding. They may hoard toys they aren't using, or concern themselves only with how things affect them, while ignoring the needs of others. They are inquisitive, especially asking questions that cannot be answered.

Sulphur is known for a number of digestive symptoms. One distinctive symptom is an empty sensation in the stomach that may or may not be associated with hunger. Often around 11 A.M., the patient has a ravenous appetite that comes on suddenly and cannot be satisfied. He often suffers indigestion after eating. Early in the morning he may be driven out of bed by a powerful, sudden urge to have a bowel movement. He tends to like strong-tasting foods and may crave spicy foods, sweets, fatty foods, and alcohol, but also may be averse to milk, meat, sweets, and fats. Bread, cold food or drinks, fats, sweets, milk, or even the sight of food may aggravate symptoms.

Usually the *Sulphur* patient is quite thirsty. He may prefer warm drinks, which may indeed make his symptoms better.

The *Sulphur* patient may be unable to get to sleep before midnight, or he may be troubled by waking up too early (3 A.M. or somewhat later is common). He is likely to feel unusually lethargic after he has overslept.

Sulphur is commonly prescribed for a wide variety of skin conditions, and rashes or other skin eruptions may accompany any condition for which the medicine is indicated. Itching is usually intense and is worse at night in warmth, and in warm beds. Scratching may relieve this temporarily but often results in increased itching and burning.

Typically, people who need *Sulphur* experience more complaints on the left than right side of the body.

What Makes *Sulphur* Symptoms

Worse: warmth, warm rooms, warmth of the bed, cold air, left side, 11 A.M., standing, washing, scratching, long sleep, changeable weather

Better: open air, warm drinks

PART 4

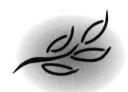

HOMEOPATHIC

RESOURCES

HOMEOPATHIC ORGANIZATIONS

National Center for Homeopathy
801 N. Fairfax #306
Alexandria, VA 22314 (703) 548-7790

This is the most important American homeopathic organization. It publishes a monthly magazine, maintains an active network of homeopathic study groups, holds annual conferences and short summer training programs for laypeople and health professionals, and provides spokespersons to the media.

International Foundation for Homeopathy
P.O. Box 7
Edmonds, WA 98020 (206) 776-4147

This organization specializes in training homeopaths. It also publishes a bi-monthly magazine and organizes an annual conference for serious students and practitioners of homeopathy.

American Institute for Homeopathy
925 E. 17th Avenue
Denver, CO 80218

Founded in 1844 and the oldest national medical society in the country, this organization admits only medical doctors and osteopaths as voting members. It publishes a journal and sponsors or cosponsors an annual conference. It also interfaces with government bodies on issues relating to the homeopathic profession.

Foundation for Homeopathic Education and Research
2124 Kittredge Street
Berkeley, CA 94704 (510) 649-8930

This organization seeks to educate the medical community and the general public about research in homeopathy. It provides speakers on homeopathic research to hospitals, medical schools, industry, and community groups.

Homeopathic Academy of Naturopathic Physicians
P.O. Box 12488
Portland, OR 97212 (503) 795-0579

This is the organization of naturopathic physicians who specialize in homeopathy. It certifies qualified naturopaths and publishes a professional journal.

S O U R C E S   O F
H O M E O P A T H I C   M E D I C I N E S

The following companies either manufacture homeopathic medicines or provide a mail-order service for them. Homeopathic medicines are commonly available also at health-food stores and pharmacies, though the following companies provide a more extensive assortment of homeopathic remedies, as well as homeopathic home medicine kits.

Biological Homeopathic Industries
11600 Cochiti SE
Albuquerque, NM 87123
(505) 293-3843

Boiron-Bornemann, Inc.
6 Campus Blvd., Building A
Newtown Square, PA 19073
(610) 325-7464
or:
98c W. Cochran
Simi Valley, CA 93065
(805) 582-9091

Boericke and Tafel
2381 Circadian Way
Santa Rosa, CA 95407
(707) 571-8202

Dolisos
3014 Rigel Road
Las Vegas, NV 89102
(702) 871-7153

Medicine from Nature
10 Mountain Springs Parkway
Springville, UT 84663
(801) 489-1500

Hahnemann Pharmacy
828 San Pablo
Albany, CA 94706 (510) 527-3003

Natra-Bio
1441 W. Smith Road
Bellingham, WA 98226
(206) 384-5656

Homeopathic Educational Services
2124 Kittredge Street
Berkeley, CA 94704 (510) 649-0294

Standard Homeopathic Company
204-210 W. 131st Street
Los Angeles, CA 90061
(310) 321-4284

Luyties Pharmacal
4200 Laclede Avenue
St. Louis, MO 63108
(314) 533-9600

RECOMMENDED BOOKS ON HOMEOPATHY

INTRODUCTORY AND FAMILY GUIDEBOOKS

*Buegel, Dale, Blair Lewis, and Dennis Chernin. *Homeopathic Remedies for Health Professionals and Laypeople.* Honesdale, PA: Himalayan, 1991.

Bruning, Nancy, and Corey Weinstein. *Healing Homeopathic Remedies.* New York: Dell, 1995.

Castro, Miranda. *The Complete Homeopathy Handbook.* New York: St. Martin's, 1990.

Cook, Trevor. *Homeopathic Medicine Today.* New Canaan, CT: Keats, 1989.

Gaier, Harald. *Encyclopedic Dictionary of Homeopathy.* London: Thorsons, 1991.

*Grossinger, Richard. *Homeopathy: An Introduction for Beginners and Skeptics.* Berkeley: North Atlantic, 1993.

*Kruzel, Thomas. *Homeopathic Emergency Guide.* Berkeley: North Atlantic, 1992.

---

* Particularly good books

*Jonas, Wayne, and Jennifer Jacobs. *Healing with Homeopathy.* New York: Warner, 1996.

Lockie, Andrew. *The Family Guide to Homeopathy.* New York: Fireside, 1993.

Lockie, Andrew, and Nicola Geddes. *The Complete Guide to Homeopathy.* New York: Dorling Kindersley, 1995.

Panos, Maesimund, and Jane Heimlich. *Homeopathic Medicine at Home.* New York: Tarcher, 1980.

Rose, Barry. *The Family Guide to Homeopathy.* Berkeley: Ten Speed Press, 1993.

*Ullman, Dana. *Discovering Homeopathy.* Berkeley: North Atlantic, 1991.

*Ullman, Dana. *The Consumer's Guide to Homeopathy.* New York: Jeremy P. Tarcher/Putnam, 1996.

*Ullman, Robert, and Judyth Reichenberg-Ullman. *Patient's Guide to Homeopathic Medicine.* Edmonds, WA: Picnic Point, 1995.

Vithoulkas, George. *Homeopathy: Medicine for the New Man.* New York: Arco, 1979.

*Whitmont, Edward C. *The Alchemy of Healing.* Berkeley: North Atlantic, 1993.

SPECIALIZED SELF-CARE BOOKS

Castro, Miranda. *Homeopathy for Pregnancy, Birth and Your Baby's First Year.* New York: St. Martin's, 1993.

Chappel, Peter. *Emotional Healing with Homeopathy.* Rockport, MA: Element, 1994.

Curtis, Susan, and Romy Fraser. *Natural Healing for Women.* London: Pandora, 1991.

*Hershoff, Asa. *Homeopathic Medicines for Musculoskeletal Healing.* Berkeley: North Atlantic, 1997.

Lessell, Colin. *The World Traveller's Manual of Homeopathy.* Walden, England: C. W. Daniel, 1993.

*Lockie, Andrew, and Nicola Geddes. *The Women's Guide to Homeopathy.* New York: St. Martin's, 1994.

*Moskowitz, Richard. *Homeopathic Medicine for Pregnancy and Childbirth.* Berkeley: North Atlantic, 1992.

*Schmidt, Michael A. *Healing Childhood Ear Infections: Prevention, Home Care, and Alternative Treatments.* Berkeley: North Atlantic, 1996.

Souter, Keith. *Homeopathy for the Third Age.* Walden, England: C. W. Daniel, 1993.

*Subotnick, Steven. *Sports and Exercise Injuries: Conventional, Homeopathic, and Alternative Treatments.* Berkeley: North Atlantic, 1991.

*Ullman, Dana. *Homeopathic Medicine for Children and Infants.* New York: Jeremy P. Tarcher/Putnam, 1992.

*Ullman, Robert, and Judyth Reichenberg-Ullman. *Ritalin-free Kids: Homeopathic Treatment of A.D.D. and other Behavioral and Learning Problems.* Rocklin, CA: Prima, 1996.

*Zand, Janet, Rachel Walton, and Bob Rountree. *Smart Medicine for a Healthier Child.* New York: Avery, 1994.

PHILOSOPHY AND METHODOLOGY

Note: Books on philosophy and methodology are primarily for students or practitioners of homeopathy, though anyone with a serious interest in the healing process can learn much from them.

*Hahnemann, Samuel. *Organon of Medicine.* New Delhi. Reprint. A newly translated edition which is considered more accurate is: *The Organon of the Medical Art.* Seattle: Birdcage, 1996.

*Kent, James Tyler. *Lectures on Homeopathic Philosophy.* Berkeley: North Atlantic, 1979. Reprint.

Koehler, Gerhard. *The Handbook of Homeopathy.* Rochester, VT: Healing Arts, 1987.

Roberts, H. A. *The Principles and Art of Cure by Homeopathy.* New Delhi: B. Jain. Reprint.

*Sankaran, Rajan. *The Spirit of Homoeopathy.* Bombay: Homeopathic Medical Publishers, 1991.

*Vithoulkas, George. *The Science of Homeopathy.* New York: Grove, 1980.

*Wright, Elizabeth Hubbard. *A Brief Study Course in Homeopathy.* St. Louis: Formur, 1977.

MATERIA MEDICA AND REPERTORIES

Note: A *materia medica* is a book that lists homeopathic medicines and the various symptoms and syndromes they are known to cure. A *repertory* is a listing of symptoms and the various medicines that have been found to cause them in overdose and cure them in homeopathic doses. It is common for people to have several *materia medica* and at least one repertory.

Most of these books are useful primarily for professional home-opaths, though many people will be able to understand and use them. By adding a *materia medica* and a repertory to your library, you can be more precise in the selection of an individualized remedy.

*Bailey, Philip. *Homeopathic Psychology: Personality Profiles of the Major Constitutional Remedies.* Berkeley: North Atlantic, 1995.
*Boericke, William. *Pocket Manual of* Materia Medica *with Repertory.* Santa Rosa: Boericke and Tafel. Reprint.
Clarke, John. *Dictionary of Practical* Materia Medica (3 volumes). Walden, England: C. W. Daniel. Reprint.
*Gibson, D. M. *Studies of Homeopathic Remedies.* Beaconsfield, England: Beaconsfield Publishers, 1987.
Hering, Constantine. *Guiding Symptoms of Our* Materia Medica (10 volumes). New Delhi: B. Jain. Reprint.
*Herscu, Paul. *The Homeopathic Treatment of Children: Pediatric Constitutional Types.* Berkeley: North Atlantic, 1991.
*Kent, James Tyler. *Lectures on Homeopathic* Materia Medica. New Delhi: B. Jain. Reprint.
*———. *Repertory of Homeopathic* Materia Medica. New Delhi: B. Jain. Reprint.
*Morrison, Roger. *Desktop Guide to Keynotes and Confirmatory Symptoms.* Berkeley: Hahnemann Publishing, 1993.
*Murphy, Robin. *Homeopathic Medical Repertory.* Pagosa Springs, CO: HANA, 1993.
*———. *Lotus* Materia Medica. Pagosa Springs, CO: HANA, 1995.
Sankaran, Rajan. *The Substance of Homoeopathy.* Bombay: Homoeopathic Medical Publishers, 1994.
*Schroyens, F. *Synthesis Repertorium.* London: Homoeopathic Book Publishers, 1993.
Tyler, Margaret. *Drug Pictures.* Walden, England: C. W. Daniel, 1952.
*Van Zandvoort, Roger. *The Complete Repertory.* Leidschendam, The Netherlands: IRHIS, 1994.
*Vermeulen, Frans. *Concordant* Materia Medica. Haarlem, The Netherlands: Merlijn Publishers, 1994.
*———. *Synoptic* Materia Medica (2 volumes). Haarlem, The Netherlands: Merlijn Publishers, 1994, 1996.
*Whitmont, Edward C. *Psyche and Substance: Essays on Homeopathy in the Light of Jungian Psychology.* Berkeley: North Atlantic, 1991.
*Zaren, Ananda. *Core Elements of the* Materia Medica *of the Mind* (2 volumes). Gottingen, Germany: Burgdorf, 1993, 1994.

SCIENCE AND RESEARCH

*Bellavite, Paolo, and Andrea Signorini. *Homeopathy: A Frontier in Medical Science.* Berkeley: North Atlantic, 1995.

Coulter, Harris L. *Homeopathic Science and Modern Medicine: The Physics of Healing with Microdoses.* Berkeley: North Atlantic, 1980.

Endler, P. C., and J. Schulte (eds.). *Ultra High Dilution: Physiology and Physics.* Boston: Kluwer Academic, 1994.

HISTORY OF HOMEOPATHY

Cook, Trevor. *Samuel Hahnemann: The Founder of Homeopathic Medicine.* Wellingborough, England: Thorsons, 1981.

*Coulter, Harris L. *Divided Legacy: A History of the Schism in Medical Thought* (4 volumes). Berkeley: North Atlantic, 1975, 1977, 1981, 1994.

*Handley, Rima. *A Homeopathic Love Story.* Berkeley: North Atlantic, 1990.

————. *In Search of the Later Hahnemann.* Beaconsfield, England: Beaconsfield Publishers, 1996.

Wood, Matthew. *The Magical Staff: The Vitalist Tradition in Western Medicine.* Berkeley: North Atlantic, 1992.

SOURCE OF HOMEOPATHIC BOOKS, TAPES, AND SOFTWARE

Most of the sources of homeopathic medicines (listed previously) are also sources of books on homeopathy, though they do not have an extensive selection.

Homeopathic Educational Services
2124 Kittredge Street
Berkeley, CA 94704 (510) 649-0294
Email: mail@homeopathic.com

INTERNET RESOURCES

http://www.homeopathic.com.
This is the Website for Homepathic Educational Services, one of America's leading homeopathic resource centers. There are more than 100 ar-

ticles on homeopathic medicine of interest to the general public and health professionals, plus a catalog of homeopathic books, tapes, medicines, and software that can be ordered.

http://www.dungeon.com/~cam/homeo.html
This Website provides a listing of various homeopathic resources and Websites throughout the world. You can subscribe, without cost, to a homeopathic discussion group, or you can access various topics by searching their table of contents.

http://antenna.n1/homeoweb/
This Website provides listings of homeopathic Internet sites and Internet addresses of key homeopathic organizations and individuals.

http://www.wolfe.net.com/~enos/ho_web/index.html
This Website is an on-line homeopathic magazine with articles, reviews, and accounts of personal experiences with homeopathy.

http://www.monmouth.com/~altvetmed/
People interested in information on homeopathic and alternative veterinarian care will be interested in this Website.

http://www.healthy.com
HealthWorld is a large site providing access to a broad range of alternative-medicine information, organizations, services, and products.

GLOSSARY

ALLOPATHY: The homeopathic term for conventional medicine. *Allos* is the Greek term for "other than" or "different from," and *pathy* means "disease" or "suffering." Allopathic medicine refers to the practice of prescribing pharmaceuticals that are chosen simply because they diminish symptoms, often because they are antagonistic to the disease process.

ANTIDOTE: A substance or experience that slows, stops, or reverses the curative action of a homeopathic medicine.

CASETAKING: The interview process used in homeopathy to determine the correct homeopathic medicine.

COMMON SYMPTOMS: Those symptoms that people typically experience with a specific disease (e.g., jaundice and lack of appetite during hepatitis). These symptoms are less important in determining the correct homeopathic medicine for the individual.

CONSTITUTION: The overall health of the person as determined by his/her heredity, life history, lifestyle, environment, and past treatments.

CONSTITUTIONAL TREATMENT: Treatment that is determined by a careful assessment of a person's constitution and present total symptomatology in an effort to stimulate the person's inner healing most deeply.

CURE: A profound overall improvement in health in which the individual achieves a sense of physical, emotional, and mental freedom.

DRUG PICTURE: The essential characteristics of a homeopathic medicine's action compiled from collected provings, accounts of poisonings, and clinical experience. Also referred to as "essence of a medicine" or a "medicine's essence."

GENERAL SYMPTOMS: Those symptoms which pertain to the person as a whole, including all psychological symptoms and those physical symptoms in which the whole body is affected (e.g., energy level, restlessness, sensitivity to cold, tiredness in the morning). Because these symptoms are representations of the body's overall response, they are considered deeper symptoms and thus are particularly important when choosing the correct homeopathic medicine.

GLOBULES: Pellet-sized sugar pills on which the potentized solution is dropped (larger than granules).

GRANULES: Small grains of sand-sized sugar pills on which the potentized solution is dropped (smaller than globules).

HEALING CRISIS: A common experience of those who use homeopathic medicines to treat chronic conditions and some acute illnesses in which some more-external symptoms initially get worse in the process of cure. (Sometimes referred to by homeopaths as "aggravation" of symptoms.)

HERING'S LAWS OF CURE: First described by Constantine Hering (1800–1880), these principles define the changes in symptoms that should be observed during a genuine curative response to treatment. The three components are (1) healing proceeds from the deeper parts within the organism necessary for survival and growth extending outward to the more superficial parts; (2) healing proceeds from the top of the person to the bottom; and (3) healing proceeds in reverse order of the symptoms' appearance in the person.

LAW OF SIMILARS: The fundamental tenet of homeopathy that states that a substance which causes a set of symptoms in a healthy person acts as a curative medicine when given to sick people who have its similar symptoms.

MATERIA MEDICA: Taken from Latin, meaning "materials of medicines." Homeopathic *materia medica*s are books that list the medicines used and the detailed indications for their application.

MODALITY: A circumstance that makes a person's overall health or a specific symptom better or worse (e.g., in weakness worse in the morning or headache better by cold applications, "worse in the morning" and "better by cold applications" are the modalities).

NOSODE: A homeopathic medicine made of material taken from diseased material, such as bacteria, viruses, and pus.

PALLIATION OF SYMPTOMS: The temporary relief of symptoms without actually curing the disease from which they originated.

PARTICULAR SYMPTOMS: Those symptoms which are local to a specific area of the body (e.g., a throbbing pain in the head, a burning pain in the stomach, an itching on the scalp).

POLYCHREST: A homeopathic medicine that has many uses.

POTENCY: The term used in homeopathy to describe the number of times a substance has been diluted and succussed (shaken) according to the strict rules of the *Homeopathic Pharmacopeia*. When an "x" is written after a number (as in 6x, 30x), it refers to the number of times one part of a medicine was diluted with nine parts of the dilutant (usually distilled water). When a "c" is written after a number (as in 6c, 30c), this refers to the number of times one part of a medicine was diluted with 99 parts of dilutant. When "lm" is written after a number (as in 6lm, 30lm), this refers to the number of times one part of a medicine was diluted with 50,000 parts of dilutant.

POTENTIZATION: The pharmaceutical process of repeated dilution with succussion (vigorous shaking) by which the homeopathic medicines are prepared.

PROVING: The procedure for giving doses of a substance to healthy subjects in order to find what it causes in overdose and thus what it has the capacity to cure when given to ill people in potentized dose.

REPERTORY: A valuable homeopathic text that is an index of symptoms and a listing of those medicines which have been found to cause and/or cure specific symptoms.

REPERTORIZATION: The process of determining the correct medicine for the person by noting his/her characteristic symptoms, by finding in a repertory which substances cause these symptoms, by determining which substances cause the greatest number of symptoms, and then by selecting the one substance that most accurately fits the whole person.

RUBRIC: A symptom that is listed in a repertory.

SIMILIA: A Greek word meaning "similar"; used in reference to the law of similars.

SIMILLIMUM: The medicine most similar to the person's totality of symptoms.

STRANGE, RARE, AND PECULIAR SYMPTOMS: These are symptoms that are unusual in people or are contradictory to what most people experience with a similar illness.

SUCCUSSION: An integral part of the homeopathic pharmaceutical process in which a medicinal substance is diluted in distilled water and vigorously shaken by striking it against a firm surface.

SUPPRESSION OF SYMPTOMS: To treat symptoms in such a way that they disappear but other more serious symptoms manifest.

SYMPTOMS: Observable or felt changes in the physical, emotional, or mental condition of a person that limit optimal health. Homeopaths believe that symptoms represent efforts of the organism to deal with an internal or external stress.

VIS MEDICATRIX NATURAE: The inherent healing power of the organism which automatically works in a self-regulating, self-organizing capacity to reestablish health, often creating various symptoms as its way of externalizing the stress to inner processes.

BIBLIOGRAPHY

Bach, Edward, and F. J. Wheeler. *The Bach Flower Remedies*. New Canaan, CT: Keats, 1977.

Bailar, J. "The Practice of Meta-Analysis." *Clinical Epidemiology* 48(1995): 149–57.

Barnard, G. P., and James Stephenson. "Fresh Evidence for a Biophysical Field." *Journal of the American Institute of Homeopathy* 62 (April 1969) 73–85. In *Monograph on Homeopathic Research,* edited by Dana Ullman. Berkeley: Homeopathic Educational Services, 1980.

———. "Microdose Paradox: A New Biophysical Concept." *Journal of the American Institute of Homeopathy* 60 (September 1967). In *Monograph on Homeopathic Research,* edited by Dana Ullman. Berkeley: Homeopathic Educational Services, 1980.

Barness, Lewis A. *Manual of Pediatric Physical Diagnosis* 5th edition. Chicago: Year Book Medical Publishers, 1981.

Bellavite, Paolo, and Andrea Signorini. *Homeopathy: A Frontier in Medical Science*. Berkeley: North Atlantic, 1995.

Bierman, June, and Barbara Toohey. *The Woman's Holistic Headache Relief Book*. Los Angeles: Jeremy P. Tarcher, 1979.

Boericke, William, and W. A. Dewey. *Twelve Tissues Salts*. New Delhi: Indian Books and Periodicals, 1914. Reprint.

Bouchayer, F. "Alternative Medicines: A General Approach to the French Situation." *Complementary Medical Research* 4(2): 4–8.

Boyd, Linn. *A Study of the Simile in Medicine.* Philadelphia: Boericke and Tafel, 1936.

Bradford, Thomas Lindsay. *The Logic of Figures or Comparative Results of Homeopathic and Other Treatments.* Philadelphia: Boericke and Tafel, 1900.

Cantekin, E. I., T. W. McGuire, and T. L. Griffith. "Antimicrobial Therapy for Otitis Media with Effusion (Secretory Otitis Media)." *Journal of the American Medical Association* 266(23): 3309–17.

Carroll, David. *The Complete Book of Natural Medicines.* New York: Summitt, 1980.

Cattell, J. McKean (ed.), *Science* 72 (1930): 256.

Cave, Ray (ed.). "Those Overworked Medical Drugs." *Time* (17 August, 1981).

Coulter, Harris L. *Divided Legacy: A History of the Schism in Medical Thought.* Vol. 1., *The Patterns Emerge: Hippocrates to Paracelsus (350 B.C.–1600 A.D.).* Vol. 2, *Progress and Regress: J. B. Helmont to Claude Bernard (1600–1850).* Washington, DC: Wehawken, 1975, 1977. Vol. 3, *The Conflict Between Homeopathy and the American Medical Association: Science and Ethics in American Medicine (1800–1914).* Berkeley: North Atlantic, 1981. Vol. 4, *The Bacteriological Era.* Washington, DC: Center for Empirical Medicine, 1994.

————. *Homeopathic Science and Modern Medicine: The Physics of Healing with Microdoses.* Berkeley: North Atlantic, 1981.

Diamont, M., et al. "Abuse and Time of Use of Antibiotics in Acute Otitis Media." *Archives in Otolaryngology* 100 (1974): 226–32.

Dubos, René. Introduction to *Anatomy of an Illness,* by Norman Cousins. New York: W. W. Norton, 1979.

Endler, P. C., and J. Schulte (eds.). *Ultra High Dilution: Physiology and Physics.* Boston: Kluwer Academic, 1994.

Feinbloom, Richard L., and Boston Children's Medical Center. *Child Health Encyclopedia.* New York: Delacorte, 1975.

Ferguson, Tom (ed.). *Medical Self-Care: Access to Health Tools.* New York: Summit, 1980.

Ferley, J. P., D. Zmirou, D. D'Admehar, et al. "A Controlled Evaluation of a Homeopathic Preparation in the Treatment of Influenza-like Syndrome." *British Journal of Clinical Pharmacology* 27 (March 1989): 329–35.

Fishman, Mark C., Andrew R. Hoffman, Richard D. Klausner, Stanley G. Rockson, and Malcolm S. Thaler. *Medicine.* Philadelphia: J. B. Lippincott, 1981.

Florey, Sir Howard W. *British Medical Journal* (1943):654.

Froom, J., et al. "Diagnosis and Antibiotic Treatment of Acute Otitis Media: Report from the International Primary Care Network." *British Medical Journal* 300 (1990): 582–86.

Galpin, Jeffrey E. (ed.). "Does Zinc Have an Effect on the Common Cold?" *Infectious Disease Alert* 3, no. 12 (1984).

Gibson, R. G., Shiela L. M. Gibson, A. D. MacNeill, and W. Watson. "Homeopathic Therapy in Rheumatoid Arthritis: Evaluation by Double-Blind Clinical Therapeutic Trial." *British Journal of Clinical Pharmacology* (May 1980): 453–59.

Graedon, Joe. *The People's Pharmacy-2*. New York: Avon, 1980.

Grossinger, Richard. *Homeopathy: An Introduction for Beginners and Skeptics.* Berkeley: North Atlantic, 1993.

Hahnemann, Samuel. *Lesser Writings.* New York: Radde, 1852.

Hastings, Arthur, James Fadiman, and James Gordon (eds.). *Health for the Whole Person.* Boulder, CO: Westview, 1980.

Hockelman, R. A., et al. (eds.). *Principles of Pediatrics.* New York: McGraw-Hill, 1978.

Hudak, Carolyn M., Paul M. Redstone, Nancy L. Hokanson, and Irene E. Suzuki. *Clinical Protocols.* Philadelphia: J. B. Lippincott, 1976.

Jacobs, Jennifer, Margarita Jimenez, Stephen Gloyd, et al. "Treatment of Acute Childhood Diarrhea with Homeopathic Medicine: A Randomized Clinical Trial in Nicaragua." *Pediatrics* 93 (May 1994): 719–25.

Jaffe, Dennis. *Healing from Within.* New York: Bantam, 1982.

Kleijnen, J., P. Knipschild, and G. ter Riet. "Clinical Trials of Homeopathy." *British Medical Journal* 302 (1991): 316–23.

Kluger, Matthew J. "Fever." *Pediatrics* 66 (November 1980): 720–24.

———. "Fever and Survival." *Science* 188 (April 1975): 166–68.

Kluger, Matthew J., and Barbara A. Rothenburg. "Fever and Reduced Iron: Their Interaction As a Host Defense Response to Bacterial Infection." *Science* 203 (26 January, 1979): 374–76.

———. "Fever, Trace Metals, and Disease." In *Fever,* edited by J. M. Lipton. New York: Raven, 1980.

Krupp, Marcus A., and Milton J. Chatton. *Current Medical Diagnosis and Treatment.* Los Altos, CA: Lange, 1982.

Lappé, Marc. *When Antibiotics Fail.* Berkeley: North Atlantic, 1986.

Levin, Alan Scott, and Merla Zellerbach. *The Type 1/Type 2 Allergy Relief Program.* Los Angeles: Jeremy P. Tarcher, 1983.

Linde, K., W. B. Jonas, D. Melchart, et al. "Critical Review and Meta-Analysis of Serial Agitated Dilutions in Experimental Toxicology." *Human and Experimental Toxicology* 13 (1994): 481–92.

McHugh, Paul. "Rattler!" *San Francisco Magazine* (May 1982): 58–63.

Nesse, Randolph M., and George C. Williams. *Why We Get Sick.* New York: Times, 1994.

Norton, Ruth (ed.). "Challenge of a Painful Pox." *Acute Care Medicine* 1, 3 (1984): 12–28.

Office of Technology Assessment. *Assessing the Efficacy and Safety of Medical Technologies.* Washington, DC: Government Printing Office, 1978.

Pantell, Robert H., James F. Fries, and Donald M. Vickery. *Taking Care of Your Child* 2nd edition. Reading, MA: Addison-Wesley, 1984.

Paradise, J. L. "Otitis Media in Infants and Children." *Pediatrics* 65, no. 5 (1980): 917.

Paterson, John. "Report on Mustard Gas Experiments." *British Homoeopathic Journal* 33, no. 1 (1943).

Pelletier, Kenneth R. *Holistic Medicine: From Stress to Optimum Health.* New York: Delacorte/Lawrence, 1979.

———. *Mind As Healer, Mind As Slayer.* New York: Delacorte/Lawrence, 1977.

Reilly, David, Morag Taylor, Neil Bettie, et al. "Is Evidence for Homeopathy Reproducible?" *Lancet* 344 (10 December, 1994): 1601–06.

Ritz, Sandra. "Bladder Infections." *Medical Self-Care* (Spring 1981): 9–14.

Sehnert, Keith. *How to Be Your Own Doctor (Sometimes).* New York: Grosset & Dunlap, 1975.

Selye, Hans. *The Stress of Life* revised edition. New York: McGraw-Hill, 1978.

Smith, Lendon. *The Encyclopedia of Baby and Child Care.* New York: Warner, 1980.

Starling, Ernest, and Sir Charles Lovatt Evans. *Principles of Human Physiology* 14th edition. London: J & A Churchill, 1968.

Ullman, Dana. *The Consumer's Guide to Homeopathy.* New York: Jeremy P. Tarcher/Putnam, 1996.

Ullman, Dana (ed). *Monograph on Homeopathic Research.* Berkeley: Homeopathic Educational Services, 1980.

Van Buchen, F. L., et al. "Therapy of Acute Otitis Media: Myringotomy, Antibiotics, or Neither?" *Lancet* 2, no. 8252 (1981): 883–87.

van Wijk, Roeland, and Frederik A. C. Wiegant. *Cultured Mammalian Cells in Homeopathy Research: The Similia Principle in Self-Recovery.* Utrecht, The Netherlands: University of Utrecht, 1994.

Vickery, Donald M., and James F. Fries. *Take Care of Yourself: A Consumer's Guide to Medical Care.* Reading, MA: Addison-Wesley, 1976.

Vithoulkas, George. *The Science of Homeopathy.* New York: Grove, 1980.

Wharton, Richard, and George Lewith. "Complementary Medicine and the General Practitioner." *British Medical Journal* 292 (7 June, 1986): 1498–1500.

Whitmont, Edward C. *Psyche and Substance: Essays on Homeopathy in the Light of Jungian Psychology.* Berkeley: North Atlantic, 1980.

INDEX

ABOUT THE AUTHORS

Dana Ullman, M.P.H., is the president of the Foundation for Homeopathic Education and Research; an elected Board member of the National Center for Homeopathy; and directs Homeopathic Educational Services, America's largest publisher and distributor of homeopathic books, tapes, and medicine kits. He serves as a member of the Advisory Council of the Alternative Medicine Center at Columbia University's College of Physicians and Surgeons; the Advisory Board of U.C. Davis's Center for Complementary and Alternative Medicine; and is a consultant to Harvard Medical School's Center to Assess Alternative Therapy for Chronic Illness.

Ullman is the author also of *The Consumer's Guide to Homeopathy* (1996); *Homeopathic Medicines for Children and Infants* (1992); *The One-Minute (or so) Healer* (1991); and *Discovering Homeopathy: Medicine for the 21st Century* (1991), which includes a foreword by Dr. Ronald W. Davey, Physician to Her Majesty Queen Elizabeth II.

Stephen Cummings, M.D., received his medical training at the University of California, Davis School of Medicine, and has been studying and practicing homeopathy for more than twenty years. He participated in the founding of the Hering Family Health Clinic, the first American homeopathic clinic in recent times and an early leader in the homeopathic renaissance of the late twentieth century. Dr. Cummings has been an editor of *Journal of Homeopathic Practice,* and currently maintains a private practice in the San Francisco Bay area.

To order, call 1-800-788-6262, or send your order to:

Jeremy P. Tarcher, Inc.
Mail Order Department
The Putnam Berkley Group, Inc.
P.O. Box 12289
Newark, NJ 07101-5289

Subtotal $ _____
Shipping and handling _____
Sales tax (CA, NJ, NY) _____
Canada GST _____
Total amount due _____

Payable in U.S. funds (no cash orders accepted). $15.00 minimum for credit card orders.
*Shipping and handling: $3.50 for one book, $1.00 for each additional book, not to exceed
$8.50.

Enclosed is my   ❏   check   ❏   money order

Please charge my   ❏   Visa   ❏   MasterCard   ❏   American Express

Card # _____   Expiration date _____

Signature as on credit card _____

Daytime phone number _____

Name _____

Address _____

City _____ State _____ Zip _____

Please allow six weeks for delivery. Prices subject to change without notice.